Current Practices in Ophthalmology

Series Editor

Parul Ichhpujani, Department of Ophthalmology, Government Medical College and Hospital, Chandigarh, India

This series of highly organized and uniform handbooks aims to cover the latest clinically relevant developments in ophthalmology. In the wake of rapidly evolving innovations in the field of basic research, pharmacology, surgical techniques and imaging devices for the management of ophthalmic disorders, it is extremely important to invest in books that help you stay updated. These handbooks are designed to bridge the gap between journals and standard texts providing reviews on advances that are now part of mainstream clinical practice. Meant for residents, fellows-in-training, generalist ophthalmologists and specialists alike, each volume under this series covers current perspectives on relevant topics and meets the CME requirements as a go-to reference guide. Supervised and reviewed by a subject expert, chapters in each volume provide leading-edge information most relevant and useful for clinical ophthalmologists. This series is also useful for residents and fellows training in various subspecialties of ophthalmology, who can read these books while at work or during emergency duties. Additionally, these handbooks can aid in preparing for clinical case discussions at various forums and examinations.

Fasika Ambachew Woreta
Rohan Bir Singh
Editors

Cornea Casebook

Springer

Editors
Fasika Ambachew Woreta
Wilmer Eye Institute
Johns Hopkins University School
of Medicine
Baltimore, MD, USA

Rohan Bir Singh
Department of Ophthalmology
Massachusetts Eye and Ear, Harvard
Medical School
Boston, MA, USA

ISSN 2523-3807 ISSN 2523-3815 (electronic)
Current Practices in Ophthalmology
ISBN 978-981-96-0494-4 ISBN 978-981-96-0495-1 (eBook)
https://doi.org/10.1007/978-981-96-0495-1

This Springer imprint is published by the registered company Springer Nature Singapore Pte Ltd.
The registered company address is: 152 Beach Road, #21-01/04 Gateway East, Singapore 189721, Singapore

To my dear friends, family, and colleagues—thank you for your unwavering support, inspiration, and collaboration. This work is a testament to your guidance and encouragement every step of the way.—Fasika

To my mother, Neena Dhaliwal, whose unwavering support and encouragement have guided me through every challenge.—Rohan

Foreword

The *Cornea Casebook*, authored by Dr. Rohan Bir Singh and Dr. Fasika Woreta, will be a welcome addition for ophthalmologists like us and our trainees. Over the past four decades, I have had the privilege of witnessing the evolution of our field, and I continue to be inspired by the dedication and innovation of my fellow ophthalmologists. This textbook is a testament to the authors' commitment to advancing our understanding of corneal disorders.

Cornea Casebook is a comprehensive and invaluable addition to the literature on corneal disorders. Drs. Singh and Woreta are highly esteemed physician-scientists and educators, with a wealth of clinical experience and a deep passion for teaching. In this textbook, they have masterfully organized a collection of case studies that span the spectrum of corneal pathology, offering readers a practical and instructive resource for understanding, diagnosing, and managing these challenging conditions.

What sets the *Cornea Casebook* apart is its emphasis on a case-based approach. Each case study presents a clinical scenario, diagnostic challenges, treatment decisions, and the outcomes. This approach allows readers to actively engage with the material, enhancing their problem-solving skills and clinical acumen. Moreover, the inclusion of high-quality clinical images and diagnostic tests adds depth to the learning experience, enabling readers to better appreciate the intricacies of corneal pathology.

Sir William Osler, who has been termed "The Father of Modern Medicine," famously opined that "he who studies medicine without books sails an uncharted sea, but he who studies medicine without patients does not go to sea at all." For people like me, who learn and remember best through experiences with challenging patients, the case-based approach offered by these authors is ideal.

In addition to its educational value, this textbook reflects the ever-evolving landscape of ophthalmology. The field of cornea and external disease has witnessed remarkable advancements in recent years, from the introduction of novel imaging technologies to the development of innovative surgical techniques. Drs. Singh and Woreta have ensured that their textbook is up to date, incorporating the latest evidence-based practices and treatment options. As such, it is not only an excellent resource for trainees and seasoned practitioners but also an essential reference for those pursuing subspecialty training in cornea and external diseases.

Furthermore, this textbook underscores the importance of collaboration in our field. Ophthalmology is a discipline that thrives on the exchange of knowledge and expertise among colleagues. The authors' willingness to share their insights and experiences in the form of case studies fosters a sense of community and encourages the continuous pursuit of excellence in patient care.

In conclusion, I wholeheartedly endorse this textbook as a remarkable contribution to the field of ophthalmology, specifically in the realm of corneal diseases. Drs. Singh and Woreta have crafted a textbook that is both informative and accessible, ensuring that readers of all levels will find value within its pages. Their dedication to advancing the understanding and management of corneal disorders is evident throughout this book, making it an indispensable resource for ophthalmologists and eye care professionals worldwide.

I commend the authors for their exceptional work, and I have no doubt that *Cornea Casebook* will serve as a beacon of knowledge and inspiration for the next generation of cornea specialists. It is a privilege to be a part of a field that is continually advancing, and this textbook exemplifies the spirit of progress and dedication that defines our profession.

William Holland Wilmer Professor
of Ophthalmology & Director
Wilmer Eye Institute at the Johns
Hopkins University School of Medicine
Baltimore, MD, USA
October 2, 2023

Peter J. McDonnell

Contents

About the Editors

Fasika Ambachew Woreta, MD, MPH is the Eugene de Juan, M.D. Professor of Ophthalmic Education and an Associate Professor of Ophthalmology at the Wilmer Eye Institute. Dr. Woreta received her M.D. degree from the Johns Hopkins University School of Medicine and her M.P.H. degree from the Johns Hopkins Bloomberg School of Public Health. Following an internship in internal medicine at The Johns Hopkins Hospital, she completed her residency in ophthalmology at the Wilmer Eye Institute. She then completed a fellowship in cornea and refractive surgery at the Bascom Palmer Eye Institute, University of Miami Miller School of Medicine. Dr. Woreta returned to Wilmer Eye Institute in 2013 to join the faculty as Assistant Chief of Service and Assistant Director of the Eye Trauma Center at Johns Hopkins Hospital. She is currently the Director of the Eye Trauma Center and Residency Program Director. She is the immediate past president of the American Society of Ophthalmic Trauma. Her clinical and research interests include complex cataract and corneal surgeries, ocular trauma, medical education, and quality improvement in healthcare delivery. She has published more than 140 peer-reviewed publications and chapters in leading ophthalmology journals.

Rohan Bir Singh, MD is a senior fellow at the Laboratory of Ocular Immunology, Transplantation and Regeneration at the Schepens Eye Research Institute of Massachusetts Eye and Ear, Harvard Medical School, Boston, MA, USA. He graduated from the Government Medical College and Hospital, Panjab University, Chandigarh, India. His research interests include the immunopathogenesis of dry eye disease, immunology of corneal graft rejection and ocular graft versus host disease, and epidemiology of ocular disorders in the United States. He is a PhD candidate at the Leiden University Medical Center, The Netherlands, specializing in corneal immunology. Dr. Singh is also a an honorary associate professor in the Division of Ophthalmology and Visual Sciences, Adelaide Medical School, University of Adelaide, Australia. He has published more than 100 peer-reviewed publications and chapters in leading ophthalmology and vision science journals.

Part I

Ocular Surface Diseases

1 Dry Eye Disease

Tianxiang Huang, Jaemyoung Sung, Alan Yee,
and Takenori Inomata

1.1 Introduction

In the last two decades, significant efforts have been made to define and conceptualize dry eye disease (DED) as a pathology, and research on its epidemiology, pathophysiology, diagnosis, and management has made immense strides. DED is the most common ocular surface disease, affecting over ten million people globally, with an estimated prevalence of 5–50% [1–3]. Unfortunately, the prevalence is thought to increase, as the trend towards an aging population and digitalized society

T. Huang · A. Yee
Department of Ophthalmology, Juntendo University Graduate School of Medicine, Tokyo, Japan

Department of Digital Medicine, Juntendo University Graduate School of Medicine, Tokyo, Japan

J. Sung
Department of Ophthalmology, Juntendo University Graduate School of Medicine, Tokyo, Japan

Morsani College of Medicine, University of South Florida, Tampa, FL, USA

T. Inomata (✉)
Department of Ophthalmology, Juntendo University Graduate School of Medicine, Tokyo, Japan

Department of Digital Medicine, Juntendo University Graduate School of Medicine, Tokyo, Japan

Morsani College of Medicine, University of South Florida, Tampa, FL, USA

Department of Hospital Administration, Juntendo University Graduate School of Medicine, Tokyo, Japan

AI Incubation Farm, Juntendo University Graduate School of Medicine, Tokyo, Japan
e-mail: tinoma@juntendo.ac.jp

F. A. Woreta, R. B. Singh (eds.), *Cornea Casebook*, Current Practices in Ophthalmology, https://doi.org/10.1007/978-981-96-0495-1_1

are inevitably linked to known risk factors for developing DED [2, 4–6]. Numerous symptoms of DED have been reported, including eye dryness, ocular discomfort, visual impairment, and generalized fatigue [7–12]. In addition, the collection of symptoms for each patient is highly heterogeneous [11, 13, 14]. These symptoms can negatively affect the quality of vision, leading to decreased work productivity and quality of life (QoL) [15–19]. However, recent reports indicate that a significant portion of patients with DED may be left undiagnosed and experience progressive loss of QoL without proper intervention [13, 20]. Such DED progression may eventually cause irreversible vision loss, corneal defects, and persistent ocular pain [21–24]. DED is also a chronic illness, and proper long-term management becomes crucial in minimizing exacerbations and further damage to the ocular surface [25, 26]. Therefore, early diagnosis, longitudinal monitoring, and appropriate intervention are imperative for preventing chronic QoL decrease attributed to DED [3, 9, 11].

Dr. Schirmer made the earliest known description of DED assessment in 1903; he detailed a novel technique for pathological tear reduction evaluation [27]. DED was formally defined in 1995 by two individual leading institutes. Dr. Lemp, leading the United States National Eye Institute (NEI) [28] and members of the Japan Dry Eye Society [29], each created a comprehensive overview of its definition, classification, and diagnostic criteria. Fast forward nearly a decade, global experts and researchers established the Dry Eye Workshop (DEWS) to improve the previous conceptualization of DED and advance the frontiers concerning examination strategies, epidemiology, basic science research, and intervention [30]. In November 2016, a renewed perspective on DED was shared by the Japan Dry Eye Society [31], which became the basis for defining and interpreting DED by the Asia Dry Eye Society (ADES) [32] centered around major Asian countries, including South Korea, China, and Japan. The latest executive summary report on DED, DEWS II [33], was released in 2017 by the Tear Film and Ocular Surface Society (TFOS). Despite extensive efforts by experts to create a single standard, DEWS has not yet reached a worldwide consensus on its definition and diagnostic criteria for DED, and many countries continue to implement independent standards for DED diagnosis and management.

The DED diagnosis and treatment discrepancy between the West and Asia appears to result from the difference in the perspectives on the primary driving mechanism. In the West, the foundation for understanding DED originates from the DEWS II definition of DED, as shown in Table 1.1 [33]. The primary mechanism proposed by DEWS II involves tear hyperosmolarity and resultant ocular surface inflammation [30, 35, 36]. Both phenomena contribute to a vicious cycle initiated by a disruption in various ocular surface corneal cells. This is followed by the destabilization of tear homeostasis and a further increase in tear hyperosmolarity [30]. The inflammatory process can be broadly separated into acute and chronic forms, where the former is characterized by rapid tear hyperosmolarity and inflammatory cytokine release attributed to acute cellular disturbances by an inciting event [37].

In contrast, the latter is thought to be an immunological sequela caused by accumulating episodes of acute inflammation [36]. In this concept of DED, initial tear hyperosmolarity is depicted as the initial trigger, and inflammation is the central

Table 1.1 Definition of dry eye disease in Western and Asian countries (Japan)

Dry Eye Workshop II (DEWS II), 2017 [15]	Dry eye is a multifactorial disease of the ocular surface characterized by a loss of homeostasis of the tear film and accompanied by ocular symptoms, in which tear film instability and hyperosmolarity, ocular surface inflammation and damage, and neurosensory abnormalities play etiological roles.
Japanese Dry Eye Society, 2016 [34]	Dry eye is a multifactorial disease leading to a decreased stability of the tear film layers, possibly accompanying ocular discomfort, visual discomfort, and ocular surface dysfunction.

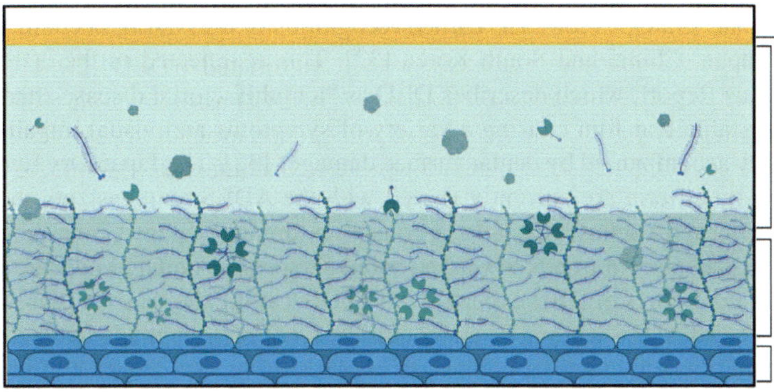

Fig. 1.1 Illustration of the tear film and outer corneal layers. The outermost layer of the anterior eye consists of the corneal epithelial cells and tear film layers, which can be further divided into the outer and inner aqueous layers (aqueous component and secretory mucins). The outer corneal epithelium comprises membrane-associated mucins and epithelial cells. (Image made by RBS using Biorender.com)

physiological process [38]. This logic supports the use of topical cyclosporine, an immunomodulatory agent, to dampen the inflammatory response occurring on the ocular surface. Western countries' perspective on DED views tear hyperosmolarity and inflammation as the primary disease elements that divide DED into two sub-types: aqueous tear-deficient dry eye (ATDDE) and evaporative dry eye (EDE). Based on this classification and its severity, a stepwise regimen was tailored to best treat the underlying mechanisms.

In contrast, the overarching view of DED in Japan stems from the definition and perspective shared by the Japan Dry Eye Society in 2016, as shown in Table 1.1 [31]. The stability of the tear film layer is thought to be at the core of the disease. As shown in Fig. 1.1, the corneal surface is composed of corneal epithelium and tear film, and the tear film is composed of lipid and aqueous layers. The aqueous layer is composed of an aqueous component and secretory mucin. The corneal epithelium comprises membrane-associated mucins and epithelial cells. The lipid layer, aqueous fluid, secretory mucins, and membrane-associated mucins are essential for maintaining tear film stability in this structure. Therefore, insufficiency in any one of these components is thought to result in tear film instability [39]. Homeostasis of these layers is believed to be central to the pathophysiology of DED in Japan, which has become the basis of tear film-oriented diagnosis (TFOD) and therapy (TFOT). TFOD evaluates DED by observing the tear film layer dynamics and fluorescein breakup patterns to delineate DED into three major subtypes: aqueous deficient DE (ADDE), decreased wettability DE (DWDE), and increased evaporation DE (IEDE) [32, 39]. TFOT is an approach to DED management that considers the subtype when selecting treatment [32, 39]. This perspective, diagnosis, and strategies for DED earned recognition in the ADES, becoming a standard in Japan, China, and South Korea [32]. This is reflected in the 2016 ADES Consensus Report, which describes DED as "a multifactorial disease characterized by unstable tear film causing a variety of symptoms and visual impairment, potentially accompanied by ocular surface damage" [32]. The Japan Dry Eye Society diagnostic criteria are currently shared with the ADES, emphasizing the TFOT and TFOD approaches, reaching a consensus among Japan, China, and South Korea. Hence, current trends toward a shared perspective on DED appear to be led by two major bodies of DED experts, with TFOS leading the West and Japan Dry Eye Society and ADES leading Asian countries. As efforts are made to create a global standard, these two expert bodies are expected to be at the center of the conversation.

The following sections discuss and compare one case representative of a traditional (Western) treatment approach to ADDE and another of a TFOT and TFOD approach to DED management from Japan.

1.2 Diagnostic Criteria of DED

1.2.1 Diagnostic Criteria in the West

In Western countries, the most prominent diagnostic standards implemented in clinical practice are derived from either the Dry Eye Syndrome Preferred Practice Pattern published by the American Academy of Ophthalmology (AAO) or the DEWS II released by the TFOS [33, 40]. Before diagnosis, it is essential to exclude conditions that can mimic DED using several triaging questions (Table 1.2). Subsequently, a subjective symptom evaluation through dedicated questionnaires, including the Ocular Surface Disease Index (OSDI) and Dry Eye Questionnaire-5 (DEQ-5), should be completed to indicate whether a patient might have DED [41–44]. A score beyond a designated cutoff value (i.e., ≥13 for OSDI and ≥6 for DEQ-5) is considered a positive examination result, triggering further clinical evaluation. The subsequent evaluation entails the assessment of homeostasis markers, as shown in Table 1.3. Any of these three markers is considered representative of disrupted homeostasis, confirming the diagnosis of DED. Once the diagnosis is

Table 1.2 Questions for the differential diagnosis of dry eye disease

How severe is the eye discomfort?
Do you have any mouth dryness or swollen glands?
How long have your symptoms lasted & was there any triggering event?
Is your vision affected and does it clear on blinking?
Are the symptoms or any redness much worse in one eye than the other?
Do the eyes itch, appear swollen or crusty, or have given off any discharge?
Do you wear contact lenses?
Have you been diagnosed with any general health conditions (including recent respiratory infections) or are you taking any medications?

Table 1.3 Markers of homeostasis in diagnosing dry eye disease

Noninvasive tear film breakup time	<10 s
Tear osmolarity	≧308 mOsm/L in either eye or interocular difference >8 mOsm/L
Corneal fluorescein staining	>5 corneal spots
	>9 conjunctival spots
	Lid margin (≧2 mm length and ≧25% width)

confirmed, specialized examinations, including meibography, lipid interferometry, and tear secretion volume measurement, should be conducted to determine the subtype and severity of DED to guide management.

1.2.2 Diagnostic Criteria in Asia

Per the newly defined definition of DED established in November 2016, the diagnostic criteria for DED were modified to assess the presence of (1) tear film breakup time (TFBUT) shorter than 5 s measured by fluorescein staining, and (2) subjective symptoms of DED, such as ocular discomfort and decline in vision [31]. This set of criteria differs significantly from the previously implemented criteria since 2006 [45], which consist of (1) tear dysfunction, (2) keratoconjunctival epithelial damage, and (3) subjective symptoms of DED. The omission of new criteria reflects the results from research that suggests tear film instability without keratoconjunctival epithelial damage to be sufficient to cause a subset of DED with symptom severity comparable to that of highly progressed ADDE [46]. Thus, the newly established diagnostic criteria in 2016 acknowledge the existence of a DED subtype defined by shortened TFBUT and subjective symptoms, allowing a sizable number of patients classified as "dry eye suspects" to receive a formal diagnosis of "short TFBUT" subtype of DED. In addition, recent studies with satisfactory results on the reliability and validity of simple DED symptom questionnaires, such as the Dry Eye-Related Quality-of-Life Score (DEQS) [47] and the Japanese version of the OSDI (J-OSDI) [7] also supported the added attention placed on subjective symptom evaluation in a primarily non-English speaking population. Recently, smartphone app-based subjective symptoms and lifestyle management for DED have been introduced in Japan [9–11, 13, 20, 48].

1.3 DED Treatment

1.3.1 Treatment in the West

In the Dry Eye Syndrome Preferred Practice Pattern released by the AAO, the treatment plan follows a four-step approach for DED management (Table 1.4) [35]. The following section describes a case scenario based on the approach primarily utilized by Western countries.

Table 1.4 Staged management and treatment recommendations for dry eye disease*†‡

Step 1
Education regarding the condition, its management, treatment, and prognosis
Modification of local environment
Education regarding potential dietary modifications (including oral essential fatty acid supplementation)
Identification and potential modification/elimination of offending systemic and topical medications
Ocular lubricants of various types (if MGD is present, consider lipid-containing supplements)
Lid hygiene and warm compresses of various types
Step 2 (If the above options are inadequate consider:)
Nonpreserved ocular lubricants to minimize preservative-induced toxicity
Tea tree oil treatment for *Demodex* (if present)
Tear conservation Punctal occlusion Moisture chamber spectacles/goggles
Overnight treatments (such as ointment or moisture chamber devices)
In-office, physical heating and expression of the meibomian glands (including device-assisted therapies, such as LipiFlow, or intense pulse light treatment)
In-office intense pulsed light therapy for MGD
Prescription drugs to manage DED§ Topical antibiotic or antibiotic/steroid combination applied to the lid margins for anterior blepharitis (if present) Topical corticosteroid (limited-duration) Topical secretagogues Topical nonglucocorticoid immunomodulatory drugs (such as cyclosporine) Topical LFA-1 antagonist drugs (such as lifitegrast) Oral macrolide or tetracycline antibiotics
Step 3 (If the above options are inadequate consider:)
Oral secretagogues
Autologous/allogeneic serum eye drops
Therapeutic contact lens options Soft bandage lenses Rigid scleral lenses

(continued)

Table 1.4 (continued)

Step 4 (If the above options are inadequate consider:)
Topical corticosteroid for longer duration
Amniotic membrane grafts
Surgical punctal occlusion
Other surgical approaches (e.g., tarsorrhaphy, salivary gland transplantation)

Reproduced with permission from Jones et al. TFOS DEWS II management and therapy report. Ocul Surf. 2017;15(3):609

DED dry eye disease, *LFA-1* lymphocyte function-associated antigen 1, *MGD* meibomian gland dysfunction

* Potential variations within the disease spectrum are acknowledged to exist between patients and the management options listed above are not intended to be exclusive. The severity and etiology of the DED state will dictate the range and number of management options selected from one or more steps.

† One or more options concurrently within each category can be considered within the step of the dry eye disease state. Options within a category are not ranked according to importance and may be equally valid.

‡ It should be noted that the evidence available to support the various management options differs and will inevitably be lower for newer management options. Thus, each treatment option should be considered in accordance with the level of evidence available at the time of management is instigated.

§ The use of prescription drugs needs to be considered in the context of individual patient presentation, and the relative level of evidence supporting their use for that specific indication, as this group of agents differs widely in mechanism of action.

1.3.1.1 Case 1

Effective management of ADDE presenting as a complication of Sjögren's syndrome using punctal plugs.

Key Points

- Characteristics of ADDE secondary to underlying Sjögren's syndrome
- Tear conservation therapy (punctal plugs) as an effective next-line treatment alternative for ADDE refractory to topical treatment

A 37-year-old female presented with bilateral ocular pain and decreased visual acuity in the left eye, who recently received a diagnosis of Sjögren's syndrome following a referral by a local dentist owing to the complaint of dry mouth. The patient had no prior significant medical history or medication at the initial ophthalmology visit. The average screen time was approximately 6 h a day with no particular exposure to dry working conditions. The best-corrected visual acuity was 20/20 and 20/200 for the right and left eyes, respectively. The fundoscopic examination was unremarkable in both eyes.

Subjective symptom evaluation through disease-specific questionnaires yielded total scores of 71 and 50 for the OSDI and DEQS, respectively. Regarding the tear evaluation, the patient's TFBUT was 2 s and 0.3 s, the tear meniscal height (TMH) was 0.2 mm (low; <0.25 mm) and 0.1 mm, and Schirmer's test yielded 4 mm/5 min (low; <5 mm/5 min) and 2 mm/5 min (low) for the right and left eyes, respectively. Corneal fluorescein staining score yielded a van Bijsterveld grading system [49] of 3 and 9 for the right and left eyes, respectively (Fig. 1.2a). No concerning findings were encountered in the patient's bilateral eyelids or meibomian glands. After a comprehensive assessment, the patient was diagnosed with ADDE.

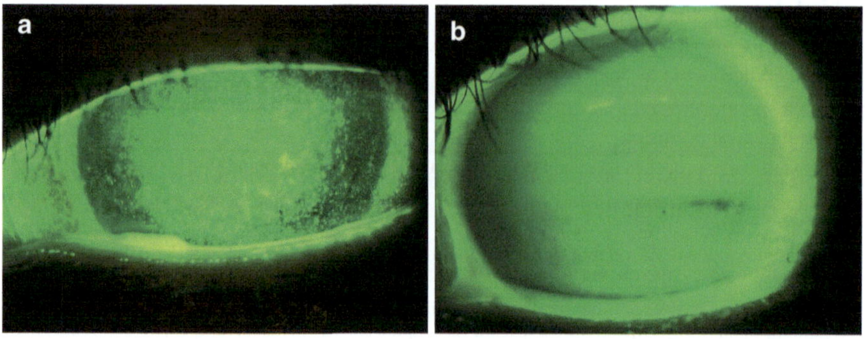

Fig. 1.2 Corneal fluorescein staining of the left eye under a blue-free barrier filter at 10× magnification. Corneal fluorescein staining during the initial examination revealed severe keratoconjunctival epithelial defects and decreased tear meniscus height (**a**). After the insertion of punctal plugs, notable improvements were observed, and the tear meniscus height returned to the normal range (**b**)

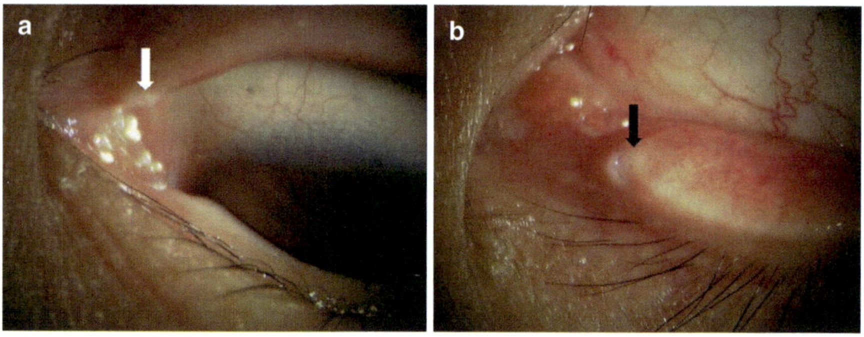

Fig. 1.3 Image of punctal plugs inserted into the left eyelid. (**a**) Upper punctal plug (white arrow). (**b**) Lower punctal plug (black arrow). Magnification, 10×

In addition to advising the patient to minimize screen time, a topical preservative-free artificial tear regimen was initiated. At the 1-month follow-up, subjective symptoms, corneal integrity, and tear secretion volume were improved in the right eye. However, the left eye did not show any improvement. Therefore, a punctal plug was placed in each of the upper and lower puncta (Fig. 1.3). The punctal plugs used were the 0.6 mm SuperFlex™ and 0.9 mm SuperFlex ™ (Manufactured by EagleVision®, United States, Distributed by WhiteMedical, Japan) for the upper lower puncta, respectively. In the subsequent follow-up examination, the visual acuity of the left eye recovered to 20/20, and the dry eye-specific questionnaire scores improved to 7 and 3 for the OSDI and DEQS, respectively. In addition, TFBUT was 7 s and 10 s, TMH was within the normal limits, and Schirmer's test yielded 14 mm/5 min and 10 mm/5 min for the right and left eyes, respectively. The corneal fluorescein staining score also improved, with a van Bijsterveld grading system of 3 and 0 for the right and left eyes, respectively (Fig. 1.2b).

Punctal plugs are effective tools for DED improvement, particularly ADDE, which is accompanied by a decrease in the tear secretion volume. As reduction in the tear secretion volume is a major component of several DED-related diseases, including Sjögren's syndrome, conjunctivochalasis, superior limbic keratoconjunctivitis, filamentary keratitis, and postoperative DED (i.e., cataract surgery and laser in situ keratomileusis) [50], punctal plug placement appears to be an effective alternative in case first-line topical artificial tears are inadequate. The mechanism of punctal plugs is relatively simple, and since they help sustain the patient's tears, fewer side effects are expected following their placement.

Punctal plugs are manufactured in various sizes and materials. Materials may affect the various characteristics of the plug, particularly its absorbability. Atelocollagen is an absorbable, thermosensitive material, while silicone is a commonly used non-absorbable alternative; however, more precaution is needed for selecting the correct diameter for each patient in the case of silicone. An ideal plug, regardless of the material, should maintain good retention, prolonged treatment effect, and low complication rates. Complications include (1) failed insertion, (2) plug loss, (3) pyogenic granuloma, (4) excessive tearing (epiphora), (5) corneal epithelial damage during insertion, (6) infectious biofilm formation, and (7) dacrocystitis [51]. SuperFlex™ plugs manufactured by EagleVision® are examples of silicone plugs that facilitate easier insertion and comparatively reduced reported rates of complications, such as pyogenic granuloma and plug extrusion. While the initial product had concerns of failed insertion and plug loss [52, 53], improvements were made in subsequent versions of the product.

1.3.2 Treatment for DED in Asia·Japan

In 2019, the Japan Dry Eye Society published guidelines for DED management with recommendations as shown in Table 1.5 [54]. Experts in Japan and surrounding countries in Asia view disruption of the tear film layers as the primary driver of DED pathogenesis. This concept has paved the way for TFOD-guided therapy, TFOT, to emerge as the predominant approach to DED management in Asia.

Table 1.5 Treatment of dry eye disease recommendations by the Japan Dry Eye Society (2019)

Strongly recommended (should be considered for everyone)	3% diquafosol sodium 2% rebamipide Hyaluronic acid
Somewhat recommended (advised, but under discretion of clinician's judgment)	Punctal plug Steroid eye drops Omega-3 fatty acids (oral)
Not recommended	NSAIDs eye drops 0.05% cyclosporine eye drops Autologous serum eye drops

NSAIDs nonsteroidal anti-inflammatory drugs

This approach starts by determining the subtype of DED by delineating which layer of the tear film or corneal epithelium is disrupted, followed by targeted therapy based on the underlying pathophysiology. Here, the fluorescein breakup pattern [39], rather than a singular focus on TFBUT, was examined in detail under corneal fluorescein staining. As shown in Table 1.6, fluorescein breakup patterns are categorized into five types, and each is indicative of disruption in specific layers of the tear film and corneal epithelium with different recommended treatments for each observed fluorescein breakup pattern [39]. The fluorescein breakup patterns were classified with reference to (1) when fluorescein breakup occurred in relation to upward movement of fluorescein-stained aqueous tears, which was observed after the patient's eye was opened. (2) where the fluorescein breakup occurs within the interpalpebral zone of the cornea and (3) the shape of the tear breakup [39].

Table 1.6 Tear film-oriented diagnosis (TFOD)-guided therapy (TFOT)

Fluorescein break up pattern	Line break	Area break	Dimple break	Spot break	Random break
Pathophysiology (severity)	Aqueous-deficient (mild to moderate)	Aqueous-deficient (severe)	Decreased wettability	Decreased wettability	Increased evaporative
Dry eye disease subtype	ADDE	ADDE	DWDE	DWDE	IEDE
Shape of break up pattern	Line-like	Area-like	Line-like	Circle-like	Indefinite
UMF after eye is opened	○	×~△	◎	◎	◎
Timing	During UMF	Immediately after eye is opened	During UMF	Immediately after eye is opened	After the cessation of UMF
Corneal portion for fluorescein breakup pattern to be seen	Lower part	Whole cornea	Central part	Central~upper part	Indefinite
Tear secretion volume	Decreased	Decreased	Normal	Mostly normal	Dependent on degree of evaporation
Corneal epithelial defect	+ ~ ++	+++	— ~ +	— ~ +	— ~ +
Disrupted tear film layer	Aqueous tear layer	Aqueous tear layer epithelium	Epithelium (membrane-associated mucin layer)	Epithelium (membrane-associated mucin layer)	Lipid layer
Recommended treatment	DQS HA PP	PP	DQS RBM	DQS RBM	AT HA DQS

ADDE aqueous deficient dry eye, *DWDE* decreased wettability dry eye, *IEDE* increased evaporation dry eye, *UMF* upward movement of fluorescein, ○ slow, ◎ quick, △ slow and limited within the lower part of the cornea, × cannot be observed, *DQS* 3% diquafosol sodium, *RBM* 2% rebamipide, *PP* Punctal plug, *HA* hyaluronic acid, *AT* artificial tears

For example, a spot break pattern is diagnosed as a spot-like shape immediately after eye opening, and at least one spot break pattern is not erased during the upward movement of fluorescein-stained aqueous tears. The spot break pattern is thought to be associated with DWDE [39].

1.3.2.1 Case 2

Effective management of the decreased wettability subtype of DED through TFOT.

Key Points

- The decreased wettability subtype is characterized by minimal keratoconjunctival epithelial damage, comparatively severe subjective symptoms, and decreased TFBUT.
- A fluorescein breakup pattern was used to deduce the instability of the tear film layer to guide therapy.

A 69-year-old female presented with a chief complaint of left-sided eye pain. The patient described the pain as severe, with difficulty opening the left eye attributed to pain upon facing strong winds. She had no major medical history. Best-corrected visual acuity was 20/16 in both eyes at the time of clinical observation. TFBUT were 1.0 s and 1.2 s for the right and left eye, respectively. The TMH was 0.3 mm and 0.5 mm in the right eye and normal in the left eye. Symptom evaluation through DED-specific questionnaires yielded OSDI and DEQS scores of 21 and 50, respectively. Corneal fluorescein scores using the van Bijsterveld grading system were 0 and 1, and Schirmer's test results were 10 mm/5 min and 10 mm/5 min for the right and left eyes, respectively. A spot break (Fig. 1.4a) was observed in the right eye. The fluorescein breakup pattern indicated severely decreased wettability of the ocular surface, and the clinician diagnosed DWDE. To counteract the decreased wettability of the patient's tear film, a regimen of topical 3% diquafosol sodium (DIQUAS ophthalmic solution 3%, Santen Pharmaceutical Co., Ltd., Osaka, Japan) [55] and 2% rebamipide (Mucosta ophthalmic suspension UD 2%, Otsuka Pharmaceutical Co., Ltd., Tokyo, Japan) [47] six times a day was initiated for the

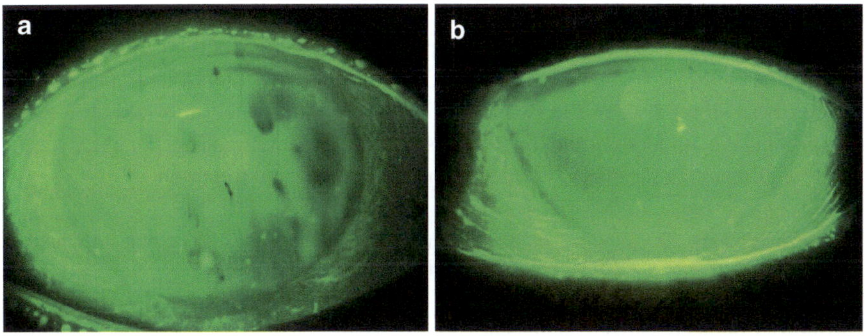

Fig. 1.4 Spot break pattern of the right eye. Examination during the initial encounter revealed a distinct spot break pattern (**a**). After 1-month of treatment with diquafosol and rebamipide, the tear film breakup time increased to over 10 s, and no pathologic break pattern was observed (**b**). Magnification, 10×

right eye. At the 1-month follow-up, TFBUT improved to >10 s in the right eye, and no pathologic fluorescein break pattern was observed (Fig. 1.4b). The OSDI and DEQS improved to 5 and 4, respectively. Diquafosol sodium (3%) acts on the P2Y2 receptors on the conjunctival epithelial and goblet cells to promote the secretion of water and mucin [46]. Although patients may experience conjunctival hyperemia or ocular irritation, these side effects typically subside upon continued application. During the initial stages of diquafosol treatment, the mucinous secretions increase in the ocular surface in a short-lived manner, requiring frequent administration (4~6/day). Diquafosol rarely attains its full effect within the first few days of administration, and it may often take weeks to months for patients to experience noticeable effects. A 2% rebamipide is another treatment option for DWDE management, which was initially approved for gastric mucosal disorders through its prostaglandin and glycoprotein synthesis-promoting effects [56]. On the ocular surface, this translated into an increase in the conjunctival goblet cell count and mucin synthesis in the corneal epithelium [57–59]. Its effect does not appear to directly increase the amount of tear secretion [60], but improvements in the corneal fluorescein staining scores and TFBUT indicate that rebamipide's effects may assist corneal wound healing by maintaining tear film stability [61]. Patients may complain of transient visual difficulties after administration owing to the opacity of the rebamipide solution [60]. Other common side effects include bitter taste, dacrocystitis, and lacrimal duct obstruction [62], which require regular monitoring for minimizing and addressing the respective complications.

1.4 Conclusion

In this chapter, we compared Asian countries centered around Japan and the West based on the similarities and differences in their definition, diagnostic criteria, and approach to the management of DED. Two case scenarios were discussed in detail to underscore the contrasting approaches chosen by the two expert bodies, in which the core concepts and treatment approaches in the West were derived from DEWS II and AAO practice guidelines, and those of Japan and nearby Asian countries were derived from the Japan Dry Eye Society and ADES reports that underscore a tear film layer-oriented (TFOD and TFOT) perspective. Sincenotable advances have been made in the past 20 years in our understanding of DED and its management, future discussion between the two expert bodies is anticipated to establish a more comprehensive understanding encompassing the two contrasting perspectives to create a global standard for DED definition, diagnosis, and treatment.

Acknowledgments The authors would like to thank the Juntendo University Graduate School of Medicine, Department of Ophthalmology for their support.

Disclosure/Conflict of Interest Statement None.

Funding This chapter was supported by JSPS KAKENHI Grant Number 20KK0207 (T.I.), the OTC Self-Medication Promotion Foundation (T.I.), and Takeda Science Foundation 2022 (T.I.).

References

1. Stapleton F, Alves M, Bunya VY, Jalbert I, Lekhanont K, Malet F, et al. TFOS DEWS II epidemiology report. Ocul Surf. 2017;15(3):334–65.
2. Inomata T, Shiang T, Iwagami M, Sakemi F, Fujimoto K, Okumura Y, et al. Changes in distribution of dry eye disease by the new 2016 diagnostic criteria from the Asia Dry Eye Society. Sci Rep. 2018;8(1):1918.
3. Heidari M, Noorizadeh F, Wu K, Inomata T, Mashaghi A. Dry eye disease: emerging approaches to disease analysis and therapy. J Clin Med. 2019;8(9)
4. Ding J, Sullivan DA. Aging and dry eye disease. Exp Gerontol. 2012;47(7):483–90.
5. Murakami S, Kohmura Y, Shiraishi Y, Aoki K, Nakata M, Hamano R, et al. Dry eye among undergraduate students studying sports-related subjects: current status and associated issues. Gazzetta Medica Italiana Archivio per le Scienze Mediche. 2019;178(3):126–31.
6. Kitazawa K, Inomata T, Shih K, Hughes JB, Bozza N, Tomioka Y, et al. Impact of aging on the pathophysiology of dry eye disease: a systematic review and meta-analysis. Ocul Surf. 2022;25:108–18.
7. Midorikawa-Inomata A, Inomata T, Nojiri S, Nakamura M, Iwagami M, Fujimoto K, et al. Reliability and validity of the Japanese version of the Ocular Surface Disease Index for dry eye disease. BMJ Open. 2019;9(11):e033940.
8. Hua R, Yao K, Hu Y, Chen L. Discrepancy between subjectively reported symptoms and objectively measured clinical findings in dry eye: a population based analysis. BMJ Open. 2014;4(8):e005296.
9. Okumura Y, Inomata T, Midorikawa-Inomata A, Sung J, Fujio K, Akasaki Y, et al. DryEyeRhythm: a reliable and valid smartphone application for the diagnosis assistance of dry eye. Ocul Surf. 2022;25:19–25.
10. Inomata T, Iwagami M, Nakamura M, Shiang T, Fujimoto K, Okumura Y, et al. Association between dry eye and depressive symptoms: large-scale crowdsourced research using the DryEyeRhythm iPhone application. Ocul Surf. 2020;18(2):312–9.
11. Inomata T, Nakamura M, Sung J, Midorikawa-Inomata A, Iwagami M, Fujio K, et al. Smartphone-based digital phenotyping for dry eye toward P4 medicine: a crowdsourced cross-sectional study. NPJ Digit Med. 2021;4(1):171.
12. Rhee J, Chan TC, Chow SS, Di Zazzo A, Inomata T, Shih KC, et al. A systematic review on the association between tear film metrics and higher order aberrations in dry eye disease and treatment. Ophthalmol Ther. 2022;11(1):35–67.
13. Inomata T, Iwagami M, Nakamura M, Shiang T, Yoshimura Y, Fujimoto K, et al. Characteristics and risk factors associated with diagnosed and undiagnosed symptomatic dry eye using a smartphone application. JAMA Ophthalmol. 2020;138(1):58–68.
14. Inomata T, Sung J. Changing medical paradigm on inflammatory eye disease: technology and its implications for P4 medicine. J Clin Med. 2022;11(11)
15. Craig JP, Nichols KK, Akpek EK, Caffery B, Dua HS, Joo C-K, et al. TFOS DEWS II definition and classification report. Ocul Surf. 2017;15(3):276–83.
16. Yamada M, Mizuno Y, Shigeyasu C. Impact of dry eye on work productivity. Clinicoecon Outcomes Res. 2012;4:307–12.
17. Uchino M, Schaumberg DA. Dry eye disease: impact on quality of life and vision. Curr Ophthalmol Rep. 2013;1(2):51–7.
18. Morthen MK, Magno MS, Utheim TP, Snieder H, Hammond CJ, Vehof J. The physical and mental burden of dry eye disease: a large population-based study investigating the relationship with health-related quality of life and its determinants. Ocul Surf. 2021;21:107–17.
19. Hanyuda A, Sawada N, Uchino M, Kawashima M, Yuki K, Tsubota K, et al. Relationship between unhealthy sleep status and dry eye symptoms in a Japanese population: the JPHC-NEXT study. Ocul Surf. 2021;21:306–12.
20. Eguchi A, Inomata T, Nakamura M, Nagino K, Iwagami M, Sung J, et al. Heterogeneity of eye drop use among symptomatic dry eye individuals in Japan: large-scale crowdsourced research using DryEyeRhythm application. Jpn J Ophthalmol. 2021;65(2):271–81.

21. Belmonte C, Nichols JJ, Cox SM, Brock JA, Begley CG, Bereiter DA, et al. TFOS DEWS II pain and sensation report. Ocul Surf. 2017;15(3):404–37.
22. Michaelov E, McKenna C, Ibrahim P, Nayeni M, Dang A, Mather R. Sjögren's syndrome associated dry eye: impact on daily living and adherence to therapy. J Clin Med. 2022;11(10)
23. Narayanan S, Redfern RL, Miller WL, Nichols KK, McDermott AM. Dry eye disease and microbial keratitis: is there a connection? Ocul Surf. 2013;11(2):75–92.
24. Baranwal VK, Satyabala K, Mishra A, Dutta AK. Sterile corneal perforations in a case of severe dry eyes. Med J Armed Forces India. 2015;71(3):290–2.
25. Jones L, Downie LE, Korb D, Benitez-Del-Castillo JM, Dana R, Deng SX, et al. TFOS DEWS II management and therapy report. Ocul Surf. 2017;15(3):575–628.
26. Messmer EM. The pathophysiology, diagnosis, and treatment of dry eye disease. Dtsch Arztebl Int. 2015;112(5):71–81. quiz 2
27. Schirmer O. Studien zur physiologie und pathologie der tranenabsonderung und tranenabfuhr. Graefes Arch Clin Exp Ophthalmol. 1903;56:197–291.
28. Lemp MA. Report of the National Eye Institute/industry workshop on clinical trials in dry eyes. CLAO J. 1995;21(4):221–32.
29. Shimazaki J. Definition and criteria of dry eye. Ganka. 1995;37:765–70.
30. The definition and classification of dry eye disease: report of the Definition and Classification Subcommittee of the International Dry Eye WorkShop (2007). Ocul Surf 2007;5(2):75–92.
31. Shimazaki J. Dry Eye Research Group. Definition and diagnosis of dry eye. http://dryeye.ne.jp/teigi/index.html. 2016.
32. Tsubota K, Yokoi N, Shimazaki J, Watanabe H, Dogru M, Yamada M, et al. New perspectives on dry eye definition and diagnosis: a consensus report by the Asia Dry Eye Society. Ocul Surf. 2017;15(1):65–76.
33. Craig JP, Nelson JD, Azar DT, Belmonte C, Bron AJ, Chauhan SK, et al. TFOS DEWS II report executive summary. Ocul Surf. 2017;15(4):802–12.
34. Shimazaki J. Definition and diagnostic criteria of dry eye disease: historical overview and future directions. Invest Ophthalmol Vis Sci. 2018;59(14):DES7–12.
35. Lemp MA, Bron AJ, Baudouin C, Benitez Del Castillo JM, Geffen D, Tauber J, et al. Tear osmolarity in the diagnosis and management of dry eye disease. Am J Ophthalmol. 2011;151(5):792–8 e1.
36. Stevenson W, Chauhan SK, Dana R. Dry eye disease: an immune-mediated ocular surface disorder. Arch Ophthalmol. 2012;130(1):90–100.
37. Luo L, Li DQ, Doshi A, Farley W, Corrales RM, Pflugfelder SC. Experimental dry eye stimulates production of inflammatory cytokines and MMP-9 and activates MAPK signaling pathways on the ocular surface. Invest Ophthalmol Vis Sci. 2004;45(12):4293–301.
38. Stern ME, Pflugfelder SC. Inflammation in dry eye. Ocul Surf. 2004;2(2):124–30.
39. Yokoi N, Georgiev GA. Tear film-oriented diagnosis and tear film-oriented therapy for dry eye based on tear film dynamics. Invest Ophthalmol Vis Sci. 2018;59(14):DES13–22.
40. Akpek EK, Amescua G, Farid M, Garcia-Ferrer FJ, Lin A, Rhee MK, et al. Dry eye syndrome preferred practice pattern(R). Ophthalmology. 2019;126(1):P286–334.
41. Schiffman RM, Christianson MD, Jacobsen G, Hirsch JD, Reis BL. Reliability and validity of the Ocular Surface Disease Index. Arch Ophthalmol. 2000;118(5):615–21.
42. Chalmers RL, Begley CG, Caffery B. Validation of the 5-Item Dry Eye Questionnaire (DEQ-5): discrimination across self-assessed severity and aqueous tear deficient dry eye diagnoses. Cont Lens Anterior Eye. 2010;33(2):55–60.
43. Okumura Y, Inomata T, Iwata N, Sung J, Fujimoto K, Fujio K, et al. A review of dry eye questionnaires: measuring patient-reported outcomes and health-related quality of life. Diagnostics (Basel). 2020;10(8)
44. Inomata T, Nakamura M, Iwagami M, Midorikawa-Inomata A, Okumura Y, Fujimoto K, et al. Comparing the Japanese version of the Ocular Surface Disease index and dry eye-related quality-of-life score for dry eye symptom assessment. Diagnostics (Basel). 2020;10(4)
45. Shimazaki J, Dry Eye Research Group. Definition and diagnosis of dry eye 2006. Atarashii Ganka (J Eye). 2006;24:181–4.

46. Yokoi N, Uchino M, Uchino Y, Dogru M, Kawashima M, Komuro A, et al. Importance of tear film instability in dry eye disease in office workers using visual display terminals: the Osaka study. Am J Ophthalmol. 2015;159(4):748–54.
47. Sakane Y, Yamaguchi M, Yokoi N, Uchino M, Dogru M, Oishi T, et al. Development and validation of the Dry Eye-Related Quality-of-Life Score questionnaire. JAMA Ophthalmol. 2013;131(10):1331–8.
48. Inomata T, Nakamura M, Iwagami M, Shiang T, Yoshimura Y, Fujimoto K, et al. Risk factors for severe dry eye disease: crowdsourced research using DryEyeRhythm. Ophthalmology. 2019;126(5):766–8.
49. van Bijsterveld OP. Diagnostic tests in the Sicca syndrome. Arch Ophthalmol. 1969;82(1):10–4.
50. Miura M, Inomata T, Nakamura M, Sung J, Nagino K, Midorikawa-Inomata A, et al. Prevalence and characteristics of dry eye disease after cataract surgery: a systematic review and meta-analysis. Ophthalmol Ther. 2022;11(4):1309–32.
51. Rumelt S, Remulla H, Rubin PA. Silicone punctal plug migration resulting in dacryocystitis and canaliculitis. Cornea. 1997;16(3):377–9.
52. Parikh NB, Francis JH, Latkany RA. Retention rate of silicone punctal plugs placed by residents in a general clinic setting. Ophthalmic Plast Reconstr Surg. 2010;26(6):400–2.
53. Balaram M, Schaumberg DA, Dana MR. Efficacy and tolerability outcomes after punctal occlusion with silicone plugs in dry eye syndrome. Am J Ophthalmol. 2001;131(1):30–6.
54. Shimazaki J, Tsubota K, Yokoi N, Watanabe H. Dry Eye Research Group. Dry Eye treatment guidelines. http://dryeye.ne.jp/for-member/guidelines/. 2019.
55. Koh S. Clinical utility of 3% diquafosol ophthalmic solution in the treatment of dry eyes. Clin Ophthalmol. 2015;9:865–72.
56. Arakawa T, Higuchi K, Fujiwara Y, Watanabe T, Tominaga K, Sasaki E, et al. 15th anniversary of rebamipide: looking ahead to the new mechanisms and new applications. Dig Dis Sci. 2005;50(Suppl 1):S3–s11.
57. Takeji Y, Urashima H, Aoki A, Shinohara H. Rebamipide increases the mucin-like glycoprotein production in corneal epithelial cells. J Ocul Pharmacol Ther. 2012;28(3):259–63.
58. Kase S, Shinohara T, Kase M, Ishida S. Effect of topical rebamipide on goblet cells in the lid wiper of human conjunctiva. Exp Ther Med. 2017;13(6):3516–22.
59. Itoh S, Itoh K, Shinohara H. Regulation of human corneal epithelial mucins by rebamipide. Curr Eye Res. 2014;39(2):133–41.
60. Kinoshita S, Oshiden K, Awamura S, Suzuki H, Nakamichi N, Yokoi N. A randomized, multicenter phase 3 study comparing 2% rebamipide (OPC-12759) with 0.1% sodium hyaluronate in the treatment of dry eye. Ophthalmology. 2013;120(6):1158–65.
61. Kinoshita S, Awamura S, Nakamichi N, Suzuki H, Oshiden K, Yokoi N. A multicenter, open-label, 52-week study of 2% rebamipide (OPC-12759) ophthalmic suspension in patients with dry eye. Am J Ophthalmol. 2014;157(3):576–83.e1.
62. Imamura H, Eguchi H, Sakamoto M, Hotta F, Tabuchi H, Kusaka S. Case report: a rare orbital abscess caused by dacryocystitis after administration of rebamipide ophthalmic suspension. Front Med (Lausanne). 2021;8:646397.

Blepharitis Associated Disorders

2

Minh Nguyen, Micah Buckmiller, Miel Sundararajan, and Parisa Taravati

2.1 Introduction

Blepharitis is a chronic inflammatory condition affecting the eyelid margin. It most commonly causes ocular surface irritation and transient vision changes secondary to dry eye but does not typically lead to permanent vision loss. However, in certain cases, it can cause significant secondary inflammation, resulting in keratoconjunctivitis, corneal ulceration, corneal neovascularization (KNV), and corneal perforation. Blepharitis can be subcategorized based on location of pathology (anterior or posterior) or based on pathophysiology (meibomian gland dysfunction (MGD), staphylococcal blepharitis, or seborrheic blepharitis) [1].

Meibomian gland dysfunction (MGD) primarily arises from the occlusion of the meibomian glands in the posterior eyelid margin. This diminishes both the quantity and quality of the lipid component of the tear film, resulting in evaporative dry eye disease. A combination of conservative measures including warm compresses, lid massage, and lid scrubs with wet cloth or medicated wipes can be used for initial treatment [2, 3]. Low-dose topical corticosteroids can also provide relief of symptoms. Moderate to severe MGD usually co-exists with an infectious process; thus, antibiotics should also be considered (see management of staphylococcal blepharitis below) [4]. Novel methods to treat MGD will be introduced elsewhere in this chapter.

Staphylococcal blepharitis is associated with *Staphylococcus aureus*. The term infectious blepharitis has been used increasingly due to the prevalence of other bacterial and parasitic pathogens (Table 2.1). This subtype of blepharitis typically affects the anterior eyelid margin, presenting with collarettes, matted lashes, papillary reaction, and mucopurulent discharge. Its sequelae vary from mild dry eye

M. Nguyen (✉) · M. Buckmiller · M. Sundararajan · P. Taravati
Department of Ophthalmology, University of Washington, Seattle, WA, USA
e-mail: minhng88@uw.edu; mcbuckm@uw.edu; mielsun@uw.edu; taravati@uw.edu

F. A. Woreta, R. B. Singh (eds.), *Cornea Casebook*, Current Practices in Ophthalmology, https://doi.org/10.1007/978-981-96-0495-1_2

Table 2.1 Common pathogenic isolates from blepharitis and their exam findings or associated disorders [4–7]

Blepharitis-associated microorganisms	Exam findings or associated disorders
Bacteria	
Staphylococcal aureus	Collarettes, periorbital impetigo
Staphylococcal epidermidis	Most common pathogen in postoperative endophthalmitis
Streptococcal spp.	Periorbital erysipelas
Moraxella lacunata	Angular blepharitis
Cutibacterium acnes (formerly *Propionibacterium acnes*)	Delayed-onset postoperative endophthalmitis
Parasites	
Demodex folliculorum	Sleeves
Phthirus pubis	Phthiriasis palpebrarum (lice infestation)

disease to more serious inflammatory diseases such as phlyctenular keratoconjunctivitis, Staphylococcal marginal keratitis, and KNV. Due to its infectious nature, cultures should be obtained on presentation to guide treatment; however, topical antibiotics (typically bacitracin or erythromycin ointment) and/or oral antibiotics (in particular, tetracyclines and macrolides) are the mainstay of bacterial blepharitis management. In the case of *Demodex* blepharitis, which is frequently associated with ocular rosacea, treatment should include tea tree oil or anti-parasitic medications [4].

Seborrheic blepharitis classically presents with scaling, oily or greasy scurf at the base of the lashes in the anterior eyelid margin, inspissated meibomian glands associated with turbid secretions on expression, and inferior punctate epithelial erosions. This causes irritation, discomfort, and evaporative dry eye disease and frequently occurs alongside MGD or staphylococcal blepharitis. In addition to the conservative therapies recommended for MGD management, clinicians have used agents such as selenium sulfide-containing ointment with great success [8].

In this chapter, we further discusses the blepharitis-associated corneal disorders in a case-based approach in order to enhance understanding of these disease entities and their relationship with blepharitis, as well as explore the recommended treatment regimens.

2.2 Case I

2.2.1 Presentation

An 82-year-old male with past ocular history of non-exudative age-related macular degeneration, pseudophakia, and glaucoma suspect status presented with a 10-day history of bilateral eye pain. He described his pain as sharp and associated with a foreign body sensation. He trialed frequent artificial tears (with preservatives) and antihistamine drops without significant symptomatic improvement. On examination, he was found to have inspissated meibomian glands, lid margin telangiectasias, reduced tear break-up time (TBUT), and diffuse punctate epithelial erosions. The clinical picture was consistent with evaporative dry eye disease related to MGD, and he was treated with preservative-free artificial tears six times daily, lubricating ointment at bedtime, and was advised to follow a regimen of warm compresses and lid scrubs. One week later, he was seen for follow-up with resolution of his ocular symptoms. On slit lamp examination, his epitheliopathy and TBUT had improved significantly.

2.2.2 Discussion

Dry eye disease (DED) is a multifactorial disease of the ocular surface with loss of homeostasis of the tear film and ocular symptoms [9]. Its prevalence varies from 5% to 50%, but only 6.8% of the US population has a clinical diagnosis of dry eye [10]. It is more common in women and with older age [11]. DED is classified into aqueous tear deficiency and evaporative disease. Possible etiologies of aqueous tear deficiency include Sjogren's syndrome, diseases of the lacrimal gland, obstruction of lacrimal gland ducts, reflex sensory/motor block, and medication side effects. On the other hand, evaporative dry eye is closely related to blepharitis, ocular surface disease, vitamin A deficiency, and contact lens wear [9, 12]. DED commonly presents with dryness, conjunctival hyperemia, excessive tearing, light sensitivity, blurred vision, and irritation of the eyes described as a gritty or burning sensation. Findings on eye examination include conjunctival injection, reduced TBUT, increased tear osmolarity, and punctate epithelial erosions.

Initial treatments for aqueous tear deficiency include modification of local environment or lifestyle (such as smoking cessation, frequent breaks while reading or working on a computer) and artificial tears. If these are insufficient, management can be escalated to frequent non-preserved artificial tears, topical cyclosporine 0.05%, lifitegrast 5%, low-dose corticosteroids, punctal plugs, eyeglasses with side shields, moisture chambers, and varenicline nasal spray [13, 14]. In severe cases, autologous serum drops, punctal cautery, or scleral lenses may be considered.

For evaporative disease, in addition to treating the ocular surface as outlined above, it is important to treat the underlying pathology. This includes achieving control of disorders of eyelids or ocular surface. Since blepharitis of all subtypes is the major cause of this disease entity, most patients should be recommended to perform frequent warm compresses, lid hygiene, and hypochlorous lid scrubs or sprays. Topical antibiotics, such as erythromycin ointment, or oral antibiotics, such as doxycycline, can also be used to address the common bacterial pathogens of infectious blepharitis. Newer technologies such as intense-pulsed-light therapy or LipiFlow (Johnson & Johnson, Irvine, California) have shown some promising results and may be included in the treatment regimen for evaporative DED related to MGD [15, 16]. Response to treatment can be determined by symptoms, physical examination, or questionnaires. Treatment is usually chronic unless a causative factor can be identified and eliminated. In the case above, symptomatic relief was achieved by treating the blepharitis with conservative measures.

2.2.3 Key Points

- Blepharitis causes evaporative dry eye disease, which is characterized by reduced tear break-up time.
- Treatment of evaporative dry eye disease should include treatment of the associated blepharitis, which may include warm compresses, lid hygiene, topical and/or systemic antibiotics, and newer technologies such as intense-pulsed-light therapy.

2.3 Case II

2.3.1 Case Presentation

A 12-year-old female with history of recurrent styes and presumed allergic conjunctivitis presented with 5 days of progressive redness, tearing, and intermittent pain in the left eye. She had recently moved to America from the Philippines, and for the past few years, she had had annual episodes of similar symptoms treated with topical olopatadine and trimethoprim/polymyxin by her home ophthalmologist. Slit lamp examination of both eyes showed several chalazia, collarettes on the lashes, conjunctival injection, and 360° of active KNV bilaterally with a few elevated, gelatinous lesions at the limbus and mid-peripheral cornea (Fig. 2.1). Corneal and conjunctival cultures were obtained, and the patient was started on topical moxifloxacin, a short taper course of fluorometholone, oral doxycyline, erythromycin, and lid scrubs. Interferon-gamma release testing was negative for latent tuberculosis. Her conjunctival culture was positive for *Staphyloccoccus aureus*, and she

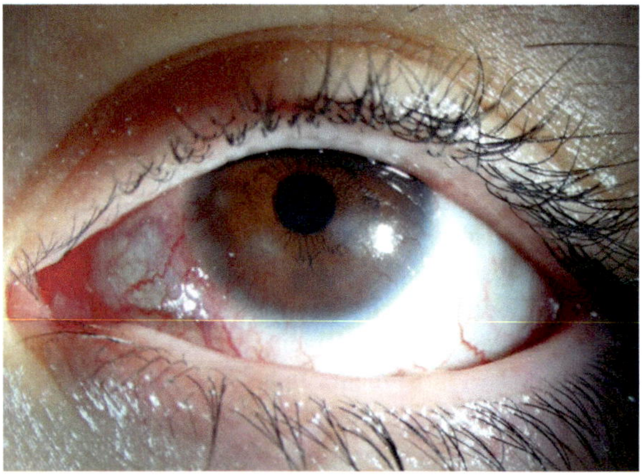

Fig. 2.1 Slit lamp photo of the left eye shows mildly injected conjunctiva, 360° of corneal neovascularization, and small, elevated, gelatinous conjunctival and corneal lesions

responded well to treatment with resolution of her symptoms. The corneal inflammatory lesions progressed to stromal scarring with time, and the KNV partially regressed.

2.3.2 Discussion

Phlyctenular keratoconjunctivitis (PKC) is an inflammation of the conjunctiva and cornea secondary to a type IV hypersensitivity reaction to a foreign protein, most commonly due to *Staphylococcus aureus* or *Mycobacterium tuberculosis* antigens [17]. Due to its frequent association with staphylococcal antigens, PKC occurs predominantly in pediatric patients who also have blepharitis and recurrent chalazia. Presenting symptoms include irritation, eye pain, redness, and light sensitivity. Examination demonstrates elevated, gelatinous, round lesions on the conjunctiva and/or cornea, which can progress to ulceration, KNV, and scarring. Since PKC is caused by an inflammatory process, topical steroid is an effective first-line therapy [18]. However, due to the recurrent nature of this disease in a younger patient population and the vision-threatening side effects associated with long-term steroids, other nonsteroidal agents such as topical cyclosporine and tacrolimus have been used as alternative or adjunctive therapy [19, 20]. In severe and refractive disease, systemic immunomodulatory therapy may be required [21].

Another important aspect of PKC management is the treatment of blepharitis to eliminate the source of antigens. This can be achieved with warm compresses, lid scrubs, and topical and/or oral antibiotics. Although oral doxycycline is classically used for blepharitis in adults, oral azithromycin or erythromycin is the antibiotic of choice in childhood PKC to avoid side effects of oral tetracyclines, such as tooth staining [22]. It is also crucial to rule out tuberculosis if there is a recent history of travel or immigration. In recurrent cases or presentations outside of the typical age group, a neoplastic etiology should be included in the differential diagnosis [23].

2.3.3 Key Points

- Phlyctenular keratoconjunctivitis (PKC) is an inflammatory condition of the conjunctiva and cornea secondary to a type IV hypersensitivity reaction.
- Treatment of PKC includes control of inflammation with topical steroid or nonsteroidal agents, as well as treatment of the associated blepharitis.

2.4 Case III

2.4.1 Case Presentation

A 7-year-old female with a history of recurrent styes presented to the Emergency Department with 2 days of blurry vision, redness, pain, photophobia, and foreign body sensation. Examination demonstrated stromal infiltrates approximately 1 mm from the limbus in both eyes, consistent with staphylococcal marginal keratitis (Fig. 2.2). This responded to treatment with topical ofloxacin, prednisolone acetate, erythromycin ointment, and a course of oral azithromycin. She was also advised to use warm compresses and lid scrubs. She was seen elsewhere four times over the subsequent years for recurrences. During each episode, her symptoms resolved with a tapering course of tobramycin-dexamethasone drops and erythromycin ointment. However, during this timeframe of infrequent monitoring, the patient developed worsening keratitis and KNV. She presented urgently after 3 years with decreased vision, and on exam, was found to have severe corneal thinning with perforation requiring placement of cyanoacrylate glue (Fig. 2.3). The patient was also treated with prednisolone acetate, moxifloxacin drops, and doxycycline. This regimen was useful in the stabilization of corneal thinning, but KNV was persistent and encroached on the pupillary axis. Notably, the patient required a long-term course of low-dose topical steroids to maintain control of inflammation.

2.4.2 Discussion

The patient in this case presented with chronic staphylococcal marginal keratitis that progressed to significant KNV, thinning, and eventual perforation. Marginal keratitis is similar to PKC in terms of etiology and its association with blepharitis (see Case II and discussion) and classically presents as a stromal infiltrate 1–2 mm from the limbus, adjacent to the eyelid margins. The most common pathogen is *Staphylococcus aureus,* but colonization of *Haemophilus*, *Moraxella,* or *Streptococcus* spp. has also been reported [24]. Chronic inflammation can then lead to KNV. The normal cornea is avascular to preserve transparency and maintain refractive functionality; however, chronic inflammation shifts the balance of pro-angiogenic versus anti-angiogenic factors to help address the immediate insult to the ocular environment, resulting in KNV [25]. Unfortunately, this has a detrimental effect on the cornea's functionality since the new blood vessels could impede the

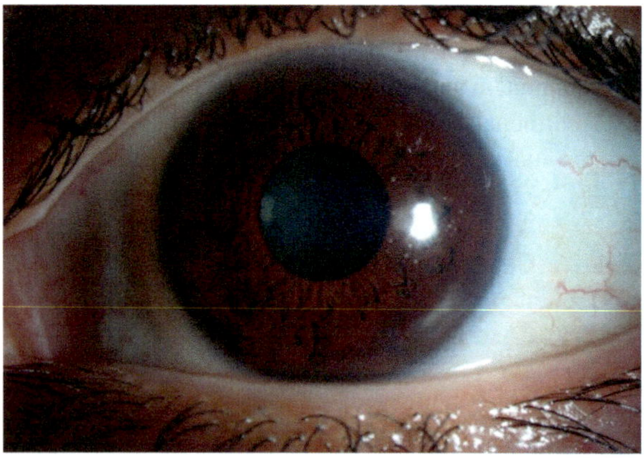

Fig. 2.2 Slit lamp photo shows a peripheral stromal infiltrate inferotemporally in the left eye

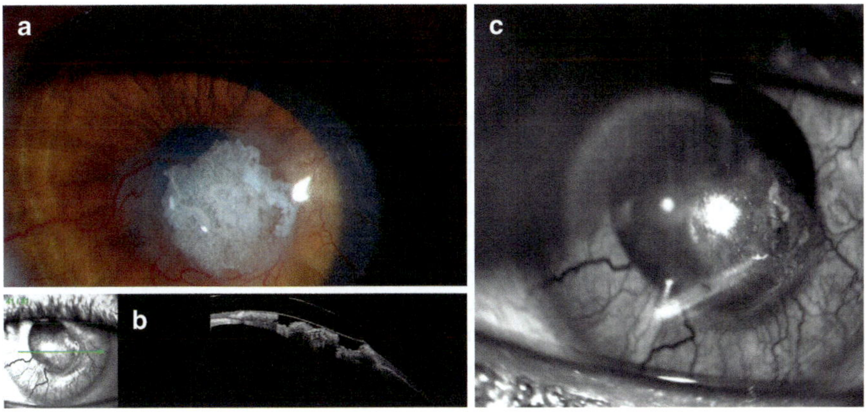

Fig. 2.3 (**a**) Corneal perforation status post placement of cyanoacrylate glue, with significant KNV approaching area of thinning. (**b**) Anterior segment OCT shows significant corneal thinning. (**c**) Infrared reflectance imaging shows the patient's left eye with neovascularization extending toward the pupillary axis. The central cornea also has an area of thinning that was glued after perforation

visual axis and induce irregular astigmatism. Hence, treatment for staph marginal keratitis and KNV should focus on efforts to decrease inflammation and slow the progression of KNV. Topical corticosteroids such as prednisolone or difluprednate drops are considered first-line therapy for active KNV [26].

Just as in the case of PKC, it is key to control the source of inflammation by treating blepharitis adequately with warm compress, lid hygiene, and topical and/or oral antibiotics. In addition, oral doxycycline has demonstrated some anti-neovascularization properties in rat models [27]. Subconjunctival or intrastromal anti-VEGF injection and mitomycin intravascular chemoembolization have also been shown to reduce KNV [28, 29]. Concomitant use of angiography-guided thermo-ablation and photodynamic therapy may also increase the success rate of medical therapies [30].

2.4.3 Key Points

- Marginal keratitis is a corneal hypersensitivity reaction, with *Staphylococcus aureus* as the most common pathogen.
- Marginal keratitis typically presents as a sterile infiltrate 1–2 mm from the limbus; however, in some cases, it can progress to significant corneal neovascularization, thinning, or perforation.
- Treatment of marginal keratitis includes control of inflammation with topical steroids, as well as treatment of the associated blepharitis.

2.5 Case IV

2.5.1 Case Presentation

A 37-year-old female with a history of facial rosacea, oral-facial-digital syndrome, and developmental delay presented with 5 days of worsening left eye pain, swelling, redness, tearing, and blurry vision. She was diagnosed elsewhere with preseptal cellulitis and was treated with oral cephalexin, trimethoprim/sulfamethoxazole, and erythromycin ointment without improvement. She was then admitted to an outside hospital for broad-spectrum intravenous antibiotic treatment, followed by outpatient treatment with oral cefpodoxime and doxycycline. The preseptal cellulitis resolved; however, in the following weeks, she experienced worsening pain and blurry vision. She was referred urgently to the ophthalmology clinic, and examination showed lid margin telangiectasias, inspissated meibomian glands, circumferential sleeves on most lashes, an epithelial defect with stromal white blood cell recruitment, and KNV (Fig. 2.4). Additionally, her face showed flushing, as well as erythematous papules and pustules. Appropriate corneal cultures were sent and demonstrated no growth of organisms. Due to persistence of the large epithelial defect and concomitant neurotrophic keratopathy, a temporary tarsorrhaphy was performed. She was managed with oral doxycycline, topical prednisolone acetate, moxifloxacin, and ivermectin. Warm compresses and lid scrubs with tea tree oil wipes were also done diligently 2–3 times a day. The corneal ulcer and KNV slowly improved (Fig. 2.5).

2.5.2 Discussion

Ocular rosacea (ORS) is the ocular manifestation of acne rosacea, a chronic dermatological inflammatory disorder [31, 32]. The cutaneous signs of rosacea are erythematotelangiectatic, phymatous skin changes, papules, and pustules, whereas ORS is classically described with lid margin thickening and telangiectasia, meibomian

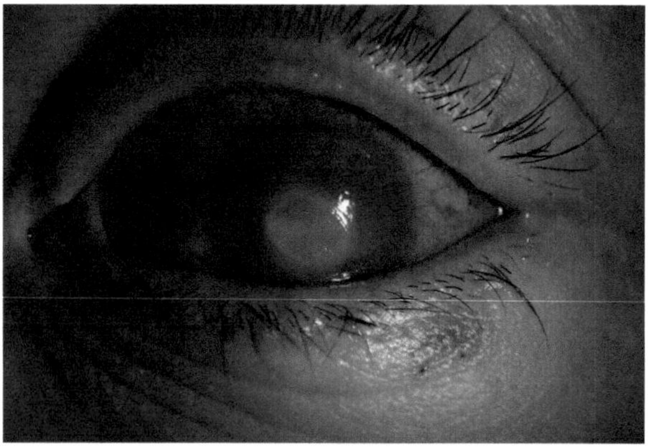

Fig. 2.4 Left eye slit lamp exam showing a central epithelial defect with dense corneal neovascularization of superiorly and inferiorly

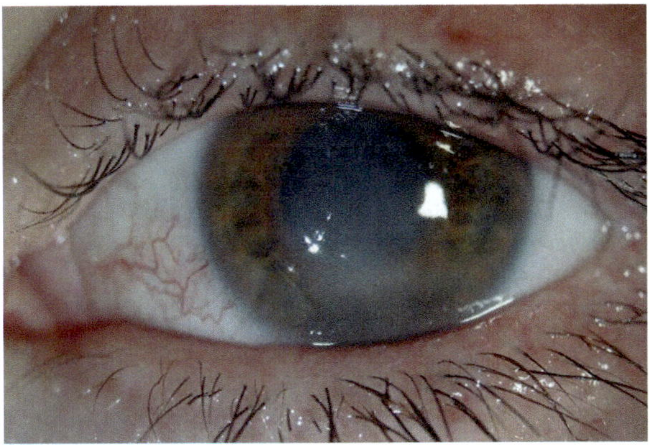

Fig. 2.5 Left eye with significant regression of superior and inferior corneal neovascularization and healing epithelial defect

gland dysfunction, and evaporative dry eye. When ORS is misdiagnosed and not treated adequately for a long period of time as in this case, more serious and potentially irreversible changes may develop, including cicatricial conjunctivitis, sterile corneal ulcer, and KNV [33].

Recent studies linking the cutaneous microbiome to inflammatory cascades in rosacea have offered more insight into the pathophysiology of this disease and its relationship with blepharitis. While *Cutibacterium acnes, Corynebacterium kroppenstedtii, Campylobacter ureolyticus,* and *Prevotella intermedia* have been isolated from the facial skin of patients with rosacea in a few studies, Demodex mites were found in most ORS cases and corresponded with the level of inflammation [34–37]. This knowledge helps guide treatment of ORS more effectively, as there is now an emphasis on managing Demodex blepharitis, in addition to topical corticosteroids and oral antibiotics. Demodex blepharitis may be treated using lid scrubs with tea tree oil or terpinen-4-ol wipes for at least 6 weeks [38, 39]. For demodicosis that is recalcitrant to these initial treatments, topical ivermectin, permethrin, lotilaner and/or oral ivermectin or metronidazole should be considered [40]. Nevertheless, ORS remains a chronic, remitting-relapsing disease requiring long-term treatment, though a gold-standard regimen has not yet been established [41, 42].

2.5.3 Key Points

- Ocular rosacea can cause lid margin thickening and telangiectasia, meibomian gland dysfunction, and evaporative dry eye.
- In some cases, ocular rosacea can progress to cicatricial conjunctivitis, sterile corneal ulceration, or corneal neovascularization.
- Ocular rosacea has been associated with Demodex blepharitis, which may be treated with tea tree oil or terpinen-4-ol wipes, topical or oral ivermectin, permethrin, lotilaner or oral metronidazole.

References

1. McCulley JP, Dougherty JM, Deneau DG. Classification of chronic blepharitis. Ophthalmology. 1982;89(10):1173–80.
2. Key JE. A comparative study of eyelid cleaning regimens in chronic blepharitis. CLAO J. 1996;22(3):209–12.
3. Stroman DW, Mintun K, Epstein AB, et al. Reduction in bacterial load using hypochlorous acid hygiene solution on ocular skin. Clin Ophthalmol. 2017;11:707–14.
4. Amescua G, Akpek EK, Farid M, Garcia-Ferrer FJ, Lin A, Rhee MK, Varu DM, Musch DC, Dunn SP, Mah FS. American Academy of Ophthalmology Preferred Practice Pattern Cornea and External Disease Panel. Blepharitis Preferred Practice Pattern®. Ophthalmology. 2019;126(1):56–93.
5. Zhu M, Cheng C, Yi H, Lin L, Wu K. Quantitative analysis of the bacteria in blepharitis with Demodex infestation. Front Microbiol. 2018;31(9):1719.
6. Wu N, Zhang H, Sun FY. Phthiriasis palpebrarum: a case of eyelash infestation with Phthirus pubis. Exp Ther Med. 2017;13(5):2000–2.
7. Fowler BJ, Miller D, Yan X, Yannuzzi NA, Flynn HW Jr. Postoperative endophthalmitis caused by Cutibacterium (formerly Propionibacterium) acnes: case series and review. Case Rep Ophthalmol. 2021;12(1):1–10.
8. Gupta PK, Periman LM, Lain E, Donnenfeld E, Hovanesian J, Kim T, Trattler W, Yeu E, Holland E. Meibomian gland dysfunction: a dermatological perspective on pathogenesis and treatment outlook. Clin Ophthalmol. 2021;15:4399–404.
9. Craig JP, Nichols KK, Akpek EK, et al. TFOS DEWS II definition and classification report. Ocul Surf. 2017;15(3):276–83.
10. Stapleton F, Alves M, Bunya VY, et al. TFOS DEWS II epidemiology report. Ocul Surf. 2017;15(3):334–65.
11. Farrand KF, Fridman M, Stillman IÖ, Schaumberg DA. Prevalence of diagnosed dry eye disease in the United States among adults aged 18 years and older. Am J Ophthalmol. 2017;182:90–8.
12. Bohm K, Djalilian A, Pflugfelder S, Starr C. Dry eye. In: Mannis M, Holland E, editors. Cornea, vol. 1. 4th ed. Philadelphia: Elsevier; 2017. p. 377–96.
13. Wirta D, Vollmer P, Paauw J, Chiu KH, Henry E, Striffler K, Nau J, ONSET-2 Study Group. Efficacy and safety of OC-01 (varenicline solution) nasal spray on signs and symptoms of dry eye disease: the ONSET-2 phase 3 randomized trial. Ophthalmology. 2022;129(4):379–87.
14. Akpek EK, Amescua G, Farid M, et al. Dry Eye Syndrome Preferred Practice Pattern®. Ophthalmology. 2019;126(1):286–334.
15. Toyos R, McGill W, Briscoe D. Intense pulsed light treatment for dry eye disease due to meibomian gland dysfunction; a 3-year retrospective study. Photomed Laser Surg. 2015;33(1):41–6.
16. Hu J, Zhu S, Liu X. Efficacy and safety of a vectored thermal pulsation system (Lipiflow®) in the treatment of meibomian gland dysfunction: a systematic review and meta-analysis. Graefes Arch Clin Exp Ophthalmol. 2022;260(1):25–39.
17. Abu el Asrar A, Geboes K, Maudgal P, et al. Immunocytological study of phlyctenular eye disease. Int Ophthalmol. 1987;10:33–9.
18. Thygeson P. The etiology and treatment of phlyctenular keratoconjunctivitis. Am J Ophthalmol. 1951;34(9):1217–36.
19. Doan S, Gabison E, Gatinel D, Duong MH, Abitbol O, Hoang-Xuan T. Topical cyclosporine A in severe steroid-dependent childhood phlyctenular keratoconjunctivitis. Am J Ophthalmol. 2006;141(1):62–6.
20. Yoon C, Kim M, Oh J. Topical tacrolimus 0.03% for maintenance therapy in steroid-dependent, recurrent phlyctenular keratoconjunctivitis. Cornea. 2018;37(2):168–71.
21. Valério Sequeira Valadares J, Bastos-Carvalho A, Pedroso Franco JM, Mourão AF, Monteiro-Grillo M. Phlyctenular keratoconjunctivitis—an atypically severe case treated with systemic biologic immunosuppressive therapy. GMS Ophthalmol Case. 2014;4:Doc02.

22. Culbertson WW, Huang AJ, Mandelbaum SH, Pflugfelder SC, Boozalis GT, Miller D. Effective treatment of phlyctenular keratoconjunctivitis with oral tetracycline. Ophthalmology. 1993;100(9):1358–66.
23. Medagoda K, Salvin KA, Mahendra BAGG. A conjunctival myxoid stromal tumor (COMST) mimicking phlyctenulosis: a case report and brief review of the literature. Am J Ophthalmol Case Rep. 2022;27:101590.
24. Cohn H, Mondino BJ, Brown SI, et al. Marginal corneal ulcers with acute beta streptococcal conjunctivitis and chronic dacryocystitis. Am J Ophthalmol. 1979;87:541–3.
25. Abdelfattah NS, Amgad M, Zayed AA, Hussein H, Abd E-BN. Molecular underpinnings of corneal angiogenesis: advances over the past decade. Int J Ophthalmol. 2016;9(5):768–79.
26. McNatt LG, Weimer L, Yanni J, Clark AF. Angiostatic activity of steroids in the chick embryo CAM and rabbit cornea models of neovascularization. J Ocul Pharmacol Ther. 1999;15(5):413–23.
27. Dan L, Shi-long Y, Miao-li L, et al. Inhibitory effect of oral doxycycline on neovascularization in a rat corneal alkali burn model of angiogenesis. Curr Eye Res. 2008;33(8):653–60.
28. Chang JH, Garg NK, Lunde E, Han KY, Jain S, Azar DT. Corneal neovascularization: an anti-VEGF therapy review. Surv Ophthalmol. 2012;57(5):415–29.
29. Mimouni M, Ouano D. Initial outcomes of mitomycin intravascular chemoembolization (MICE) for corneal neovascularization. Int Ophthalmol. 2022 Aug;42(8):2407–16.
30. Yoon HJ, Kim MK, Seo KY, Ueta M, Yoon KC. Effectiveness of photodynamic therapy with verteporfin combined with intrastromal bevacizumab for corneal neovascularization in Stevens-Johnson syndrome. Int Ophthalmol. 2019;39(1):55–62.
31. Gallo RL, Granstein RD, Kang S, et al. Standard classification and pathophysiology of rosacea: the 2017 update by the National Rosacea Society Expert Committee. J Am Acad Dermatol. 2018;78:148–55.
32. Alexis AF, Callender VD, Baldwin HE, et al. Global epidemiology and clinical spectrum of rosacea, highlighting skin of color: review and clinical practice experience. J Am Acad Dermatol. 2019;80:1722–9.
33. Erzurum SA, Feder RS, Greenwald MJ. Acne rosacea with keratitis in childhood. Arch Ophthalmol. 1993;111:228–30.
34. Thompson KG, Rainer BM, Antonescu C, et al. Comparison of the skin microbiota in acne and rosacea. Exp Dermatol. 2020;30:1375. https://doi.org/10.1111/exd.14098.
35. Rainer BM, Thompson KG, Antonescu C, et al. Characterization and analysis of the skin microbiota in rosacea: a case–control study. Am J Clin Dermatol. 2020;21:139–47.
36. Dursun R, Durmaz K, Oltulu P, Ataseven A. Demodex positive discoid lupus erythematosus: is it a separate entity or an overlap syndrome? Dermatol Ther. 2020;33:e13394.
37. Deeks ED. Ivermectin: a review in rosacea. Am J Clin Dermatol. 2015;16(5):447–52.
38. Cheng A, Sheha H, Tseng S. Recent advances on ocular Demodex infestation. Curr Opin Ophthalmol. 2015;26:295–300.
39. Gao Y, Di Pascuale M, Elizondo A, Tseng S. Clinical treatment of ocular demodecosis by lid scrub with tea tree oil. Cornea. 2007;26:136–43.
40. Elston CA, Elston DM. Demodex mites. Clin Dermatol. 2014;32:739–43.
41. Travis R, Seitzman G. Ocular rosacea. Curr Opin Ophthalmol. 2020;31(6):503–7.
42. Thiboutot D, Anderson R, Cook-Bolden F, et al. Standard management options for rosacea: the 2019 update by the National Rosacea Society Expert Committee. J Am Acad Dermatol. 2020;82:1501–10.

Limbal Stem Cell Deficiency

3

Sara AlShaker, Yishay Weill, and Clara C. Chan

3.1 Introduction

3.1.1 Definition and Classification

Limbal stem cell deficiency (LSCD) is an ocular surface disorder caused by a disruption of the homeostasis and transparency of the corneal epithelium [1, 2]. This is governed by the quantity and quality of the stem cells in the basal layer of the limbal epithelium [1].

The diagnosis of LSCD is primarily clinical and includes the classic pattern of late corneal epithelium fluorescein staining and conjunctivalization [2, 3]. Additional diagnostic tools that can assist with diagnosis include impression cytology (presence of goblet cells on the cornea), anterior segment ocular coherence tomography (thinned epithelial layer with hyper-reflective conjunctiva overlying the hyporeflective cornea), and in vivo confocal microscopy (limbal stem cell drop out) [4]. Sequelae of LSCD include corneal scarring, keratinization, symblerpharon formation, and loss of fornices. There are many etiologies for LSCD, and they can

S. AlShaker
Department of Ophthalmology and Vision Sciences, University of Toronto, Toronto, ON, Canada

Department of Ophthalmology, College of Medicine, King Saud University, Riyadh, Saudi Arabia

Y. Weill
Department of Ophthalmology and Vision Sciences, University of Toronto, Toronto, ON, Canada

Shaare Zedek Medical Center, Hebrew University of Jerusalem, Jerusalem, Israel

C. C. Chan (✉)
Department of Ophthalmology and Vision Sciences, University of Toronto, Toronto, ON, Canada

F. A. Woreta, R. B. Singh (eds.), *Cornea Casebook*, Current Practices in Ophthalmology, https://doi.org/10.1007/978-981-96-0495-1_3

be divided into hereditary (i.e., aniridia), acquired nonimmune-related (i.e., chemical burn, contact lens wear), and acquired immune-related (i.e., Stevens–Johnson syndrome (SJS), ocular-involving mucous membrane pemphigoid (MMP)) [2].

3.1.2 Approach to Limbal Stem Cell Deficiency

The management of LSCD is based on staging and determining if the process is unilateral or bilateral. LSCD can be categorized based on the location of the affected corneal epithelium (peripheral, central 5 mm, or the entire cornea) and the extent of limbal stem cell involvement (<50%, 50%–100%, 100%) [5]. Patients who have chronic inflammation and suffer from conjunctival deficiency in addition to LSCD have the worst prognosis (e.g., SJS, MMP, recent chemical injury) [6].

A stepwise approach is used to manage LSCD. Regardless of disease stage, it is crucial to eliminate any offending agent(s) or inciting factor(s) (e.g., soft contact lens wear, benzalkonium chloride (BAK) preservative exposure, glaucoma drops) causing surface toxicity. The ocular surface environment must simultaneously be optimized. Aggressive optimization includes application of non-preserved lubricants, nutritional support (i.e., autologous serum tears, omega-3 fatty acid supplementation, vitamin A ointment), anti-inflammatory agents (both topical and systemic), and lid margin disease management. Some forms of mild-moderate LSCD can be reversed following ocular surface and tear film optimization alone [7]. Prior to any limbal stem cell rehabilitation procedure, preexisting glaucoma requires consideration of an early glaucoma tube shunt implantation in order to minimize toxic topical therapies. Any lid abnormalities (e.g., entropion, lash misdirection, lagophthalmos) also should be addressed. The patient should also undergo a scleral contact lens trial as modern devices, if well tolerated, can obviate the need for any additional more invasive surgery [8, 9]. In patients with decreased vision and/or pain due to LSCD and who have failed or declined scleral contact lens wear, limbal stem cell transplantation (autologous or allogeneic with systemic immunosuppression) can be considered.

In unilateral LSCD, sequential sectoral conjunctival epitheliectomy (SSCE) [10], simple limbal epithelial transplantation (SLET) [11], or conjunctival limbal autograft (CLAU) [12] are treatment options [5]. Harvesting donor tissue from the fellow healthy eye, as long as there is no history of injury or soft contact lens wear is very safe [13, 14]. Amniotic membrane transplantation (stromal side up) which does not provide any additional stem cells can be used as an adjunct in these cases to assist with the proliferation of epithelium growing from the remaining functioning limbal stem cells.

In bilateral cases, if there is a suitable living donor, then a living-related conjunctival limbal allograft (LR-CLAL, which provides 50% coverage of the limbus at 12 and 6 o'clock) can be done [15, 16].

If no living donor is available or if a patient does not want any surgery on their healthy fellow eye, then a keratolimbal allograft (KLAL, using deceased donor tissue to cover the limbus 360°) can be performed [17, 18]. Combination of living and deceased donor tissue can be used to supply limbal stem cells 360° and to supply extra healthy conjunctiva in the form of the Cincinnati procedure [19] and Modified Cincinnati procedure [20]. Anytime that allograft tissue is used, systemic immunosuppression (e.g., oral prednisone, tacrolimus, mycophenolate) is required due to the vascular and highly antigenic nature of the transplanted limbus [21–23].

Once the epithelium has stabilized after the limbal stem cell transplantation procedure, if there is residual deeper corneal scarring limiting the vision, then a deep anterior lamellar keratoplasty (DALK) or penetrating keratoplasty (PKP) is done. Should the stem cell transplant or corneal transplant fail, then the Type 1 Boston keratoprosthesis can be used. It can also be considered for patients with bilateral LSCD and contraindications to systemic immunosuppression [24]. Surface keratinization is a contraindication for limbal stem cell transplantation and a Type 2 Boston keratoprosthesis may be needed [25].

3.2 Cases

3.2.1 Case 1

- Optimization of the ocular surface in patients with SJS is crucial and requires intensive and multifaceted long-term treatment.
- Conservative management in SJS with scleral contact lenses can provide a good visual outcome.
- SJS-related LSCD can eventually result in significant visual loss despite aggressive treatment.

A 20-year-old male with a history of medication-induced SJS presented to our center. He had previously underwent cadaveric and living donor stem cell transplants in the right eye (OD).

On presentation, he had only minimal light perception vision in the right eye, and his best-corrected vision (BCVA) in the left eye (OS) was 20/40 with a Prosthetic Replacement of the Ocular Surface Ecosystem (PROSE) contact lens (Boston Centre for Sight, Boston, MA) which was eventually changed to the EyePrintPRO™ scleral lens (EyePrintPro, Lakewood, CO) for better comfort (Fig. 3.1). On examination, he had significant inflammation of the conjunctiva in both eyes. The cornea in the right eye was opaque with extensive neovascularization, while the left cornea had 360° of conjunctivalization sparing the central visual axis (Fig. 3.2). The remainder of the examination was unremarkable.

The diagnosis of LSCD secondary to SJS in both eyes with exhaustion of the previously performed limbal stem cell transplant was made.

Since the patient maintains good functional vision in his left eye, all efforts to optimize and maintain a healthy ocular surface were initiated. The patient was started on

- Warm compresses, lid hygiene, omega-3 fatty acid supplementation
- Preservative-free artificial tears 4 times daily
- Vitamin A ointment

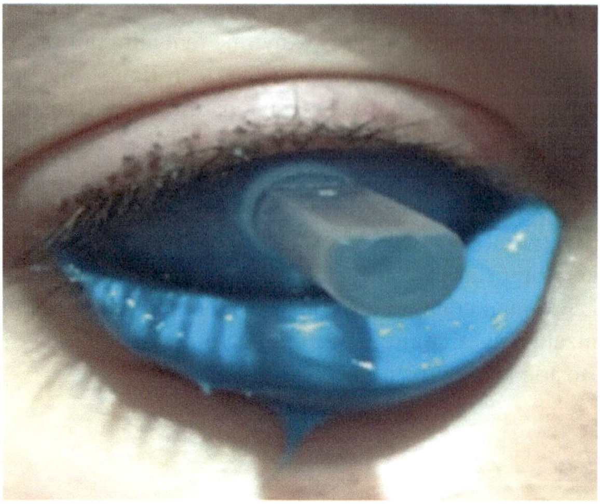

Fig. 3.1 The EyePrintPRO™ contact lens is fitted using a custom impression mold. This 3-dimensional model of the entire ocular surface is scanned and software is then used to design a custom-fitted hard contact lens device

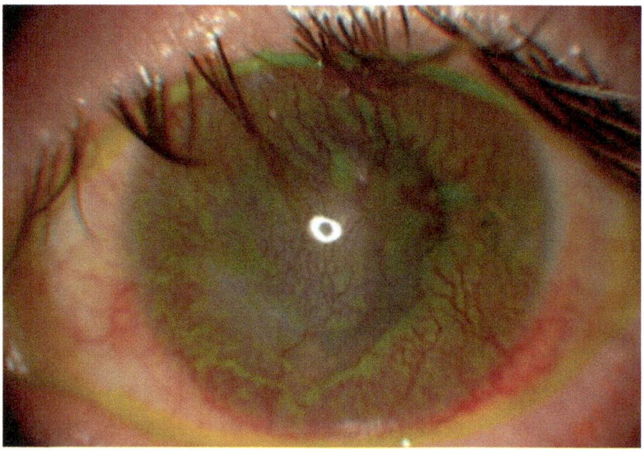

Fig. 3.2 Slit lamp photograph of a patient with Stevens–Johnson Syndrome's left eye showing 360° of conjunctivalization sparing the central 3 mm

- 40% autologous serum tears
- Topical cyclosporine 0.05% (Restasis, Allergan, Irvine, CA, USA)
- Topical prednisolone 1% drops once daily as needed for inflammation flares
- 100 mg oral doxycycline daily

Regular lengthy discussions at each follow-up visit with the patient are essential to achieve compliance with such a laborious daily regimen. The patient has maintained a BCVA of 20/30–20/40 in his left eye with the EyePrintPRO contact lens for the past 8 years.

Unfortunately, his right eye developed an infectious keratitis and corneal perforation complicated by endophthalmitis and intractable pain necessitating evisceration.

3.2.2 Case 2

- Ocular surface rehabilitation plays an important role in setting the scene for the successful management and long-term control of limbal stem cell deficiency.
- The use of commercially available dehydrated amniotic membrane can be a useful adjunct in re-establishing the limbal epithelial stem cell niche in mild to moderate cases of LSCD when there remains more than 50% of the healthy limbal stem cells.

A 71-year-old female presented with gradual decrease in vision in her right known amblyopic eye over 3 months. She had a 10-year history of soft contact lens wear. Her BCVA was 20/200 OD and 20/40 OS. On exam, the eyelids showed significant meibomian gland dysfunction. The right eye had corneal scarring with late fluorescein staining, subepithelial fibrosis, and Salzmann-like nodules (Fig. 3.3). The rest of the exam was unremarkable.

A diagnosis of limbal stem cell deficiency secondary to chronic soft contact lens wear and ocular surface disease was made.

Therapy to optimize the ocular surface was initiated as follows:

- Warm compresses, lid hygiene, omega-3 fatty acid supplementation
- Preservative-free artificial tears 4 times daily
- Serum tears 40% four times daily
- Doxycycline 100 mg daily
- Cyclosporine 0.5% (Restasis, Allergan, Irvine, CA, USA) twice daily
- A mild steroid twice daily (lotemax, loteprednol 0.5% suspension, Bausch & Lomb, Vaughan, ON, Canada)

After 3 months of ocular surface optimization, a superficial keratectomy was performed combined with the placement of a 9-mm dehydrated amniotic

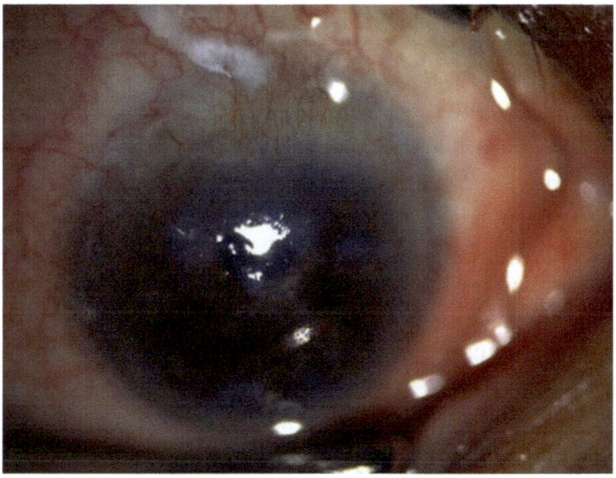

Fig. 3.3 Slit lamp photograph of a 71-year-old female right eye showing conjunctivalization superiorly and areas of subepithelial fibrosis from limbal stem cell deficiency (LSCD). Etiologies for her LSCD included decades of soft contact lens wear and severe ocular surface disease due to dry eye, rosacea, and meibomian gland dysfunction

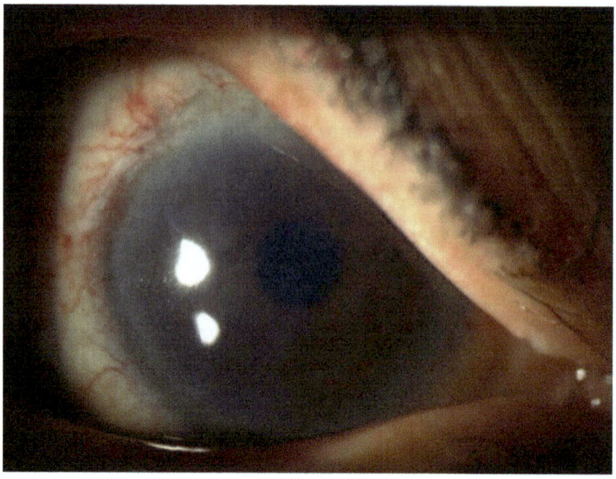

Fig. 3.4 Postoperative slit lamp photograph 6 months after superficial keratectomy and dissolved dehydrated amnion membrane. There is clear stable epithelium with crisp light reflex and residual mild limbal stem cell deficiency superiorly not involving the visual axis

extracellular matrix disc (BioDOptix, Labtician, Oakville, ON, Canada). Tobradex (tobramycin 0.3%-dexamethasone 0.1% suspension, Novartis, Dorval, QC, Canada) was prescribed followed by a course of Maxidex (dexamethasone 0.1% suspension, Novartis, Dorval QC) steroid taper. Pathology confirmed the presence of goblet cells within the corneal epithelium, which confirms the diagnosis of LSCD and loss of the conjunctival-corneal barrier allowing conjunctival goblet cells to cross over to the corneal epithelium.

Postoperatively, the vision improved to 20/60 in the right eye. There was still some evidence of mild limbal stem cell deficiency (Fig. 3.4). The patient was educated on the importance of continuing therapy to maintain a healthy ocular surface and avoiding soft contact lens wear. We also referred her for scleral contact lens fitting, which unlike soft contact lenses, can help improve the visual acuity without stressing the limbal stem cells given the design of the lens which vaults over and does not physically disturb the limbus.

3.2.3 Case 3

- Bilateral total LSCD requires a detailed work up to confirm the diagnosis.
- A multidisciplinary approach is essential for successful limbal stem cell transplantation which includes the assessment of suitable relatives (for blood type and optimal HLA matching) and systemic perioperative and long-term immune suppression.
- In the case of bilateral severe LSCD, the most common choices for stem cell transplant include a living-related conjunctival limbal allograft (CLAL) or a keratolimbal allograft (KLAL) if there is no significant available or willing living donor. Prognosis is better if any conjunctival inflammation is first controlled and any systemic underlying disease treated.

A 48-year-old female was referred with total LSCD which developed over the course of 2 years. A detailed systemic work up including dermatologic, internal medicine, and whole-body scans (PET and mammography) were all normal. Conjunctival biopsies from both eyes showed fibrin deposits along the basement membrane, suggestive of ocular lichen planus [26]. There were no immune antibody or complement deposits, which are classically seen in mucous membrane pemphigoid (MMP, previously ocular cicatricial pemphigoid (OCP)). A diagnosis of total LSCD secondary to ocular lichen planus was made and the patient was started on systemic high-dose oral steroids as well as immune-modulating therapy in the form of Rituximab by the dermatology team. Her ocular inflammation did not stabilize until she began monthly intravenous immunoglobulin (IVIG) infusion treatments. She was then referred to our center to consider options for limbal stem cell transplantation.

Her visual acuity was light perception OD and hand motions OS due to inability to open her eyes due to severe photophobia. Her conjunctiva was hyperemic but without any symblephara. There was near total limbal stem cell deficiency with conjunctivalization over the cornea (Figs. 3.5 and 3.6). The rest of the ocular exam, although limited, appeared normal.

As this was a bilateral process, a stem cell transplant in the form of an allograft was considered. The options included a cadaveric keratolimbal allograft (KLAL) or living-related conjunctival limbal allograft (LR-CLAL). However, the patient had no living-related donors that would be suitable or willing to donate tissue. Hence a KLAL surgery for the left eye was planned. As rituximab targets B-cells only, systemic immune suppression was revised to the following regimen:

- High-dose oral prednisone (up to 1 mg/kg) as a bridging therapy.
- Oral mycophenolate mofetil (MMF, CellCept), a nucleotide inhibitor, which targets T and B cells.
- Oral tacrolimus, a calcineurin inhibitor which inhibits T cells signal transduction and reduces IL-2 transcription.
- Intravenous simulect (Basiliximab), an IL-2 receptor monoclonal antibody, inhibiting T cells on day of transplant and on day 4.

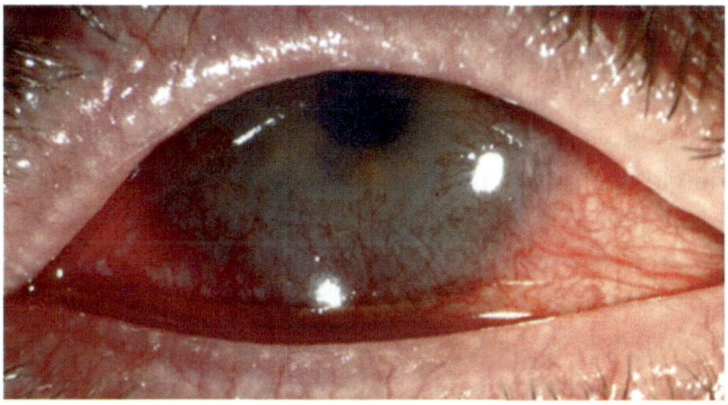

Fig. 3.5 Photo of the right eye showing hyperemic inflamed conjunctiva and superficial conjunctivalization of the cornea

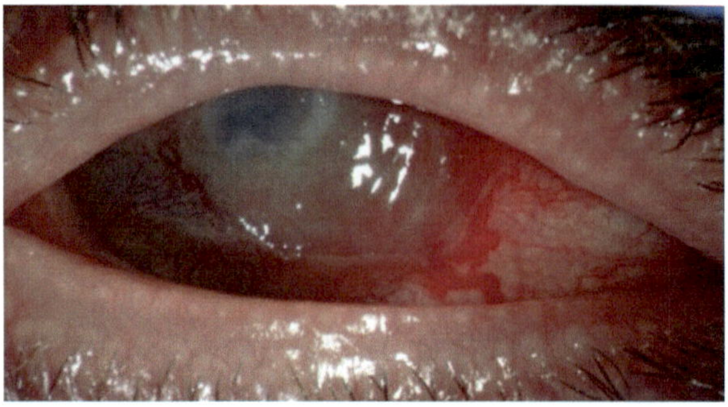

Fig. 3.6 The left eye shows a persistent epithelial defect with corneal haze and conjunctivalization

- Doxycycline 100 mg orally once daily for its anti-MMP properties.
- Intravenous immunoglobulin infusions on day of transplant and at day 7 to help reduce HLA sensitivity.

Topical therapies to control local inflammation:

- Topical steroids in the form of lotemax.
- Cequa (cyclosporine ophthalmic solution 0.09%, SunPharma, Brampton, ON, Canada).

The patient underwent KLAL surgery with fresh frozen amniotic membrane transplantation (AMT) and a temporary tarsorrhaphy in the left eye (Fig. 3.7). Her uncorrected visual acuity at 5 months postoperatively was 20/40 OS. The three KLAL segments were stable without any signs of rejection, the cornea was relatively clear with mild haze and the ocular surface was stable with no evidence of limbal stem cell deficiency recurrence or epithelial defects (Fig. 3.8).

3.2.4 Case 4

- Patients with severe bilateral LSCD, where a living donor family member is available, a LR-CLAL has possible lower rejection rates and improved graft survival [27].
- Following LR-CLAL, patients require long-term immunosuppression to prevent graft rejection and failure.

A 29-year-old female with progressive LSCD secondary to aniridia was referred due to declining visual acuity and constant pain in her left eye from chronic recurrent epithelial defects. She had glaucoma in both eyes, with the right eye being controlled with medical therapy and the left having undergone multiple glaucoma surgeries including goniotomy, trabeculectomy, and finally, insertion of a glaucoma drainage device (Baerveldt, Abbott Medical Optics Inc., Santa Ana, CA). She also had undergone cataract extraction with intraocular lens implantation in both eyes.

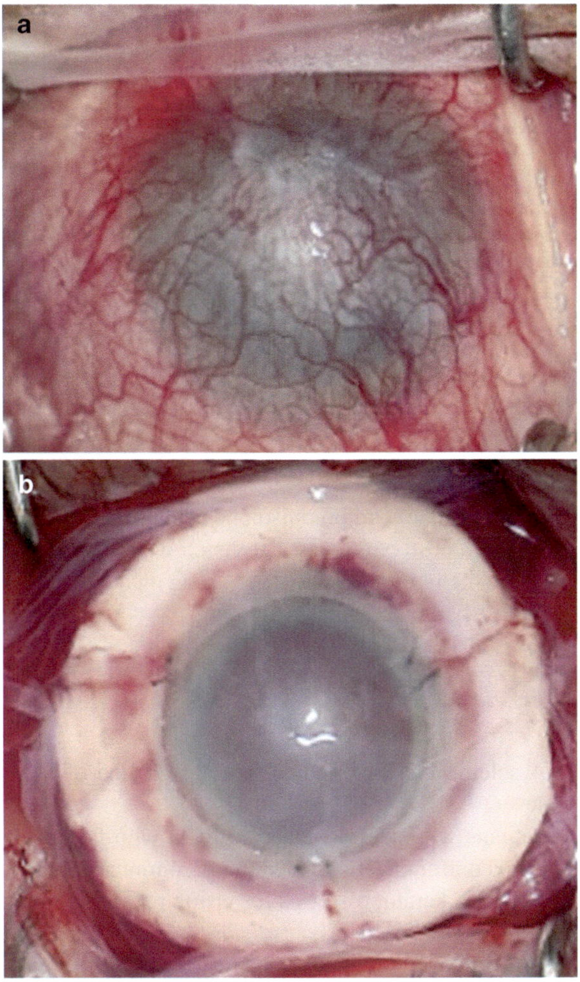

Fig. 3.7 (**a** and **b**): Intraoperative photographs of the left eye at the beginning (**a**) and end of the surgery (**b**). Note the extensive conjunctivalization and scarring at the beginning of the case. A 360° conjunctival peritomy and superficial keratectomy were performed followed by KLAL segments placement, secured with sutures at the limbus and fibrin tissue glue for the base to cover the whole limbal circumference. Finally, a layer of fresh frozen amniotic membrane is draped over and sutured

Her uncorrected visual acuity (UCVA) was 20/300 OD and counting fingers OS. On examination, the right eye showed inferior and superior corneal conjunctivalization with late staining, sparing the visual axis. The left eye demonstrated an opaque and conjunctivalized cornea.

Due to her recurrent epithelial defects, she could no longer tolerate her scleral contact lens. The patient's sister was willing to serve as a limbal stem cell donor and had no contraindications. A LR-CLAL was planned from the sister's left eye to the recipient's left eye.

The patient underwent an uneventful LR-CLAL in the left eye with two 3-clock-hours of allograft tissues secured at the superior and inferior limbus and placement of fresh-frozen amniotic membrane (Fig. 3.9). Postoperatively, the patient was treated with systemic prednisone and mycophenolate that were slowly tapered in coordination with a nephrologist. Topical moxifloxacin (Alcon, Mississauga,

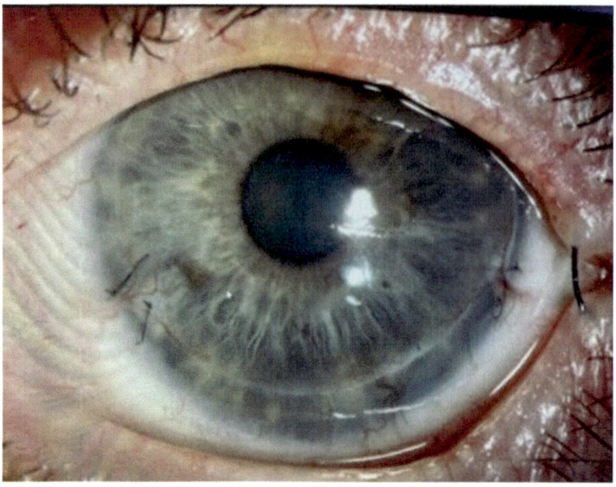

Fig. 3.8 Postoperative month 5 following left eye keratolimbal allograft (KLAL) and amniotic membrane transplant. The segments appear white with no signs of rejection and the cornea is clear. A temporary tarsorrhaphy is still in place temporally

Ontario, Canada) and prednisolone acetate 1% four times daily were administered. At 1 month postoperatively, her vision was still counting fingers due to the retained amniotic membrane. The LR-CLAL segments were well integrated and the eye was quiet with a stable epithelial surface.

3.2.5 Case 5

- A scleral lens trial should be the first line of treatment even for patients with severe LSCD.
- Patients with severe bilateral LSCD who fail a scleral contact lens trial and/or have contraindications to systemic immune suppression can benefit from a Type 1 Boston keratoprosthesis for vision rehabilitation.

An 83-year-old female with a history of SJS-related LSCD was referred for evaluation due to decreased visual acuity in the left eye. Her past ocular history included superficial keratectomy with amniotic membrane transplantation in both eyes and previous cataract extraction with intraocular lens implantation in both eyes. On presentation, her BCVA was 20/300 and 20/200 in the right and left eyes, respectively. On examination, there were 360° of conjunctivalization and late staining observed in both eyes with a relatively clear central cornea in the right eye. Symblephara and severe dryness were also noted in both eyes with early keratinization changes noted in the right eye.

Optimization of the ocular surface was initiated as a first step. The following regimen was prescribed:

- Warm compresses, lid hygiene, omega-3 fatty acid supplementation
- Preservative-free artificial tears 4 times daily
- Vitamin A ointment before bed

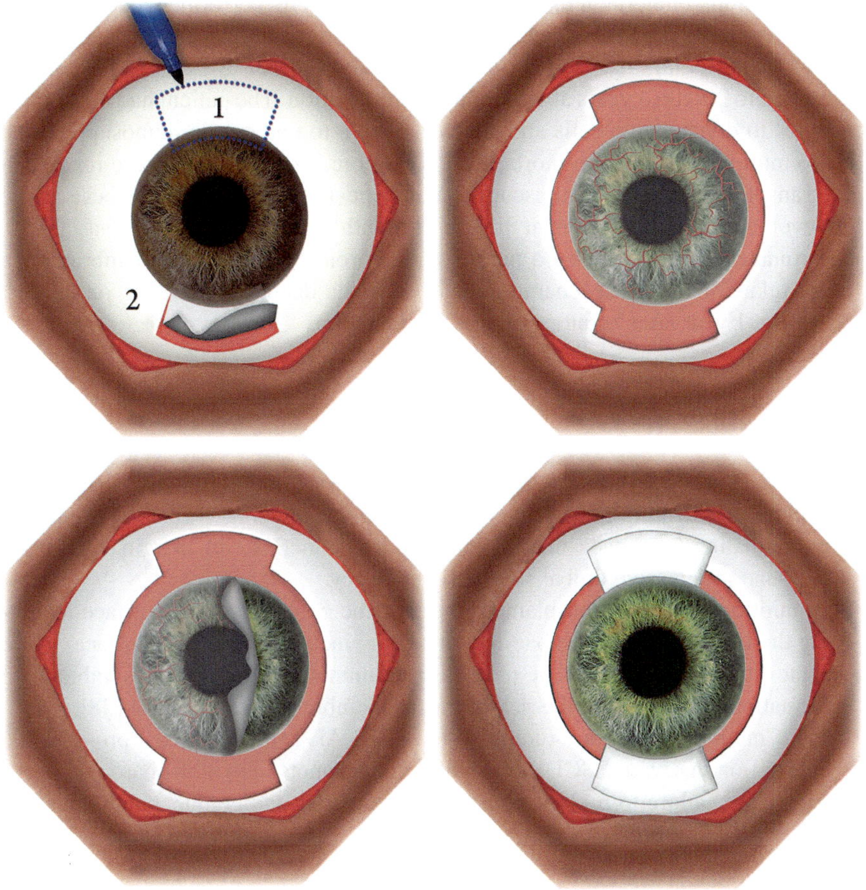

Fig. 3.9 Steps of conjunctival limbal allograft surgery (LR-CLAL). (*Top left*) 3 clock hours of superior and inferior conjunctival limbal allografts are marked and excised deep to sclera taking care to include at least 1 mm past the limbus. These are stored in a petri dish of optisol corneal storage medium (Chiron Ophthalmics, Irvine, California) or balanced salt solution for future use. (*Top right*) 360° conjunctival peritomy is done on the recipient eye. (*Bottom left*) Superficial keratectomy in the recipient eye with complete removal of all layers of hypertrophic epithelium leaving a clear Bowman's membrane layer visible. (*Bottom right*) The LR-CLAL pieces are secured at the recipient's superior and inferior limbus using 10-0 nylon or vicryl sutures and the base of the pieces secured to bare sclera using fibrin tissue glue. Amniotic membrane graft can also then be secured to the ocular surface using interrupted or a running 10-0 nylon or vicryl suture (not shown). (Medical illustration by Darya Asadi)

- 40% autologous serum tears 4 times daily
- Topical cyclosporine 0.05% (Restasis, Allergan, Irvine, CA, USA) twice daily
- Topical prednisolone 1% drops once daily
- 100 mg oral doxycycline daily

In addition, bilateral temporal tarsorrhaphies were performed. Next, scleral lenses were attempted but failed due to corneal erosions and irritation.

Her vision continued to deteriorate gradually and her BCVA in the left eye decreased to 20/400 4 years after her initial presentation. The patient had no suitable relatives to donate stem cells and she was unable to undergo immunosuppression due to multiple systemic co-morbidities. Therefore, she was not eligible for a stem cell transplant and underwent pseudophakic Type-1 Boston Keratoprosthesis in the left eye instead. The vision at her third-month postoperative visit was 20/50. Unfortunately, she developed a para-foveal choroidal neovascular membrane due to age-related macular degeneration and her vision declined to 20/100 on her last follow-up, 1 year after keratoprosthesis implantation.

3.2.6 Case 6

- Steven–Johnson Syndrome-Toxic Epidermal Lysis (SJS-TEN) is a debilitating condition with long-term sequelae owing to the ongoing chronic conjunctival inflammation, advanced meibomian gland dysfunction, lid margin keratinization, and progressive limbal stem cell deficiency.
- Amniotic membrane transplantation across the complete ocular surface including the lid margins, the bulbar and tarsal conjunctiva, and cornea surface, in the acute stages is essential in reducing inflammation, preventing symblephara formation, and reducing the risk of mucus membrane keratinization [28].
- The Cincinnati procedure (combination of KLAL and LR-CLAL) provides the best option in severe LSCD cases with large amounts of symblepharon and ocular surface failure to replace both limbal stem cells and conjunctival deficiency [19, 20].

This patient developed Steven Johnson Syndrome-Toxic Epidermal Lysis (SJS-TEN) at age 35 years old secondary to a sulfa-containing medication (Septra, trimethoprim-sulfamethoxazole). An amniotic membrane transplant was not performed at the time of the acute disease as it had not been a popularized technique yet. Over the years, the chronic features of the disease including cicatrization, keratinization of the lid margins, and progressive LSCD led to perforation and phthisis of the left eye after repeated corneal transplantations (~7 in total). He maintained a visual acuity of 20/40 to 20/60 in the right eye with a scleral lens (Fig. 3.10). However, similar to the left eye, the ongoing friction from the keratinized lid margin over the years (despite mucous membrane grafts performed by the oculoplastics team) led to worsening of the conjunctivalization and limbal stem cell deficiency. As the corneal neovascularization started to grow over the visual axis, a superficial keratectomy combined with amniotic membrane transplantation was performed. However, a nonhealing corneal epithelial defect developed postoperatively with corneal melt and perforation which necessitated an emergency penetrating keratoplasty. This transplant was maintained for years on autologous serum tears, acyclovir prophylaxis (to address a herpetic component), and with the aid of a scleral lens.

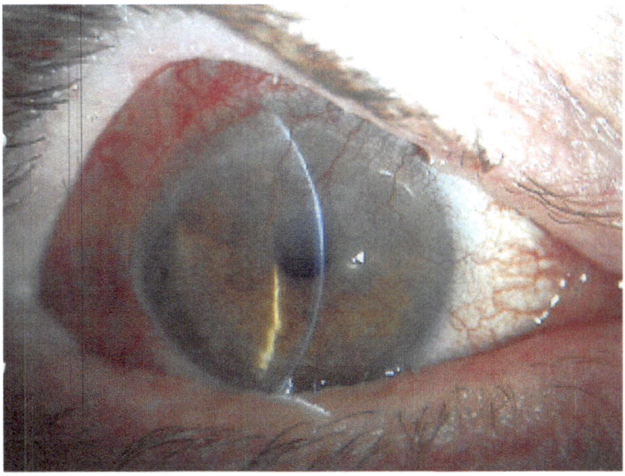

Fig. 3.10 Neovascularization, corneal haze, and conjunctival injection of the right eye in the early stages of the disease

Eventually, the central epithelium started to break down resulting in nonhealing epithelial defects, corneal melts, and repeated transplantations. The patient also developed chronic glaucoma, and given the sulfa allergy, he was limited to three classes of topical glaucoma drops, which was not sufficient to control his intraocular pressure. An endoscopic cyclophotocoagulation (ECP) was performed by the glaucoma team at the same time as a penetrating keratoplasty.

As repeated transplants would result in a similar course of failure given the LSCD, a stem cell transplantation was necessary in this monocular patient. Given the severity of the disease, a combined LR-CLAL and KLAL (Cincinnati) procedure (Fig. 3.11) was planned to give the best chance of success.

The patient underwent the Cincinnati procedure after an extensive workup in conjunction with the renal transplant team and initiation of systemic immune suppression.

The patient maintained functional vision (20/80 pinholing to 20/30) after the procedure. However, his glaucoma worsened requiring a glaucoma drainage device (Baerveldt, Abbott Medical Optics Inc., Santa Ana, CA) combined with ECP. The tube was placed in the pars plana due to a shallow anterior chamber. This surgery was performed in conjunction with the retina and cornea teams as it required a temporary intraoperative keratoprosthesis, a pars plana vitrectomy (PPV) to allow the pars plana placement of the glaucoma device followed by a new penetrating keratoplasty. His CLAL and KLAL segments continued to provide a healthy supply of stem cells for the new corneal transplant.

3.3 Conclusion

In tackling the complex mission of treating LSCD patients, a systematic stepwise approach should be followed. The etiology of LSCD should be identified, laterality confirmed, and extent assessed [2].

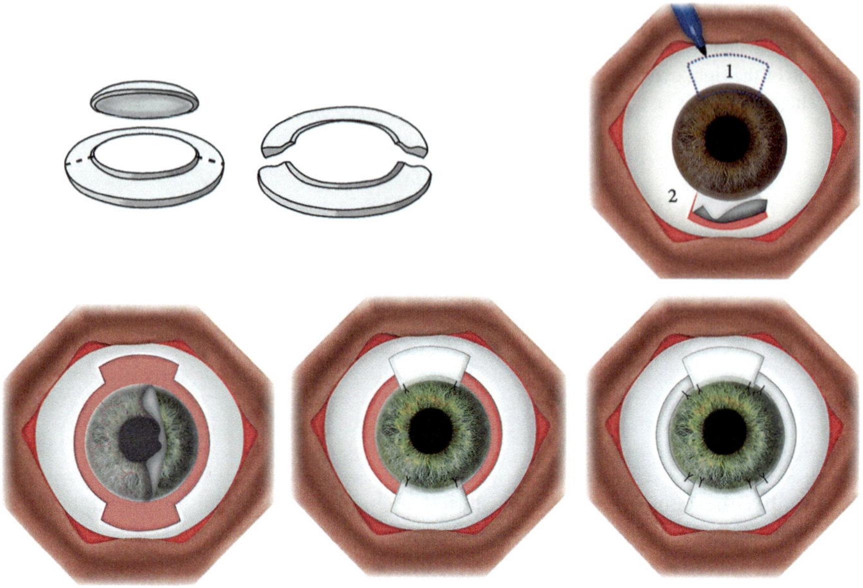

Fig. 3.11 The Cincinnati procedure combines a living-related conjunctival limbal allograft (LR-CLAL) and a deceased donor keratolimbal allograft (KLAL). (*Top left*) Donor KLAL lenticules are recovered from one cadaveric corneoscleral rim with the central 7.5 mm of cornea removed by trephination. (*Top right*) Retrieval of two conjunctival limbal grafts from the donor's eye at the 12- and 6-o'clock meridians is performed. (*Bottom from left to right*) Preparation of the recipient's corneal bed is performed by removing all the scar and conjunctivalized tissue. The LR-CLAL donor tissue is secured to the recipient using 10-0 nylon sutures at the limbus and tissue glue. Finally, the KLAL lenticules are secured to the recipient limbus using 10-0 nylon sutures and tissue glue. (Medical illustration by Darya Asadi)

In cases where sufficient limbal stem cells remain and the conjunctiva is uninflamed and healthy, discontinuing offending factors, treating comorbid ocular conditions, and administering medical treatments to optimize the ocular surface, may be sufficient to reverse LSCD [7]. If LSCD is not reversed, a scleral CL trial should be attempted which can delay or obviate the need for more invasive surgery [9].

In all LSCD cases, regardless of severity and laterality, once scleral CL and medical treatments fail to improve symptoms of decreased vision and/or pain, surgical options should be explored. In LSCD cases with severe limbal stem cell damage but with relatively healthy conjunctiva, LR-CLAL for bilateral disease or CLAU (preferred over SLET at our center) for unilateral disease can be attempted [5]. KLAL is performed if there is no living donor or if a patient does not want any surgery on their healthy fellow eye. In severely injured and inflamed eyes, where both limbal stem cells and conjunctiva are severely impaired, a Cincinnati procedure with systemic immunosuppression may offer superior long-term results to stabilize the ocular surface and reform the fornices [19]. In patients in which systemic immunosuppression is contraindicated, a keratoprosthesis may be suitable to improve and maintain vision [29].

Lastly, it is crucial to have a good multidisciplinary team to manage glaucoma, lid abnormalities as well as a transplant specialist (i.e. nephrologist) to assist with the management of systemic immunosuppression needed whenever allograft tissue is used.

References

1. Hamrah P, Sahin A. Limbus and corneal epithelium. Ocular surface disease: cornea, conjunctiva and tear film. Amsterdam: Elsevier; 2013.
2. Deng SX, Borderie V, Chan CC, et al. Global consensus on definition, classification, diagnosis, and staging of Limbal stem cell deficiency. Cornea. 2019;38:364–75.
3. Biber JM. Classification of ocular surface disease. In: Holland EJ, Mannis MJ, Lee WB, editors. Ocular surface disease: cornea, conjunctiva and tear film. New York: Elsevier; 2013.
4. Jeng BH. Diagnositc techniques in ocular surface disease. In: Edward J. Holland, MJ Mannis, W. Barry Lee, ed. Ocular surface disease: cornea, conjunctiva and tear film, New York: Elsevier, 2013.
5. Deng SX, Kruse F, Gomes JAP, et al. Global consensus on the management of limbal stem cell deficiency. Cornea. 2020;39:1291–302.
6. Chan CC, LoVerde L, Qiang J, et al. Incidence, risk factors, and surgical management of Boston Type 1 keratoprothesis corneal melts, leaks, and extrusions. Cornea. 2016;35:1049–56.
7. Kim BY, Riaz KM, Bakhtiari P, et al. Medically reversible limbal stem cell disease: clinical features and management strategies. Ophthalmology. 2014;121:2053–8.
8. Nguyen MTB, Thakrar V, Chan CC. EyePrintPRO therapeutic scleral contact lens: indications and outcomes. Can J Ophthalmol. 2018;53:66–70.
9. Garg A, Trinh T, Wong BM, et al. Prosthetic replacement of the ocular surface ecosystem for limbal stem cell deficiency: a case series. Eye Contact Lens. 2022;48:493.
10. Dua HS. Sequential Sectoral Conjunctival Epitheliectomy (SSCE). In: Holland EJ, Mannis MJ, editors. Ocular surface disease medical and surgical management. New York: Springer; 2002.
11. Sangwan VS, Basu S, MacNeil S, et al. Simple limbal epithelial transplantation (SLET): a novel surgical technique for the treatment of unilateral limbal stem cell deficiency. Br J Ophthalmol. 2012;96:931–4.
12. Holland EJ, Schwartz GS. The evolution of epithelial transplantation for severe ocular surface disease and a proposed classification system. Cornea. 1996;15:549–56.
13. Eslani M, Cheung AY, Kurji K, et al. Long-term outcomes of conjunctival limbal autograft in patients with unilateral total limbal stem cell deficiency. Ocul Surf. 2019;17:670–4.
14. Kreimei M, Sorkin N, Einan-Lifshitz A, et al. Long-term outcomes of donor eyes after conjunctival limbal autograft and allograft harvesting. Can J Ophthalmol. 2019;54:565–9.
15. Kwitko S, Marinho D, Barcaro S, et al. Allograft conjunctival transplantation for bilateral ocular surface disorders. Ophthalmology. 1995;102:1020–5.
16. Elham Ghahari AB-R, Djalilian AR. Living-Related Conjunctival–Limbal Allograft (lr-CLAL) transplantation. In: Holland EJ, Mannis MJ, editors. Ocular surface disease: cornea, conjunctiva and tear film. New York: Elsevier; 2013.
17. Holland EJ. Epithelial transplantation for the management of severe ocular surface disease. Trans Am Ophthalmol Soc. 1996;94:677–743.
18. Clara C, Chan EJH. Keratolimbal Allograft. In: Holland EJ, Mannis MJ, editors. Ocular surface disease: cornea, conjunctiva and tear film. New York: Elsevier; 2013.
19. Biber JM, Skeens HM, Neff KD, et al. The cincinnati procedure: technique and outcomes of combined living-related conjunctival limbal allografts and keratolimbal allografts in severe ocular surface failure. Cornea. 2011;30:765–71.

20. Chan CC, Biber JM, Holland EJ. The modified Cincinnati procedure: combined conjunctival limbal autografts and keratolimbal allografts for severe unilateral ocular surface failure. Cornea. 2012;31:1264–72.
21. Holland EJ, Mogilishetty G, Skeens HM, et al. Systemic immunosuppression in ocular surface stem cell transplantation: results of a 10-year experience. Cornea. 2012;31:655–61.
22. Movahedan A, Cheung AY, Eslani M, et al. Long-term outcomes of ocular surface stem cell allograft transplantation. Am J Ophthalmol. 2017;184:97–107.
23. Mimouni MCE, Kim SJ, Schiff J, Cardella C, Tinckam KJ, Slomovic AR, Chan CC. Outcomes of keratolimbal allograft from ABO compatible donors for severe bilateral limbal stem cell deficiency. Ocular Surf. 2022;27:48.
24. Aldave AJ, Kamal KM, Vo RC, et al. The Boston type I keratoprosthesis: improving outcomes and expanding indications. Ophthalmology. 2009;116:640–51.
25. Lee R, Khoueir Z, Tsikata E, et al. Long-term visual outcomes and complications of Boston keratoprosthesis type II implantation. Ophthalmology. 2017;124:27–35.
26. Ruiz-Lozano RE, Hernandez-Camarena JC, Valdez-Garcia JE, et al. Ocular involvement and complications of lichen planus, lichen planus pigmentosus, and lichen planopilaris: a comprehensive review. Dermatol Ther. 2021;34:e15137.
27. Cheung AY, Eslani M, Kurji KH, et al. Long-term outcomes of living-related conjunctival limbal allograft compared with keratolimbal allograft in patients with limbal stem cell deficiency. Cornea. 2020;39:980–5.
28. Cheung CS, Ali A, Chew HF. Successful treatment of acute ocular-involving toxic epidermal necrolysis using amniotic membrane suture fixated to custom designed symblepharon rings. Cornea. 2016;35:578–81.
29. Aravena C, Bozkurt TK, Yu F, et al. Long-term outcomes of the Boston Type I keratoprosthesis in the management of corneal limbal stem cell deficiency. Cornea. 2016;35:1156–64.

Exposure Keratopathy

4

Caroline Y. Yu, Mark A. Greiner, Mark Fisher,
and Erin M. Shriver

4.1 Introduction

Exposure keratopathy (EK) is a potentially visually devastating condition that occurs when there is compromise of ocular surface protection [1–3]. The eyelids and periocular adnexa play a vital role in preserving ocular surface health not only as a physical barrier for the cornea but also by maintaining a normal tear film composition [3]. Furthermore, blinking plays an important role in meibomian gland function, the lacrimal pump, and tear distribution, and an incomplete or infrequent blink rate can contribute to not only meibomian gland dysfunction but also aqueous tear deficiency [4, 5]. Therefore, loss of normal periocular anatomy, compromise of eyelid apposition to the globe, and abnormal eyelid function can leave the avascular corneal epithelium vulnerable to trauma, desiccation, and secondary infection, with long-term complications including scarring, denervation, microbial keratitis, ulceration, and perforation [3].

EK can occur for a number of reasons, including paralytic, mechanical, and neurotrophic etiologies [1, 2, 6–9]. Paralytic causes of facial nerve dysfunction can arise in the postoperative or postradiation setting, but can also be secondary to compression, trauma, medication side effects, and congenital conditions such as Möbius syndrome [10, 11]. Changes to periocular anatomy such as globe position, and periocular sclerosing conditions can also lead to EK [12]. While globe proptosis can lead to lagophthalmos, enophthalmos can also cause EK due to poor eyelid

C. Y. Yu · M. A. Greiner · E. M. Shriver (✉)
Department of Ophthalmology and Visual Sciences, University of Iowa Hospitals and Clinics, Iowa City, IA, USA
e-mail: erin-shriver@uiowa.edu

M. Fisher
Divison of Plastic and Reconstructive Surgery, Department of Surgery, University of Iowa Hospitals and Clinics, Iowa City, IA, USA

F. A. Woreta, R. B. Singh (eds.), *Cornea Casebook*, Current Practices in Ophthalmology, https://doi.org/10.1007/978-981-96-0495-1_4

apposition to the globe. Additionally, sclerosing conditions such as ocular cicatricial pemphigoid (OCP), chemical eye injury, thermal burns, and systemic conditions can cause cicatricial changes to not only the eyelid but also other periocular structures that can lead to EK [13, 14]. Abnormal eyelid position such as ectropion and lateral canthal disinsertion as well as complications from prior eyelid surgery can also contribute to EK [7, 15]. Abnormal corneal innervation such as in neurotrophic keratopathy and trigeminal neuralgia can exacerbate EK, via both impaired lacrimal gland secretion and blink regulation as well as decreased epithelial turnover [16].

Diagnosis of EK should include examination for signs of corneal desiccation such as punctate epithelial erosions (PEEs), corneal sensation, tear film stability, lid malposition, lagophthalmos, facial nerve function, proptosis, and enophthalmos. Supportive care for patients with EK should include frequent application of preservative-free artificial tears and lubricating ointment, but may also consist of moisture chambers, punctal plugs, and temporary tarsorrhaphy [2]. Long-term treatment will vary based on the underlying cause of exposure and can include medical management of systemic conditions, contact lens, permanent tarsorrhaphy, surgical correction of the eyelid or globe malposition, and corneal neurotization [14, 17–24].

In the following pages, the management of several cases of EK due to mechanical, paralytic, and neurogenic causes is reviewed in depth.

4.2 Cases

4.2.1 Case 1: Cicatricial Upper and Lower Eyelid Retraction Secondary to Thermal Burn

4.2.1.1 Highlights

- *Cicatricial changes affecting not only the eyelid but also the lower face and neck can contribute to EK.*
- *Prior to surgical management, underlying systemic sclerosing conditions such as ocular cicatricial pemphigoid (OCP) must be addressed as surgery can exacerbate the cicatrizing process.*
- *Surgical planning is dependent on the degree of anterior and posterior lamellar scarring and horizontal eyelid laxity.*

A 42-year-old female presented with third-degree thermal burns to her face, scalp, neck, and body secondary to a cooking accident. On initial bedside exam soon after her injury, there was inferotemporal epithelial sloughing in her left eye secondary to direct thermal injury, but no lagophthalmos or exposure keratopathy. She underwent skin grafting for her facial burn injuries, including placement of split-thickness skin grafts. However, less than 1 month following her accident, she developed worsening bilateral injection with inferior PEEs, cicatricial changes to her split-thickness facial skin grafts, and bilateral lagophthalmos. Her external exam showed anterior lamellar shortening with contracture of the skin grafts overlying her eyelid and mandibular regions leading to bilateral upper and lower eyelid retraction (Fig. 4.1a). Notably, there was relative sparing of the posterior lamellae. Initial management consisted of moisture chambers [25], around the clock topical lubricating ointments, and prophylactic antibiotic drops. Due to concern for progressive corneal epithelial irregularity at follow-up, bandage contact lenses were attempted to be placed in both eyes but were unable to be successfully retained due to her severe upper and lower eyelid retraction. Therefore, she was taken to the operating

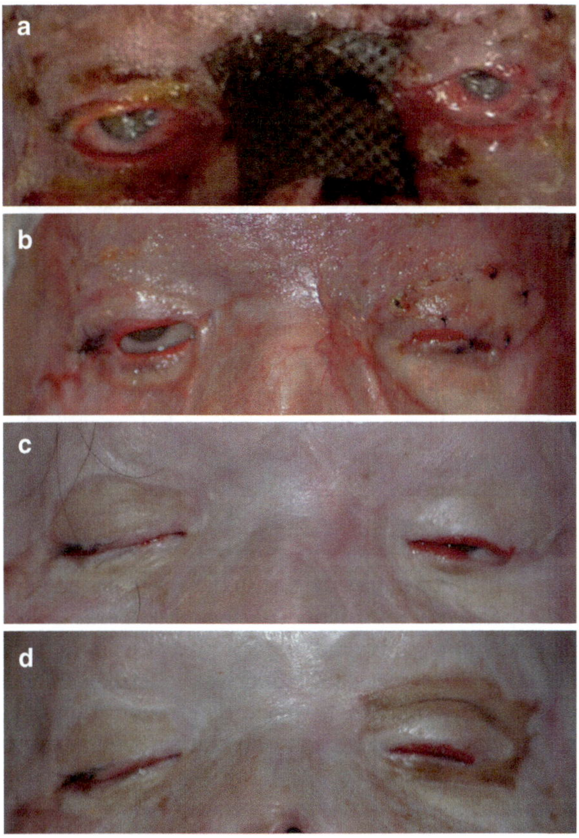

Fig. 4.1 External photographs of a 42-year-old patient with severe cicatricial bilateral eyelid retraction and exposure keratopathy from thermal injury. (**a**) Severe lagophthalmos 2 months after her initial injury with exposure keratopathy and inability to retain bandage contact lenses due to eyelid cicatricial changes. (**b**) Recurrent right lower eyelid cicatricial ectropion and lagophthalmos 3 months after full-thickness skin grafting and lateral tarsal strip, demonstrating right lower eyelid ectropion exacerbated by mouth opening, consistent with anterior lamellar shortening. Left upper eyelid demonstrates healing skin graft with sutures in place and intact left lateral tarsorrhaphy. (**c**) Recurrent left lower lid ectropion and lagophthalmos with inferior displacement of the lateral canthus 18 months after initial injury. (**d**) Improvement in lagophthalmos at follow-up 2 years following the initial accident after multiple anterior lamellar lengthening procedures including release of neck and facial cicatrix

room urgently for release of cicatrix of the bilateral upper and lower eyelids, full-thickness skin graft to her bilateral upper and lower eyelids, bilateral lower lid lateral tarsal strips, bilateral medial and lateral tarsorrhaphies, and amniotic graft membrane placement to her bilateral corneas (Fig. 4.1b).

She experienced improvement in her ocular surface initially, but approximately 3 months following this procedure, she developed recurrent left-sided lagophthalmos with significant cicatricial ectropion and increased corneal epithelial irregularity without frank epithelial breakdown as well as progression in her neck contracture (Fig. 4.1c). She was taken back to the operating room for release of cicatrix of the left lower eyelid with placement of a full-thickness skin graft and permanent left lateral tarsorrhaphy. Her postoperative course has involved close follow-up by oculoplastics, cornea, and plastic surgery, as she has continued to require interval surgical cicatricial releases from both upper and lower lids, full-thickness skin grafting, and release of cicatricial bands from her buccal, mandibular, and cervical regions (Fig. 4.1d). After her most recent follow-up visit, her corneal epithelium was intact with only trace PEEs, her uncorrected visual acuity was stable at 20/40 in the right eye and 20/60 in the left eye, and there was no visually significant corneal scarring.

This patient's case highlights the importance of a multi-disciplinary approach to patients with severe cicatricial contractions. Not only were there multiple points of contracture that needed to be addressed, but there was also a paucity of donor sites. Therefore, collaboration between multiple specialties, including oculoplastics, cornea, plastic surgery, and burn surgery, is important to optimal surgical outcomes.

With respect to periocular reconstruction, surgical planning is dependent on the extent of anterior and posterior lamellar involvement. Because this patient's eyelid retraction was primarily related to anterior lamellar cicatricial changes, repair has been focused on anterior lamellar lengthening procedures, namely, full-thickness skin grafts. Full-thickness skin grafts are preferred over split-thickness skin grafts for reconstruction in the periocular area due to improved aesthetic outcomes and a lower rate of postoperative contracture [26]. Common donor sites for periocular reconstruction include the upper eyelid, pre and postauricular, supraclavicular, and inner brachial regions but can vary depending on the available donor sites. In this patient's case, skin grafts were primarily harvested from the thighs due to the wide extent of her injury. Other options for anterior lamellae lengthening include free or pedicled flaps, local advancement flaps, and suborbicularis oculi fat (SOOF) lift.

Lastly, performing a thorough release of cicatricial bands is essential. Identifying both the various directions of contracture present, as well as achieving an appropriate depth such that unscarred tissue is reached is critical to achieve optimal outcomes [27]. Release of cicatricial bands in the eyelid must be done with care to avoid transection of the levator palpebrae superioris as well as to preserve the septum, when possible, to minimize extension of the cicatrix posteriorly. Additionally, horizontal tightening of the lower lid with anchoring medially and laterally should be considered as this can help to stabilize the lower lid position. Cicatricial changes can also be seen in the setting of trauma, inflammatory skin diseases, herpes zoster, prior surgery or laser treatment, OCP, and systemic sclerosing conditions. In general, any ongoing systemic cicatricial processes such as scleroderma and OCP should be stabilized medically before attempting surgery, as surgery can exacerbate the underlying sclerosing process [28]. However, rapid decompensation of the cornea epithelium despite maximum medical therapy is an indication for urgent surgical intervention.

4.2.2 Case 2: Thyroid Eye Disease

4.2.2.1 Highlights

- *EK in TED is multifactorial and can be caused by globe position, eyelid retraction, and a decreased blink rate.*
- *Management of EK in TED includes medical and surgical options with varying efficacy at addressing proptosis and eyelid retraction.*

A 75-year-old Caucasian female with a 19-year history of Graves' disease presented with bilateral ocular discomfort and tearing. She denied a history of tobacco use and endorsed worsening redness, irritation, and tearing as well as increased prominence of her eyes since undergoing radioactive iodine ablation 2 years prior. The exam was notable for a visual acuity of 20/20 bilaterally, no afferent pupillary defect, full-color vision, some limitation of abduction bilaterally, Hertel exophthalmometry of 29 mm and 30 mm in her right and left eye, respectively, and right greater than left upper eyelid retraction with an incomplete blink bilaterally. There were PEEs and conjunctival injection bilaterally, consistent with mild exposure keratopathy.

She was diagnosed with thyroid eye disease and started on intravenous methylprednisolone infusions as described in the European Group on Graves' Orbitopathy (EUGOGO) guidelines [29]. During her infusions, she had subjective improvement in her ocular irritation symptoms and diplopia but endorsed recurrence of her symptoms shortly after completion of her steroid infusions. Due to the development of a new left optic nerve hyperemia as well as persistent poorly controlled dry eye symptoms and diplopia, staged bilateral three-wall orbital decompressions (Fig. 4.2a) followed by strabismus surgery were performed (Fig. 4.2b). Correction of her vertical misalignment led to improvement in her strabismus but worsened left lower lid retraction (Fig. 4.2c). Due to persistent bilateral upper eyelid retraction, lagophthalmos, and EK, a bilateral upper eyelid full-thickness blepharotomy was performed and resulted in significant improvement in her symptoms initially (Fig. 4.2c).

However, this patient's disease course was unique as she experienced multiple episodes of TED reactivation over the subsequent years. She underwent multiple eyelid retraction repairs due to recurrent EK, including a left lower eyelid retractor recession with ear cartilage graft placement, a left lateral canthoplasty, a repeat left upper eyelid blepharotomy, and a small left lateral tarsorrhaphy (Fig. 4.2d). Seven years after initial diagnosis, she once again experienced a flare with new bilateral lagophthalmos, temporal injection, left greater than right corneal epithelial irregularity, and increased proptosis following an adjustment in her levothyroxine dosing (Fig. 4.2e). Following medical optimization of her thyroid levels, she completed a

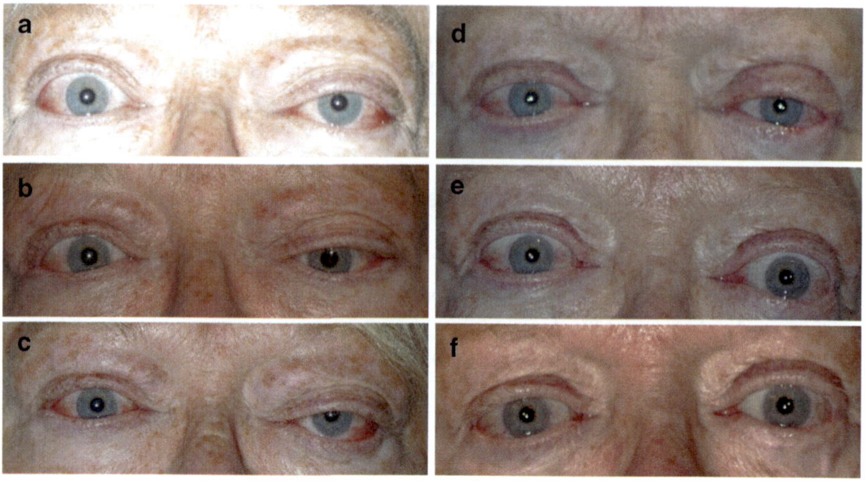

Fig. 4.2 Exposure keratopathy in a patient with longstanding Graves' disease and thyroid eye disease (TED) over the course of 11 years. (**a**) Bilateral proptosis and upper eyelid retraction prior to decompression (**b**) Strabismus following bilateral 3-wall decompression (**c**) Exacerbation of lower eyelid retraction following strabismus repair (**d**) Improvement in eyelid contour and height following multiple eyelid procedures to correct bilateral upper and lower eyelid retraction (**e**) Recurrence of proptosis and eyelid retraction 7 years after initial diagnosis. (**f**) Stable improvement in proptosis and eyelid retraction 18 months following completion of teprotumumab infusions

course of teprotumumab. After completion of teprotumumab, her proptosis decreased bilaterally, her diplopia stabilized, and her exam showed only rare PEEs in her right eye and no PEEs in the left eye. At her most recent follow-up 14 months after completion of teprotumumab infusions, she has had sustained improvement in her proptosis and has had no recurrence of lagophthalmos or EK on exam (Fig. 4.2f).

This patient with chronic thyroid eye disease demonstrates several important points. EK in TED is multifactorial and can be caused by globe position (as it relates to proptosis and strabismus), eyelid retraction, and a decreased blink rate [12, 30]. Depending on disease activity and the presence of vision-threatening exam findings, management of patients with TED will vary. Nonsurgical options include topical lubrication, smoking cessation, corticosteroids, biologic medications, orbital radiation, and teprotumumab [29, 31–33]. Most recently, teprotumumab, an insulin-like growth factor-1 (IGF-1R) inhibitor, was approved for the treatment of TED, with initial studies showing efficacy for improvement in proptosis and diplopia for patients with acute, active TED [32, 34].

Surgery has traditionally been performed in a staged fashion and delayed until the patient is in the fibrotic, stable disease stage unless there is a vision-threatening concern to avoid exacerbation of underlying inflammation and improve outcome predictability. The recommended sequence for surgical repair in TED patients has traditionally been orbital decompression followed by strabismus repair followed by eyelid surgeries for optimal patient outcomes. Eyelid retraction in TED tends to involve the posterior lamellae more than the anterior lamellae [3, 12]. For upper eyelid retraction, multiple surgical techniques have been described, including full-thickness blepharotomy, recession of Müller's muscle and/or the levator, spacer grafts, and levator lengthening by marginal myotomy [35]. Surgical options for correction of lower eyelid retraction include recession of the capsulopalpebral fascia with or without the use of spacers, suborbicularis oculi fat (SOOF) lift, and midface suspension [36]. Botulinum toxin and fillers can be used as nonsurgical eyelid weights to temporarily correct eyelid position in patients who are unable to or do not wish to undergo surgery [23, 37]. Lastly, regular follow-up with thyroid function monitoring is important for TED patients as a subset of patients develop recurrent inflammation and periocular changes years after disease onset [38].

4.2.3 Case 3: Facial Nerve Palsy

4.2.3.1 Highlights

- *Facial nerve palsy can lead to both paralytic and mechanical lagophthalmos, and surgical management should address both components.*
- *Myriad surgical options exist and can be broadly divided into static and dynamic techniques.*
- *Patients with longstanding facial nerve palsy can develop recurrence of lagophthalmos and exposure keratopathy over time and thus should have long-term ophthalmic follow-up.*

An 84-year-old woman was referred for right-sided facial nerve palsy. Her past medical history included a history of surgical resection of a right parotid gland tumor followed by radiation treatment 60 years prior. The patient subsequently developed postradiation-related squamous cell carcinoma in the right infra-auricular area. The malignancy was invasive into the right temporal bone and extensive local resection was performed, which included sacrifice of the right facial nerve. A left anterolateral thigh flap, right facial suspension, and placement of a right upper eyelid 1.2-g gold weight were performed at the time of resection (Fig. 4.3a). Postoperatively, the vision in her right eye remained stable at 20/150 and her exam showed 2 mm of lagophthalmos with decreased corneal sensation but a good Bell's phenomenon and minimal corneal exposure. Two years after her initial gold weight placement, she developed extrusion of the weight and underwent a right lower eyelid fascia lata sling and replacement of the right upper eyelid weight with a 1.6-g gold weight. Five years following her resection, she developed worsening vision to 20/400 on the right with an exam notable for right lower eyelid ectropion with right punctal ectropion, PEEs distributed in the inferior third of the cornea, a new Salzmann nodule inferotemporally, as well as previously documented foveal involving geographic atrophy on her dilated exam. However, due to other medical co-morbidities, she elected for conservative management and was recommended to increase the frequency of her topical lubrication regimen. Despite compliance with this topical regimen, her follow-up exam showed a visual decline to count fingers in the right eye with severe epitheliopathy, right lower eyelid ectropion, right-sided

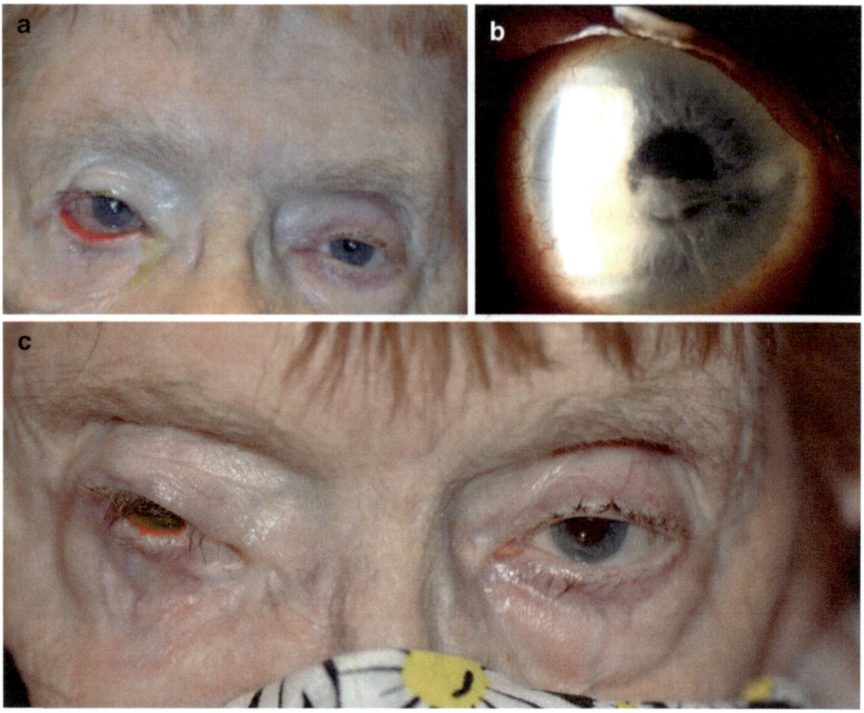

Fig. 4.3 External photographs of an 86-year-old patient with right facial nerve palsy resulting in severe epitheliopathy. (**a**) Right lower eyelid mechanical and paralytic ectropion. (**b**) Stromal scarring and an irregular epithelial ridge in the inferior half of the right cornea associated with circumferential pannus as a result of 6 mm of lagophthalmos. (**c**) Improved right lower eyelid position and apposition following midface advancement, lateral tarsal strip, and permanent lateral and medial tarsorrhaphy. Slit lamp exam showed an intact corneal epithelium and inactive corneal neovascularization

midface ptosis, and a poor Bell's reflex (Fig. 4.3b). As her lower eyelid ectropion was both paralytic and mechanical in etiology, surgical repair included a right midface advancement by adjacent tissue to address the mechanical component and a right lateral tarsal strip with permanent medial and lateral tarsorrhaphy to address the paralytic component (Fig. 4.3c). At her postoperative visits, her vision and symptoms have remained stable at hand motion at 1 foot without epithelial defects or active corneal neovascularization on a daily regimen of preservative-free artificial tears every 2 hours and bacitracin-polymyxin ointment 3 times a day.

Facial nerve palsy can occur for several reasons, including idiopathic, traumatic, iatrogenic, infectious, and compressive etiologies, typically secondary to parotid gland or cerebellopontine angle tumors as well as acoustic neuromas. Ophthalmic examination of patients with facial nerve palsy should include evaluation for abnormal upper or lower eyelid excursion, the degree of facial nerve palsy, lagophthalmos, degree of Bell's phenomenon, corneal sensation, tear function, midface position, and evidence of synkinesis or aberrant regeneration [39].

Management of patients with EK secondary to facial nerve palsy is guided by the expected duration and degree of facial nerve dysfunction, severity of corneal disease, and underlying cause. In the acute setting, conservative management is often recommended initially as some patients may recover some facial nerve function spontaneously. For patients with complete facial nerve paralysis from Bell's palsy, some evidence shows that timely facial nerve decompression may improve the likelihood of complete recovery but there is limited evidence available [40]. Nonsurgical options include topical lubrication, goggles, moisture chambers, tape tarsorrhaphy, chemical tarsorrhaphy with botulinum toxin, temporary tarsorrhaphy [18], magnetic tarsorrhaphy [41], and scleral contact lenses [21, 42]. Surgical management can be divided broadly into static and dynamic techniques. As patients can develop lagophthalmos due to a combination of upper eyelid retraction and lower eyelid laxity, static options focus on addressing eyelid and midface position to reduce lagophthalmos. There are several static techniques including temporary and permanent tarsorrhaphy [17, 20, 43], lower eyelid tightening and suspension [44, 45], upper eyelid loading such as via gold or platinum weight [19] or filler placement [23], levator lengthening [46], lateral tarsal strip, spacer graft placement, müllerectomy [47], fascia lata sling placement [48], and midface elevation [49]. Dynamic techniques include facial reanimation procedures, which are usually performed in collaboration with other specialties, and include temporalis transposition [50], free muscle grafts with cross-nerve innervation [50, 51], and cross-over or interpositional nerve grafts [52].

As with this patient, recurrence of lagophthalmos is not infrequent as patients develop tissue atrophy, upper eyelid retraction, loss of orbicularis tone, and gravitational tissue descent over time. Permanent tarsorrhaphies can affect patients' visual function and cosmesis but are a good option in patients with baseline poor visual acuity. Eyelid weights are usually well tolerated, but a subset of patients may experience allergic reaction or implant extrusion. From the ophthalmologic perspective, referring patients to facial reanimation specialists can be considered, but not all patients are good candidates for facial reanimation, and current reanimation procedures often do not produce a significant improvement in blink [53]. Ultimately, it is not uncommon for patients to require multiple procedures over time and thus patients should have regular eye exams long term.

4.2.4 Case 4: Neurotrophic Keratopathy

4.2.4.1 Highlights

- *Scleral contact lenses can be an effective therapeutic method for both ocular surface protection as well as visual rehabilitation, but not all patients are good candidates.*
- *Surgical correction of eyelid malposition can improve contact lens fit and long-term tolerance.*
- *Corneal neurotization and cenergemin are promising treatments to improve corneal sensation.*

A 61-year-old male with a history of herpes zoster keratouveitis complicated by neurotrophic keratopathy of the left eye presented for decreased visual acuity in his left eye. His best-corrected vision was 20/50 + 2 in the left eye on presentation, and his exam showed dense inferior PEEs, decreased corneal sensation, and temporal stromal scarring with mild thinning paracentrally (Fig. 4.4a). Corneal topography showed significant irregular astigmatism (Fig. 4.4b). For both visual rehabilitation and corneal protection, a scleral contact lens was recommended. Due to his irregular corneal contour secondary to stromal scarring, he ultimately underwent fitting with an EyePrintPro®, a type of custom imprint 3D scanned scleral contact lens. At his follow-up, the best corrected visual acuity with the contact lens in his left eye was 20/20 and the exam showed minimal PEEs.

Contact lenses can be an effective nonsurgical therapeutic option in patients with longstanding exposure keratopathy. Types of contact lenses include bandage contact lenses, which are typically soft contact lenses and should be used for short-term therapy only, and scleral contact lenses. Scleral lenses rest on the sclera and vault over the cornea (Fig. 4.4c). This provides both the benefit of a more stable fit over

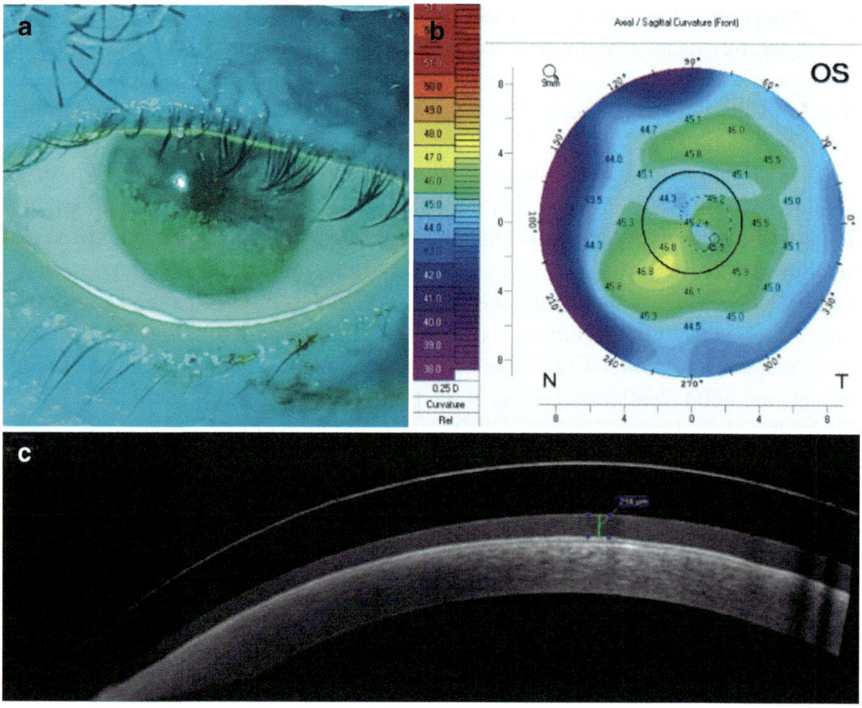

Fig. 4.4 41-year-old male with postherpetic neurotrophic keratopathy managed with a scleral contact lens. (**a**) Initial exam showed dense inferior PEEs, temporal stromal scarring, and decreased corneal sensation. (**b**) Corneal topography with irregular astigmatism and relative temporal steepening, corresponding to the area of stromal scarring. (**c**) Anterior segment optical coherence tomography shows the scleral contact lens fit over the patient's cornea with a liquid interface between the lens and cornea

irregular corneal shapes as well as providing a liquid interface that maintains ocular surface lubrication. Scleral contact lenses come in various sizes and include variations such as the PROSE [41] and EyePrintPro® [54]. Surgical correction of concurrent eyelid malpositions can be effective in improving contact lens fit and long-term tolerance [55]. While scleral contact lenses can be an effective method of managing ocular surface disease especially in patients with neurotrophic keratopathy and compromised blink dynamics (i.e., facial nerve palsy), patients with a low endothelial cell count, glaucoma drainage devices, and poor personal hygiene habits may not be good candidates for a scleral contact lens. Additionally, scleral contact lenses can be cost prohibitive as insurance coverage for contact lens-related fees can be difficult to obtain.

While this patient did well with a scleral contact lens, some patients may require further interventions. Other options include topical autologous or allogenic serum tears, tarsorrhaphy, amniotic membrane graft, and conjunctival flaps [3, 56]. Corneal neurotization and topical treatment with topically applied recombinant human nerve growth factor are promising therapies for patients with recalcitrant neurotrophic disease, but exposure should be addressed concurrent with or prior to considering these treatments [56, 57].

4.3 Conclusion

As these cases demonstrate, patients with EK should undergo a thorough history, exam, and workup to determine the underlying etiology as this is essential for guiding management. In some cases, if persistent exposure keratopathy is anticipated despite topical lubrication, treatment with contact lens, tarsorrhaphy, and other temporizing measures can be helpful. Finally in many cases such as CN V and VII palsies, patients often benefit from a multidisciplinary team approach, including cornea, oculoplastics, optometry, plastic surgery, and otolaryngology. Ultimately, prompt diagnosis and treatment of the underlying etiology are critical to improving visual outcomes in patients with EK.

Acknowledgments The authors are grateful to Christine Sindt OD, FAAO for assistance in the writing of this manuscript.

Author Disclosures CYY, MAG, and MF have no financial disclosures. EMS has served as an Advisor for Horizon Therapeutics and Tarsus Pharmaceuticals.

References

1. Wolkow N, Chodosh J, Freitag SK. Innovations in treatment of lagophthalmos and exposure keratopathy. Int Ophthalmol Clin. 2017;57(4):85.
2. Jammal H, Khader Y, Shihadeh W, Ababneh L, AlJizawi G, AlQasem A. Exposure keratopathy in sedated and ventilated patients. J Crit Care. 2012;27(6):537–41.
3. Mannis MJ, Holland EJ. Cornea. 4th ed. Elsevier Health Sciences, New York; 2010.

4. Wan T, Jin X, Lin L, Xu Y, Zhao Y. Incomplete blinking may attribute to the development of meibomian gland dysfunction. Curr Eye Res. 2016;41(2):179–85.
5. Rodriguez JD, Lane KJ, Ousler GW III, Angjeli E, Smith LM, Abelson MB. Blink: characteristics, controls, and relation to dry eyes. Curr Eye Res. 2018;43(1):52–66.
6. Miedziak AI, Gottsch JD, Iliff NT. Exposure keratopathy after cosmetic CO2 laser skin resurfacing. Cornea. 2000;19(6)
7. Daut PM, Steinemann TL, Westfall CT. Chronic exposure keratopathy complicating surgical correction of ptosis in patients with chronic progressive external ophthalmoplegia. Am J Ophthalmol. 2000;130(4):519–21.
8. Singh S, Das AV, Ali MH. Ocular involvement in facial nerve paralysis: risk factors for severe visual impairment and ocular surface exposure in 1870 patients. Orbit. 2022:1–6.
9. McMonnies CW. Incomplete blinking: Exposure keratopathy, lid wiper epitheliopathy, dry eye, refractive surgery, and dry contact lenses. Cont Lens Anterior Eye. 2007;30(1):37–51.
10. Lopez-Valverde G, Jarrin-Hernandez E, Cruz-Gonzalez F, Mateos-Sanchez E. Möbius syndrome: surgical treatment for eyelid dysfunction. Case Rep Ophthalmol. 2013;4(3):229–33.
11. Nowak-Gospodarowicz I, Różycki R, Rękas M. Quality of life in patients with unresolved facial nerve palsy and exposure keratopathy treated by upper eyelid gold weight loading. Clin Ophthalmol. 2020;14:2211–22.
12. Bahn RS. Graves' ophthalmopathy. N Engl J Med. 2010;362(8):726–38.
13. Brodovsky SC, McCarty CA, Snibson G, Loughnan M, Sullivan L, Daniell M, et al. Management of alkali burns: an 11-year retrospective review. Ophthalmology. 2000;107(10):1829–35.
14. Elner VM, Mauffray RO, Fante RG, Harris M, Morton AD, Hassan AS. Comprehensive midfacial elevation for ocular complications of facial nerve palsy. Arch Facial Plast Surg. 2003;5(5):427–33.
15. Shriver EM, Erickson BP, Kossler AL, Tse DT. Lateral canthal tendon disinsertion: clinical characteristics and anatomical correlates. Ophthal Plast Reconstr Surg. 2016;32(5):378.
16. Müller LJ, Marfurt CF, Kruse F, Tervo TMT. Corneal nerves: structure, contents and function. Exp Eye Res. 2003;76(5):521–42.
17. Cosar CB, Cohen EJ, Rapuano CJ, Maus M, Penne RP, Flanagan JC, et al. Tarsorrhaphy: clinical experience from a cornea practice. Cornea. 2001;20(8):787–91.
18. Ellis MF, Daniell M. An evaluation of the safety and efficacy of botulinum toxin type A (BOTOX) when used to produce a protective ptosis. Clin Exp Ophthalmol. 2001;29(6):394–9.
19. Razfar A, Afifi AM, Manders EK, Myers EN, Johnson JT, Ferris RL, et al. Ocular outcomes after gold weight placement and facial nerve resection. Otolaryngol Head Neck Surg. 2009;140(1):82–5.
20. Trivedi D, McCalla M, Squires Z, Parulekar M. Use of cyanoacrylate glue for temporary tarsorrhaphy in children. Ophthal Plast Reconstr Surg. 2014;30(1):60–3.
21. Chahal JS, Heur M, Chiu GB. Prosthetic replacement of the ocular surface ecosystem scleral lens therapy for exposure keratopathy. Eye Contact Lens. 2017;43(4)
22. Ziai K, Thomas S, Weller C, Lighthall JG. Corneal neurotization in the setting of facial paralysis: a comprehensive review of surgical techniques. J Craniofac Surg. 2021;32(6):2210–4.
23. Mancini R, Taban M, Lowinger A, Nakra T, Tsirbas A, Douglas RS, et al. Use of hyaluronic acid gel in the management of paralytic lagophthalmos: the hyaluronic Acid gel "gold weight". Ophthal Plast Reconstr Surg. 2009;25(1):23–6.
24. Alsuhaibani AH, Carter KD, Policeni B, Nerad JA. Orbital volume and eye position changes after balanced orbital decompression. Ophthal Plast Reconstr Surg. 2011;27(3):158–63.
25. Airiani S, Braunstein RE, Kazim M, Schrier A, Auran JD, Srinivasan BD. Tegaderm transparent dressing (3M) for the treatment of chronic exposure keratopathy. Ophthal Plast Reconstr Surg. 2003;19(1)
26. Rathore DS, Chickadasarahilli S, Crossman R, Mehta P, Ahluwalia HS. Full thickness skin grafts in periocular reconstructions: long-term outcomes. Ophthal Plast Reconstr Surg. 2014;30(6):517–20.
27. Goel A, Shrivastava P. Post-burn scars and scar contractures. Indian J Plast Surg. 2010;43(Suppl):S63–71.

28. Heiligenhaus A, Shore JW, Rubin PAD, Foster CS. Long-term results of mucous membrane grafting in ocular cicatricial pemphigoid: implications for patient selection and surgical considerations. Ophthalmology. 1993;100(9):1283–8.
29. Bartalena L, Kahaly GJ, Baldeschi L, Dayan CM, Eckstein A, Marcocci C, et al. The 2021 European Group on Graves' Orbitopathy (EUGOGO) clinical practice guidelines for the medical management of Graves' orbitopathy. Eur J Endocrinol. 2021;185(4):G43–67.
30. Ribeiro SF, Shekhovtsova M, Duarte AF, Velasco Cruz AA. Graves lower eyelid retraction. Ophthal Plast Reconstr Surg. 2016;32(3):161–9.
31. Yu CY, Keen JA, Shriver EM. Teprotumumab: a major advance in the treatment of thyroid eye disease management. Adv Ophthalmol Optom. 2022;
32. Douglas RS, Kahaly GJ, Patel A, Sile S, Thompson EHZ, Perdok R, et al. Teprotumumab for the treatment of active thyroid eye disease. N Engl J Med. 2020;382(4):341–52.
33. Bartley GB, Fatourechi V, Kadrmas EF, Jacobsen SJ, Ilstrup DM, Garrity JA, et al. Clinical features of Graves' ophthalmopathy in an incidence cohort. Am J Ophthalmol. 1996;121(3):284–90.
34. Smith TJ, Kahaly GJ, Ezra DG, Fleming JC, Dailey RA, Tang RA, et al. Teprotumumab for thyroid-associated ophthalmopathy. N Engl J Med. 2017;376(18):1748–61.
35. Kazim M, Gold KG. A review of surgical techniques to correct upper eyelid retraction associated with thyroid eye disease. Curr Opin Ophthalmol. 2011;22(5):391–3.
36. Tao JP, Aakalu VK, Wladis EJ, Sobel RK, Freitag SK, Foster JA, et al. Bioengineered acellular dermal matrix spacer grafts for lower eyelid retraction repair: a report by the American Academy of Ophthalmology. Ophthalmology. 2020;127(5):689–95.
37. Costa PG, Saraiva FP, Pereira IC, Monteiro MLR, Matayoshi S. Comparative study of Botox® injection treatment for upper eyelid retraction with 6-month follow-up in patients with thyroid eye disease in the congestive or fibrotic stage. Eye. 2009;23(4):767–73.
38. Patel P, Khandji J, Kazim M. Recurrent thyroid eye disease. Ophthal Plast Reconstr Surg. 2015;31(6):445–8.
39. Rahman I, Sadiq SA. Ophthalmic management of facial nerve palsy: a review. Surv Ophthalmol. 2007;52(2):121–44.
40. Lee SY, Seong J, Kim YH. Clinical implication of facial nerve decompression in complete Bell's Palsy: a systematic review and meta-analysis. Clin Exp Otorhinolaryngol. 2019;12(4):348–59.
41. Barmettler A, Nissanka N, Rosenblatt MI, Rao R, Lipson D, Lelli GJ Jr. Magnetic systems for tarsorrhaphy. Ophthal Plast Reconstr Surg. 2014;30(4):305–8.
42. Gire A, Kwok A, Marx DP. PROSE treatment for lagophthalmos and exposure keratopathy. Ophthal Plast Reconstr Surg. 2013;29(2)
43. Kitchens J, Kinder J, Oetting T. The drawstring temporary tarsorrhaphy technique. Arch Ophthalmol. 2002;120(2):187–90.
44. Sendul SY, Cagatay HH, Dirim B, Demir M, Acar Z, Olgun A, et al. Effectiveness of the lower eyelid suspension using fascia lata graft for the treatment of lagophthalmos due to facial paralysis. Biomed Res Int. 2015;2015:759793.
45. May M, Hoffmann DF, Buerger GF, Soll DB. Management of the paralyzed lower eyelid by implanting auricular cartilage. Arch Otolaryngol Head Neck Surg. 1990;116(7):786–8.
46. Guillou-Jamard M-R, Labbé D, Bardot J, Benateau H. Paul Tessier's technique in the treatment of paralytic lagophthalmos by lengthening of the levator muscle: evaluation of 29 cases. Ann Plast Surg. 2011;67(6)
47. Hassan AS, Frueh BR, Elner VM. Müllerectomy for upper eyelid retraction and lagophthalmos due to facial nerve palsy. Arch Ophthalmol. 2005;123(9):1221–5.
48. Rose EH. Autogenous fascia lata grafts: clinical applications in reanimation of the totally or partially paralyzed face. Plast Reconstr Surg. 2005;116(1):20–32; discussion 3–5.
49. Chung JE, Yen MT. Midface lifting as an adjunct procedure in ectropion repair. Ann Plast Surg. 2007;59(6):641.
50. Frey M, Giovanoli P, Tzou C-HJ, Kropf N, Friedl S. Dynamic reconstruction of eye closure by muscle transposition or functional muscle transplantation in facial palsy. Plast Reconstr Surg. 2004;114(4):865–75.

51. Shindo M. Facial reanimation with microneurovascular free flaps. Facial Plast Surg. 2000;16(04):357–60.
52. Tate JR, Tollefson TT. Advances in facial reanimation. Curr Opin Otolaryngol Head Neck Surg. 2006;14(4)
53. Biglioli F, Zago M, Allevi F, Ciprandi D, Dell'Aversana Orabona G, Pucciarelli V, et al. Reanimation of the paralyzed lids by cross-face nerve graft and platysma transfer. J Craniomaxillofac Surg. 2018;46(3):521–6.
54. Silverman JIM, Huffman JM, Zimmerman MB, Ling JJ, Greiner MA. Indications for wear, visual outcomes, and complications of custom imprint 3D scanned scleral contact lens use. Cornea. 2021;40(5):596–602.
55. Chahal HS, Estrada M, Sindt CW, Boehme JA, Greiner MA, Nerad JA, et al. Scleral contact lenses in an academic oculoplastics clinic: epidemiology and emerging considerations. Ophthal Plast Reconstr Surg. 2018;34(3):231–6.
56. Pflugfelder SC, Massaro-Giordano M, Perez VL, Hamrah P, Deng SX, Espandar L, et al. Topical recombinant human nerve growth factor (cenegermin) for neurotrophic keratopathy: a multicenter randomized vehicle-controlled pivotal trial. Ophthalmology. 2020;127(1):14–26.
57. Swanson MA, Swanson RD, Kotha VS, Cai Y, Clark R, Jin A, et al. Corneal neurotization: a meta-analysis of outcomes and patient selection factors. Ann Plast Surg. 2022;88(6):687–94.

Neurotrophic Keratopathy

5

Pier Luigi Surico, Chiara De Gregorio, Tommaso Mori, and Antonio Di Zazzo

Neurotrophic keratopathy (NK) is a degenerative rare disease characterized by a reduced or absent corneal sensitivity and an impairment of corneal nerves [1]. The trophism and transparency of the cornea, which lacks blood and lymphatic vessels, is mainly due to its extensive innervation from the ophthalmic branch of the trigeminal nerve [2]. Any trauma, infection, surgery, systemic, or local congenital diseases may damage corneal nerves and cause neurotrophic keratopathy (NK). Impairment or loss of corneal sensory innervation is responsible for corneal epithelial defects, ulcer, and perforation. The epidemiology of NK is still uncertain. As a rare disease, its estimated prevalence is less than 30/100,000 individuals [3].

Every ocular or systemic condition altering corneal sensory innervation, which runs from the cornea itself to the pontine trigeminal nucleus, can result in NK (Table 5.1).

In animal models, ocular nerve injury causes morphologic alterations of epithelial cells with epithelial thinning and breakdown [4–6]. Numerous theories have been postulated to elucidate the pathogenesis of NK. These include the desiccation of the corneal surface resulting from reduced lacrimal secretions, as tear secretion is reliant on nerve stimuli [7]. Moreover, it is suggested that impaired corneal sensitivity could lead to a decrease in protective blink reflexes, abnormal metabolism of epithelial cells, rendering them more susceptible to trauma, drying, and infection. Another contributory factor could be the absence of trophic support from corneal nerve fibers [8].In most cases it is probably a combination of these factors, with a neurotrophic deficit playing a major role.

The diminishment of tear fluid secretion and the decline in epithelial cell vitality can lead to decreased levels of neurotrophins on the ocular surface, particularly

P. L. Surico · C. De Gregorio · T. Mori · A. Di Zazzo (✉)
Department of Ophthalmology, Corneal Rare Disease Center,
Campus Bio-Medico University Hospital Foundation, Rome, Italy
e-mail: pierluigi.surico@unicampus.it; chiara.degregorio@unicampus.it; tmori@ucsd.edu

F. A. Woreta, R. B. Singh (eds.), *Cornea Casebook*, Current Practices in Ophthalmology, https://doi.org/10.1007/978-981-96-0495-1_5

Table 5.1 NK etiology

Ocular diseases	Medications	Ocular surgery	Nonocular surgery	Others
Herpes infection (simplex and zoster) Other infections (e.g., Acanthamoeba) Chemical and physical burns Contact lens abuse Chronic ocular surface injury or inflammation Irradiation to eye or adnexa Limbal stem cell deficiency (LSCD)	Topical anesthetic abuse Chronic use of topical medications with benzalkonium chloride (BAK) Drug toxicity (e.g., glaucoma eyedrops, NSAIDs)	Corneal refractive surgery Corneal transplantation Collagen cross-linking for keratoconus Vitrectomy Laser photocoagulation	Neurosurgical procedures or trauma damaging trigeminal nerve (e.g. for acoustic neuroma or trigeminal neuralgia)	Stroke Aneurysm Multiple sclerosis Intracranial tumors Diabetes Leprosy Vitamin A deficiency Drugs (antipsychotics and narcoleptics) Congenital hypoplasia of trigeminal nerve; Congenital syndromes (Ryley-Day syndrome; Goldenhar-Gorlin syndrome; Mobius syndrome; Familial corneal hypoaestesia)

Adapted from Dua et al. [1]

NGF (nerve growth factor). NGF plays a crucial role in the development and survival of sympathetic and sensory neurons, as well as providing trophic support following neuronal injuries [9]. In its healthy state, the cornea typically contains NGF, which plays a regulatory role in the proliferation and differentiation of epithelial cells. Furthermore, NGF seems to participate in interactions between the epithelium and stroma that promote stromal healing and remodeling. However, when NGF availability is diminished, it can lead to compromised nerve and corneal functions [10].

The diagnosis should be based on a very accurate review of the medical and surgical history of the patients.

The ocular surface symptoms could be mild or absent since the corneal sensitivity is impaired in these patients. A decrease in visual acuity is sometimes reported particularly in the advanced stages of the disease. This makes early diagnosis a challenge for clinicians. At the slit lamp examination, the clinical patterns can range from subtle ocular surface irregularities (e.g., punctate keratopathy) to ulcers and perforation. NK is usually graded in three different stages according to the "Mackie classification" [11]:

(a) Stage I is characterized by epithelial irregularity most commonly in the form of punctate keratopathy without epithelial defect.
(b) Stage II is defined by recurrent or persistent epithelial defects (PED) without stromal involvement. The PED is usually oval in shape and its margins are characteristically smooth and rolled due to impaired epithelial healing. Descemet's folds and anterior chamber inflammation may be observed.
(c) Stage III is characterized by stromal involvement leading to corneal ulcer, melting, and perforation.

It is important to perform an extensive evaluation of the ocular surface including eyelids exam, corneal staining with fluorescein, Schirmer test, and corneal sensitivity which can be assessed with corneal esthesiometers (e.g., Cochet-Bonnet contact aesthesiometer, CRCERT-Belmonte noncontact aesthesiometer). In vivo confocal microscopy can be additionally used to study the affected structure of the subbasal nerves.

Treating NK remains a challenge for ophthalmologists although several approaches have been suggested based on the severity of the disease. Bandage contact lenses and lubricating eye drops are commonly used for early stage NK, while amniotic membrane transplantation (AMT), topically applied autologous serum, and blood derivates, in different concentrations of serum tears, and tarsorrhaphy have been widely used for advanced stages of the disease as well as more complex and invasive surgical approaches like corneal neurotization [12]. More recently, the introduction of a topical recombinant human nerve growth factor (rhNGF) has provided a promising new approach to the management of the disease [13]. Nerve Growth Factor eye drops are currently approved by the FDA and EMA to treat patients with NK [14–16].

5.1 Case 1

- Corneal nerve alterations in post-herpetic disease: don't forget to test corneal sensitivity.

A 78 male with history of stroke and myocardial infarction was referred to the Cornea Service. He was diagnosed with Herpes Zoster keratitis in the left eye and treated with Acyclovir 800 mg 1 tablet three times a day, and steroid eye drops. Bandage contact lens was subsequently applied to help with the healing of the epithelial defect together with preservative-free artificial tears.

Corneal sensitivity was assessed by Cochet-Bonnet esthesiometer, resulting in marked corneal hypoesthesia in all of the corneal quadrants, confirming the suspect of possible post-herpetic NK (Stage III).

At 8 months after the diagnosis of the infection, the slit lamp exam showed a corneal ulcer measuring 4.8 × 5 mm characterized by typical oval shape and rolled margin (Fig. 5.1a). He was started with rhNGF eye drops (Cenegermin 0.002%) with the standard regimen of 6 times per day for 8 weeks. After 4 weeks of therapy,

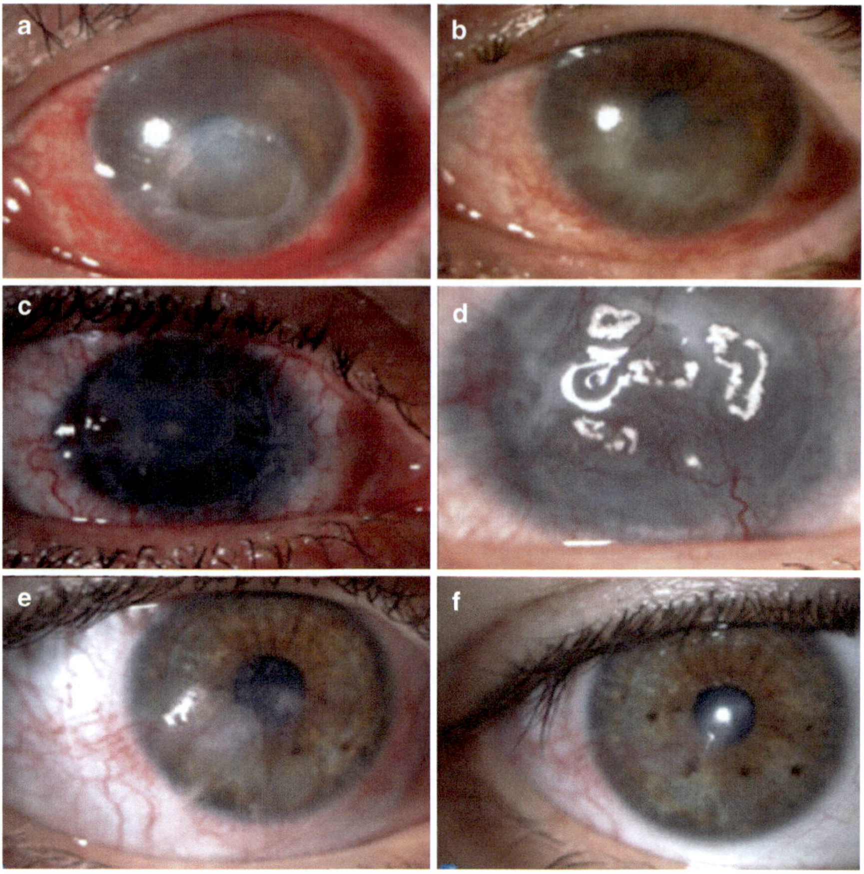

Fig. 5.1 Slit lamp images obtained before (**a**, **c**, **e**) and after (**b**, **d**, **f**) the 8-week treatment with topical rhNGF, respectively in case 1, case 2, and case 3

corneal sensitivity increased and the patient reported symptoms of ocular discomfort and mild ocular pain which is one of the most common minor side effects of the rhNGF eye drops. The ulcer was reduced to a minimal epithelial defect that was completely healed at the end of the 8 weeks therapy (Fig. 5.1b). The patient was followed-up also at 6 months and 1 year without recurrences and with improvement of the ocular discomfort symptoms.

5.2 Case 2

- NK can be a rare but possible complication of penetrating keratoplasty (PK).

A 31-year-old male came to Cornea Department with an history of penetrating trauma in the right eye 7 years before, resulting in a globe rupture. He underwent vitreoretinal surgery for retinal detachment and penetrating corneal transplant (PK) and amniotic membrane transplantation (AMT). Visual acuity of the right eye was light perception. At the slit lamp examination, a frank epithelial defect measuring 3x5 mm was detected (Fig. 5.1c). A 360 degrees corneal graft neovascularization was present. Severe hypoesthesia was assessed in all the quadrants of the graft. NK was diagnosed and the patient was started with Cenegermin 6 times per day for 8 weeks. He gradually improved and at the end of the treatment, the epithelial defect was significantly reduced and remained stable over the following visits (Fig. 5.1d). Neovascularization and peripheral sterile infiltrates were attributed to the presence of the continuous graft suture.

5.3 Case 3

- Carefully review the history of the patient: it can tell you the diagnosis!
- Exposure keratopathy can mask an underlying neurotrophic component.

A 30-year-old woman came to Cornea Department for ocular discomfort symptoms and blurry vision in the right eye. She had previously undergone surgery to remove an acoustic neuroma causing right facial (VII) and vestibulocochlear (VIII) nerve paralysis. The patient was also complaining waxing and waning pain and hypersensitivity in the right side of the face, consistent with a trigeminal involvement from the acoustic neurinoma. His visual acuity was 20/40 and 20/20, respectively, in the right and left eye. At the slit lamp examination, he showed a paracentral diffuse epithelial defect with superficial neovascularization in the right eye (Fig. 5.1e). NK suspect was confirmed by the severe hypoesthesia assessed with Cochet-Bonnet esthesiometer. In addition to preservative-free lubricants, the patient was started with Cenegermin for 8 weeks 6 times per day. The epithelial defect due to exposure keratopathy with a neurotrophic component was successfully healed (Fig. 5.1f) and the patient experienced improvement in his ocular symptoms.

The following three cases (Cases 4, 5, and 6), previously reported by our group [17], had stage 3 (corneal ulcer involving subepithelial stroma) neurotrophic keratopathy (NK) in one eye. These patients had not responded to conventional nonsurgical treatments and were subsequently treated with topical rhNGF (recombinant human nerve growth factor). Cenergemin eye drops were administered six times a day for 8 weeks. The patients were evaluated at various intervals, including baseline (before starting enegermin), weekly for 8 weeks, and monthly thereafter (Fig. 5.2).

- NGF is often effective in treating advanced NK nonresponding to conventional medical treatments.
- Ocular pain following NGF topical therapy can be associated with corneal nerves restoration and healing.

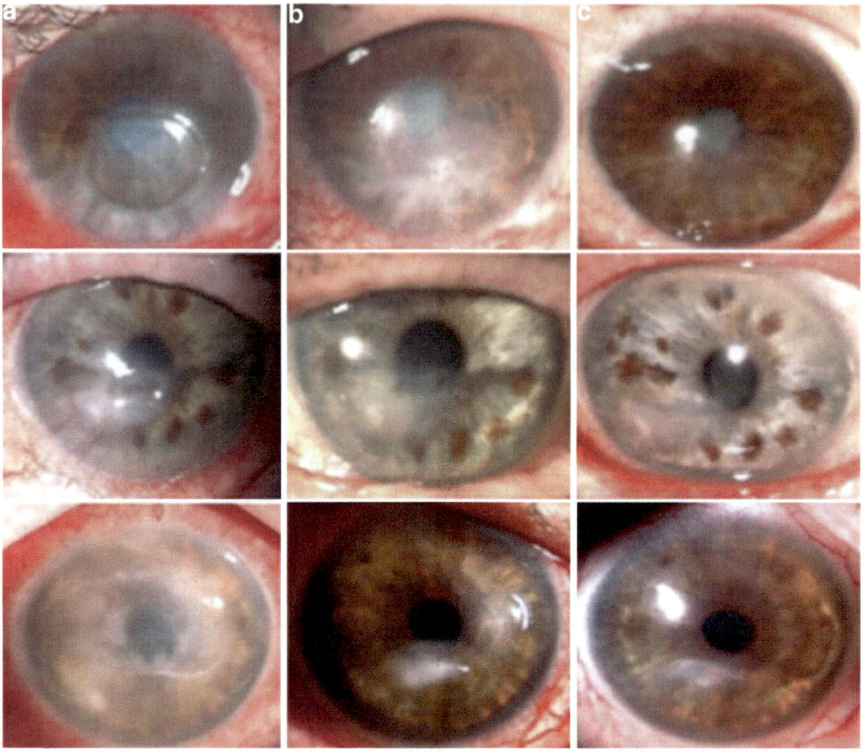

Fig. 5.2 Slit lamp images (**a**) at the start, (**b**) 4 weeks, and (**c**) 8 weeks following rhNGF topical therapy for stage III NK in case 4, case 5, and case 6, respectively, from top to bottom. (Copyright of the author A. Di Zazzo)

5.4 Case 4

A 75-year-old man with a history of herpes simplex virus (HSV) keratitis. He presented with a central corneal ulcer measuring 4.8 mm × 5 mm in the left eye. The corneal sensitivity was absent, as measured by Cochet-Bonnet aesthesiometer. The best-corrected visual acuity was hand motion.

5.5 Case 5

An 84-year-old woman also had a previous diagnosis of HSV keratitis. She had a 7 mm × 5 mm ulcer in the lower right cornea. Corneal sensitivity was nearly absent, tear secretion was severely reduced (Schirmer test type 1: 2 mm/5′), and best-corrected visual acuity was hand motion.

5.6 Case 6

A 67-year-old man who had experienced recurrent epithelial and stromal immune keratitis. After 1 month, he developed a central corneal ulcer measuring 4.2 mm × 6 mm in the right eye. He had severe sensitivity impairment and best-corrected visual acuity of hand motion.

In Cases 4, 5, and 6, the complete healing of the corneal ulcers was achieved within the standard 8-week Cenegermin treatment period. In patient 4, corneal ulceration healed showing progressive improvement since day 5 of treatment. Patient 5 had corneal epithelium growth starting at day 7, and complete recovery occurred when the therapy was completed. In case 6, persistent epithelial defect resolved after 35 days of treatment, although healing began rapidly within 3 days of starting rhNGF eye drops. In all patients, the initial signs of healing were the advancement of epithelial cells from the margin toward the center of the ulcer and the occurrence of mild-to-moderate conjunctival hyperemia accompanied by mild pain and photophobia. After completing the treatment, the follow-up period was 8–9 months. The three eyes maintained a stable, healed corneal epithelium throughout the follow-up period, with no recurrence of epithelial defects.

Corneal sensitivity improved and returned to normal limits in patients 1 and 2 after the complete healing of their corneal ulcers. Patient 6 experienced an improvement from anesthesia to hypoesthesia. The visual acuity of patients 1 and 2 improved from hand motion to counting fingers at a distance of 0.3 m, while patient 3 improved from hand motion to counting fingers at a distance of 1 m. These improvements in sensitivity and BCVA were observed after the ulcers had healed and were maintained throughout the entire follow-up period.

The main adverse event related to treatment was ocular pain. Two days after starting Cenegermin, all patients reported symptoms of ocular surface discomfort, including abnormal sensation in the eye, excess tearing, photophobia, eyelid and ocular pain, and irritation. These symptoms are believed to be associated with the therapeutic actions of rhNGF, which restores corneal innervation and sensitivity. No systemic adverse events were observed.

References

1. Dua HS, Said DG, Messmer EM, et al. Neurotrophic keratopathy. Prog Retin Eye Res. 2018;66:107–31. https://doi.org/10.1016/J.PRETEYERES.2018.04.003.
2. Bonini S, Rama P, Olzi D, et al. Neurotrophic keratitis. Eye (Lond). 2003;17:989–95. https://doi.org/10.1038/SJ.EYE.6700616.
3. Bian Y, Ma KK, Hall NE, et al. Neurotrophic keratopathy in the United States: an intelligent research in sight registry analysis. Ophthalmology. 2022;129:1255–62. https://doi.org/10.1016/J.OPHTHA.2022.06.019.
4. Li Y, Ma X, Li J, et al. Corneal denervation causes epithelial apoptosis through inhibiting NAD+ biosynthesis. Invest Ophthalmol Vis Sci. 2019;60:3538–46. https://doi.org/10.1167/IOVS.19-26909.
5. Beuerman RW, Schimmelpfennig B. Sensory denervation of the rabbit cornea affects epithelial properties. Exp Neurol. 1980;69:196–201. https://doi.org/10.1016/0014-4886(80)90154-5.

6. Ferrari G, Chauhan SK, Ueno H, et al. A novel mouse model for neurotrophic keratopathy: trigeminal nerve stereotactic electrolysis through the brain. Invest Ophthalmol Vis Sci. 2011;52:2532–9. https://doi.org/10.1167/IOVS.10-5688.
7. Belmonte C, Gallar J. Cold thermoreceptors, unexpected players in tear production and ocular dryness sensations. Invest Ophthalmol Vis Sci. 2011;52:3888–92. https://doi.org/10.1167/IOVS.09-5119.
8. Ruiz-Lozano RE, Hernandez-Camarena JC, Loya-Garcia D, et al. The molecular basis of neurotrophic keratopathy: diagnostic and therapeutic implications. A review. Ocul Surf. 2021;19:224–40. https://doi.org/10.1016/J.JTOS.2020.09.007.
9. Sacchetti M, Lambiase A. Neurotrophic factors and corneal nerve regeneration. Neural Regen Res. 2017;12:1220–4. https://doi.org/10.4103/1673-5374.213534.
10. Bonini S, Aloe L, Bonini S, et al. Nerve growth factor (NGF): an important molecule for trophism and healing of the ocular surface. Adv Exp Med Biol. 2002;506:531–7. https://doi.org/10.1007/978-1-4615-0717-8_75.
11. Saad S, Abdelmassih Y, Saad R, et al. Neurotrophic keratitis: frequency, etiologies, clinical management and outcomes. Ocul Surf. 2020;18:231–6. https://doi.org/10.1016/J.JTOS.2019.11.008.
12. Di Zazzo A, Coassin M, Varacalli G, et al. Neurotrophic keratopathy: pros and cons of current treatments. Ocul Surf. 2019;17:619–23. https://doi.org/10.1016/J.JTOS.2019.09.002.
13. Lambiase A, Rama P, Bonini S, et al. Topical treatment with nerve growth factor for corneal neurotrophic ulcers. N Engl J Med. 1998;338:372–3. https://doi.org/10.1056/NEJM199804233381702.
14. Bonini S, Lambiase A, Rama P, et al. Phase I trial of recombinant human nerve growth factor for neurotrophic keratitis. Ophthalmology. 2018;125:1468–71. https://doi.org/10.1016/J.OPHTHA.2018.03.004.
15. Bonini S, Lambiase A, Rama P, et al. Phase II randomized, double-masked, vehicle-controlled trial of recombinant human nerve growth factor for neurotrophic keratitis. Ophthalmology. 2018;125:1332–43. https://doi.org/10.1016/J.OPHTHA.2018.02.022.
16. Pflugfelder SC, Massaro-Giordano M, Perez VL, et al. Topical recombinant human nerve growth factor (cenegermin) for neurotrophic keratopathy: a multicenter randomized vehicle-controlled pivotal trial. Ophthalmology. 2020;127:14–26. https://doi.org/10.1016/J.OPHTHA.2019.08.020.
17. Di Zazzo A, Varacalli G, Mori T, et al. Long-term restoration of corneal sensitivity in neurotrophic keratopathy after rhNGF treatment. Eur J Ophthal. 2020; https://doi.org/10.1177/1120672120953343.

Pterygia

6

Brad Feldman, Brian Thai, Mark Romero, and Olivia Dutton

6.1 Case 1: Nasal Pterygium

6.1.1 Summary

- Surgical removal of a pterygium may be deemed necessary once conservative treatment with drops is no longer effective at managing symptoms or when the pterygium has extended far enough onto the cornea to induce progressive astigmatism.
- A common surgical approach is excision with conjunctival autograft and fibrin sealant. This approach minimizes the recurrence rate but can still be performed relatively quickly.

6.1.2 Presentation and Diagnosis

A 55-year-old male presented with a chief complaint of irritation in his left eye. The irritation was accompanied by blurred vision, redness, dryness, foreign body sensation, and a burning sensation. The patient reported that in the past he had used

B. Feldman (✉) · O. Dutton
Philadelphia Eye Associates, Philadelphia, PA, USA

Sidney Kimmel Medical College of Thomas Jefferson University, Philadelphia, PA, USA
e-mail: bfeldman@phillyeye.com

B. Thai
Philadelphia Eye Associates, Philadelphia, PA, USA

M. Romero
Philadelphia Eye Associates, Philadelphia, PA, USA

Warren Alpert Medical School of Brown University, Providence, RI, USA

F. A. Woreta, R. B. Singh (eds.), *Cornea Casebook*, Current Practices in Ophthalmology, https://doi.org/10.1007/978-981-96-0495-1_6

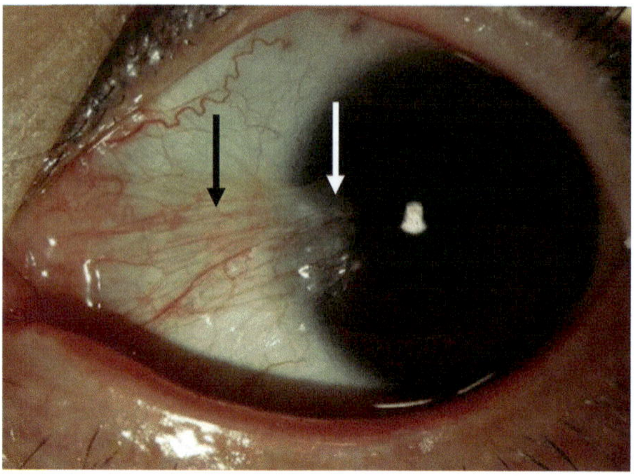

Fig. 6.1 Nasal pterygium with fibrovascular body (black arrow) over conjunctiva and head (white arrow) extending onto the cornea approximately 3mm. (Hwang et al. [1])

artificial tears to relieve the symptoms but stopped several months ago due to increasing and persistent discomfort. Of note, he grew up in Southeast Asia and immigrated to the United States in his twenties. He currently works outside in a landfill but has never consistently worn sunglasses.

Slit lamp examination of the left eye revealed a vascularized, elevated, wing-shaped, intrapalpebral growth on the nasal conjunctiva extending onto the cornea (Fig. 6.1). Corneal topography demonstrated significant nasal irregularity and asymmetric flattening along the horizontal meridian. There were over 1.5 diopters of astigmatism along the vertical meridian.

6.1.3 Management

Pterygia are wing-shaped growths of the bulbar conjunctiva that typically arise intrapalpebrally and extend onto the cornea. Histologically, pterygia consists of an accumulation of degenerated subepithelial tissue that exhibits elastotic degeneration with H&E staining. Ultraviolet radiation is a key risk factor for the development of pterygia. It is important to differentiate pterygia from ocular surface squamous neoplasms, which typically grow faster and display characteristic features such as feeder vessels and either a characteristic papilliform, gelatinous, or leukoplastic appearance.

Most pterygia that induce discomfort can be successfully managed with topical agents such as artificial tears, cyclosporine, or short courses of corticosteroids. However, some pterygia, especially large, thick, or elevated lesions, will cause persistent symptoms despite topical agents and will benefit from excision. Pterygia that induce visually significant astigmatism often necessitate earlier surgical intervention, as delaying surgery while the pterygia extend further into the visual axis may result in extensive scars, irregularity, and poorer postoperative visual outcomes.

In this case, the decision was made to pursue pterygium excision with conjunctival autograft using fibrin sealant while under IV sedation. The pterygium was excised by first peeling and avulsing the head of the pterygium from the cornea with toothed forceps. Next, the body of the pterygium was removed with sharp and blunt dissection with Westcott scissors. After removing the body, a careful dissection and excision of any remaining tenon's layer was performed over the exposed sclera and from below the free conjunctival edges. After measuring the size of the resultant tissue defect, a caliper and marking pen were used to define the size and shape of tissue that needed to be removed from the superior conjunctiva. A thin graft was achieved by first ballooning the pre-marked superior conjunctiva with subconjunctival lidocaine with epinephrine. This separated the tissue planes and made it easier to perform careful blunt and sharp dissection of the graft without causing a button hole. The limbal conjunctival tissue was excised last and was included in the autograft. The autograft tissue was then placed over the bare sclera nasally with the limbal graft edge oriented such that it lay adjacent to the nasal limbus. The graft was secured using fibrin sealant. Once secured, attention was directed superiorly where the remaining loose retracted superior conjunctival tissue was advanced to the superior limbus and secured with additional fibrin sealant.

The technique of conjunctival autograft is not new. It was described in 1965 by Jose Barraquer, and there was a resurgence of interest in the technique in the 1980's. Compared to simply excising the pterygium and closing the conjunctiva with a suture, the autograft technique leads to a significant decrease in recurrence, from a rate of 10–80% down to 3.33–16.7%. Many theorize that the conjunctival graft directly inhibits fibrovascular growth toward the cornea. The limbal autograft tissue may also play a role in inhibiting fibrovascular invasion of the cornea [2].

A relatively newer approach to conjunctival autografting is the use of fibrin sealant rather than sutures. Fibrin sealant can be applied quickly, decreasing surgical time, and may be less inflammatory than sutures [3, 4. 5].

Another popular technique in recent times has been the use of an amniotic membrane to cover the scleral defect following careful excision of the pterygium and tenon's layer. The amniotic membrane is harvested from placenta and consists of an epithelial basement membrane and an avascular stromal layer. When placed on the ocular surface, it has demonstrated anti-inflammatory properties which may lead to decreased scar formation. Amniotic membrane may also help promote re-epithelialization. In pterygium surgery, amniotic tissue is placed with the stromal side facing down against the bare sclera, and it is secured with either sutures or fibrin sealant. While the technique utilizing amniotic membrane has shown better results than simple conjunctival closure, a 2016 Cochrane review comparing amniotic membrane grafting with conjunctival autografting found a 47% decreased rate of recurrence in the conjunctival autografted eyes as compared to the amniotic membrane grafted eyes [6].

A more intensive technique to limit recurrence and improve cosmesis has been described by Dr. Lawrence Hirst. It is referred to as the "P.E.R.F.E.C.T", or pterygium extended removal followed by extended conjunctival transplant technique for treating pterygium. As the name suggests, the technique involves extensive removal of the conjunctiva and tenon's layer, including over the medial or lateral rectus. Afterward, a conjunctival autograft is performed in a manner similar to the previously described techniques. According to published literature, this technique has been found to greatly reduce rates of recurrence, with reports of recurrence rates lower than 1% [7]. The main drawbacks to the P.E.R.F.E.C.T. technique are the length and difficulty of the surgery. On average, the P.E.R.F.E.C.T. technique takes nearly an hour to complete. Typical pterygium excision with conjunctival autograft using fibrin sealant can be successfully performed in about 15 min.

6.2 Case 2: Recurrent Pterygium

6.2.1 Summary

- Recurrent pterygia are more difficult to remove and have higher complication rates compared to primary pterygia.
- Surgical options include excision with conjunctival autograft or amniotic membrane, the adjunctive use of mitomycin C, and the consideration of an extensive tenon's excision approach.

6.2.2 Presentation and Diagnosis

A 34-year-old patient who previously underwent pterygium surgery 1 year prior using the simple conjunctival closure technique in the left eye presented with a regrowth and recurrence of neovascularization, tissue thickening, and fibrosis along the conjunctiva and cornea nasally where the pterygium had previously been excised (Fig. 6.2). The patient noticed the growth over the prior few months and there was increasing redness in the eye along with light sensitivity and moderate eye discomfort. There was also diplopia and discomfort in far-left lateral gaze.

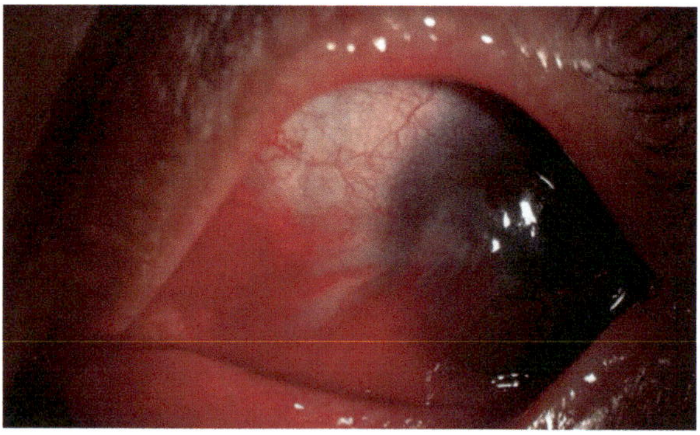

Fig. 6.2 Recurrent nasal pterygium of the left eye. Note the thick fibrovascular band of tissue that may restrict abduction in far lateral gaze. (Chen et al. [8])

6.2.3 Management

The diagnosis of recurrent pterygium was made and the patient was counseled about their options. Surgery was advised given the aggressive growth and worsening symptoms. The technique selected was an excision of the recurrent pterygium with both conjunctival autografts using fibrin sealant and the application of mitomycin C. The risks of surgery were discussed at length. These included worsening diplopia from extraocular muscle damage or restrictive scars, recurrence of the pterygium, poor cosmesis, resultant conjunctival and corneal scar, redness, dry eye or irritation, unpredictable refractive outcome, and irregular astigmatism. In addition, a special consent was signed regarding the off-label use of mitomycin C and the risks posed by its use.

Mitomycin C is approved by the FDA as an anti-neoplastic agent and was approved by the FDA in 2012, in the form of Mitosol®, solely for use as an adjunct for ab externo trabeculectomy surgery. Mitomycin C is an alkylating agent that inhibits DNA-dependent RNA synthesis. In ophthalmology, it is widely used to prevent fibrosis by inhibiting fibroblastic proliferation following glaucoma, refractive, ocular surface neoplasm, and pterygium surgeries. In fact, the first reported ophthalmic use of mitomycin C was for the treatment of recurrent pterygia in Japan in 1969 [9]. The risks of mitomycin C use include scleritis, scleral melting, iritis, persistent epithelial defects, corneal edema, corneal melt, photophobia, and pain. While serious complications of mitomycin C use are uncommon it should always be used with caution [4, 10].

The surgery was uncomplicated but lengthy due to the difficulty in identifying clear tissue planes from the extensive fibrovascular scarring. During surgery, the medial rectus was identified and tagged with a suture so that it could be avoided while the scar and tenon's layer were excised. After completing the excision, a cellulose sponge soaked in 0.02% MMC was placed on the scleral bed and against the edges of resected tissues for 3 min and then removed. The area was thoroughly rinsed with 30 ml of balanced salt solution. A large thin conjunctival autograft was then fashioned from the superior conjunctiva. This was grafted over the scleral defect using fibrin sealant.

At 3 months follow-up, there was some retraction and injection of the patch graft. A decision was made to give a 0.25 ml subconjunctival injection of 40 mg/ml triamcinolone in the area of the patch graft. One month following this steroid injection, the injection had resolved and there was no further progression of graft retraction. At 1 year, there was limited neovascularization over the nasal conjunctiva, and there was no evidence of further conjunctival or corneal recurrence. There was full resolution of the diplopia and abduction deficit.

Recurrent pterygiums are more likely after primary excision using a bare sclera technique but may occur after any type of pterygium excision [11]. Significant progress has been made in preventing pterygium recurrence through enhanced surgical techniques such as extensive tenon's excision, conjunctival autografting, amniotic membrane placement, and adjunctive therapies to inhibit inflammation or fibrosis such as topical or injectable steroids and the use of mitomycin C. Beyond surgical techniques, other risk factors for recurrence include the severity of initial pterygium, pre-operative ocular inflammation, and ocular demodex infestations [11].

The surgical approaches and goals for excision of recurrent pterygium are similar to those of primary pterygium, but the surgery can be considerably more complex given the loss of distinct tissue planes and the development of thick scar.

Another risk of recurrent pterygium excision is strabismus from either muscle disinsertion, muscle damage, or cicatricial restriction. Cicatricial restriction may develop over time from loss of conjunctival tissue, development of thick fibrovascular scar, and loss of the fornix. Postoperative strabismus is challenging to fully correct surgically [12].

6.3 Case 3: Double-Headed Pterygium

6.3.1 Summary

- Pterygia that present on both the nasal and temporal sides of an eye, so-called "double-headed pterygium" can pose a management challenge due to the lack of adequate superior conjunctiva for creating two appropriately sized patch grafts.
- Options for managing large double-headed pterygia may include a single-side autograft with either simple closure or amniotic membrane on the contralateral side, split autografts, or sequential delayed autografts.

6.3.2 Presentation and Diagnosis

A 40-year-old male complained of red discoloration in the temporal and nasal regions of his right eye. He had first noticed this several years earlier but it had progressively worsened over the prior few months and he felt his vision was diminished. He denied any prior ocular surgery. He worked as a groundskeeper at a public garden and spent a significant amount of his days outdoors without sunglasses. Examination revealed large pterygia both nasally and temporally in the right eye. On topography, these pterygia were inducing significant horizontal flattening and there was marked irregularity of the placido disc image. Based on these findings, a decision was made to proceed with surgical excision.

6.3.3 Management

The technique selected for surgery was excision with conjunctival grafting with a split superior autograft. This technique was chosen because of its reported low recurrence rate and anticipated improved cosmesis using autografts as compared to simple closure or amniotic membranes. The nasal side of the pterygium measured 6.2 mm in height along the limbus and the temporal side measured 5.5 mm along the limbus. The nasal pterygium and associated tenon's layer were excised by first avulsing the head of the pterygium with forceps and then dissecting the pre-marked edges of the pterygium with Wescott scissors. After excision of the nasal pterygium, careful dissection of the underlying tenon's layer was performed, including under the free conjunctival edges. The same surgical procedure was followed for the temporal pterygium. The largest possible superior conjunctival graft was then harvested and split in half along the vertical meridian. This tissue was placed over the bare sclera temporally and nasally. In order to fully cover each side, the grafts were not oriented with the harvested superior limbal tissue at the temporal or nasal limbus. Both grafts were secured with fibrin sealant.

At 1 year follow-up, there was minimal scarring in the areas of the patch grafts and no evidence of recurrence. The measured corneal astigmatism decreased from 2.5D to <1.0D despite nasal and temporal corneal scars, and there was a significant decrease in topographical flattening and placido disc irregularity.

Double-headed pterygia are very challenging since there typically isn't adequate conjunctival tissue for grafting in a manner that maintains the limbal orientation of the graft tissue. In cases of very large double-headed pterygia, such as "kissing pterygia," there is inadequate remaining superior conjunctiva to fully patch the defects (Fig. 6.3). Multiple surgical approaches have been reported, including the split graft approach without maintenance of limbal orientation as described in the case above [14]. Another technique involves using amniotic membrane and mitomycin C; either for both sides or unilaterally with an autograft on the contralateral side [15]. Alternatively, some surgeons will perform a single-side autograft and then delay addressing the contralateral pterygium until the superior conjunctiva regenerates to the point that a repeat autograft can be harvested [16]. Interestingly, despite the common teaching that autografts should be avoided in glaucoma patients who may need trabeculectomy, it has been shown that conjunctiva at the harvest site typically regenerates if the underlying tenon's layer is left intact [17]. Of all possible techniques to address double-headed pterygia, it is likely that the most successful is extensive Tenon's dissection and autograft followed by repeat extensive Tenon's dissection and autograft. However, this approach requires two lengthy surgeries and two periods of postoperative pain and recovery, making it more burdensome for patients [18].

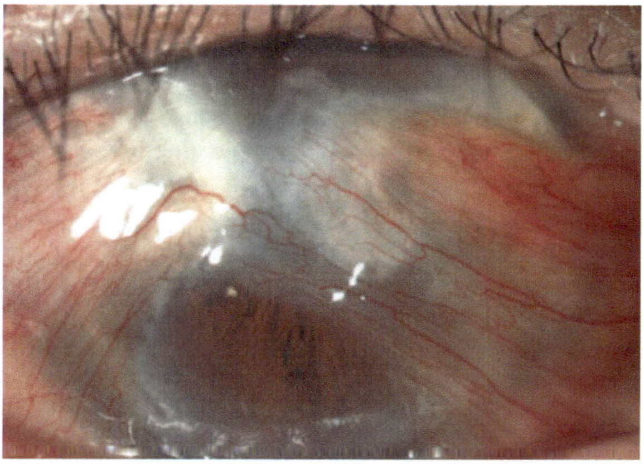

Fig. 6.3 Severe double-headed pterygium, with so-called "kissing" pterygia. Given the size of these pterygia, there would not be adequate superior conjunctival tissue to perform full autografts. (Yong et al. [13])

6.4 Case 4: Pterygium and Cataract

6.4.1 Summary

- Pterygia and cataracts often co-exist and a decision needs to be made in each case whether the pterygium needs to be excised before the cataract surgery.
- Failure to remove a significant pterygium ahead of cataract surgery or failure to wait for the cornea to stabilize after pterygium excision will result in unfavorable refractive outcomes.

6.4.2 Presentation and Diagnosis

A 67-year-old man presented with progressive vision loss and chronic redness in the left eye. He was no longer able to drive safely due to blurriness and glare. The Snellen best-corrected visual acuity in the left eye measured 20/200. Slit lamp examination revealed a nasal pterygium extending 4.5 mm onto the cornea. Additionally, there was a 3–4+ posterior subcapsular cataract in the central visual axis.

6.4.3 Management

The patient anticipated the need for cataract surgery and was eager for a quick fix. A long discussion took place about the importance and timing of pterygium excision in addition to cataract surgery. A pterygium excision with conjunctival autograft using fibrin sealant was performed in the left eye without complication. Two months later, phacoemulsification cataract surgery with placement of an intraocular lens was performed resulting in an uncorrected visual acuity of 20/50 and a best-corrected visual acuity of 20/25 (the vision was limited by residual corneal scars and corneal irregularity). At 1 year, the refraction was stable and there was no evidence of pterygium recurrence.

Pterygium and cataracts often co-exist, especially among patients over 50 years old. It is helpful to check refraction, keratometry, and topography in these patients to assess the amount of astigmatism and irregularity induced by their pterygia. When the pterygium is the primary cause of vision loss, the decision to perform an excision is straightforward; the pterygium is removed and then the cataract is dealt with in the more distant future as it progresses. However, when there is a visually significant cataract and a co-existing pterygium, the decision-making is more complicated. The ophthalmologist must determine whether the pterygium is visually significant, likely to progress to the point of visual significance, or likely to interfere with accurate intraocular power calculations. When the pterygium affirmatively meets any of these criteria, it should be excised prior to cataract extraction if possible. Proceeding with cataract surgery first and then removing the pterygium will too often lead to refractive surprises and undesirable uncorrected visual acuity.

During the initial healing period following pterygium excision, the cornea is unstable with stromal and epithelial changes that affect the corneal shape. After removing a pterygium, keratometry, biometry, and cataract surgery should be delayed at least 6 weeks, or until the eye has stable topographical findings. Eyes that are healing after the removal of large pterygia may take well over 3 months to achieve corneal stability. The delay can be challenging for these patients who may not have had any visual improvement after the initial pterygium excision. It is imperative to have clear pre-operative discussions with these patients to ensure that they understand the logic behind their delayed surgery and visual recovery.

References

1. Hwang H, Cho K, Rand G, Chuck R, Kwon J. Optimal size of pterygium excision for limbal conjunctival autograft using fibrin glue in primary pterygia. BMC Ophthalmol. 2018;18(1) https://doi.org/10.1186/s12886-018-0790-6.
2. Rubinfeld RS, Pfister RR, Stein RM, et al. Serious complications of topical mitomycin-C after pterygium surgery. Ophthalmology. 1992;99(11):1647–54. https://doi.org/10.1016/s0161-6420(92)31749-x.
3. Yüksel B, Unsal SK, Onat S. Comparison of fibrin glue and suture technique in pterygium surgery performed with limbal autograft. Int J Ophthalmol. 2010;3(4):316–20. https://doi.org/10.3980/j.issn.2222-3959.2010.04.09.
4. Hall RC, Logan AJ, Wells AP. Comparison of fibrin glue with sutures for pterygium excision surgery with conjunctival autografts. Clin Experiment Ophthalmol. 2009;37(6):584–9. https://doi.org/10.1111/j.1442-9071.2009.02105.x.
5. Hirst LW, Smallcombe K. Double-headed pterygia treated with P.E.R.F.E.C.T for PTERYGIUM. Cornea. 2017;36(1):98–100. https://doi.org/10.1097/ICO.0000000000001036.
6. Clearfield E, Muthappan V, Wang X, Kuo IC. Conjunctival autograft for pterygium. Cochrane Database Syst Rev. 2016;2(2):CD011349. Published 2016 Feb 11. https://doi.org/10.1002/14651858.CD011349.pub2.
7. Sarkar P, Pterygium TK. StatPearls [Internet]. Treasure Island: StatPearls Publishing; 2022. [Updated 2022 Feb 21]. Available from: https://www.ncbi.nlm.nih.gov/books/NBK558907/.
8. Chen D, Liu X, Long Q, Wang Z, Li Y. Effects of excimer laser phototherapeutic keratectomy in limbal-conjunctival autograft transplantation for recurrent pterygium: a retrospective case control study. BMC Ophthalmol. 2019;19(1) https://doi.org/10.1186/s12886-019-1248-1.
9. Kunitomoro N, Mori S. Studies on pterygium: Part 4, a treatment of pterygium by Mitomycin-C installation. Acta Soc Ophthalmol Jpn. 1969;67:601–7.
10. Anduze AL, Burnett JM. Indications for and complications of mitomycin-C in pterygium surgery. Ophthalmic Surg Lasers. 1996;27(8):667–73.
11. Ghiasian L, Samavat B, Hadi Y, Arbab M, Abolfathzadeh N. Recurrent pterygium: a review. J Curr Ophthalmol. 2022;33(4):367–78. Published 2022 Jan 6. https://doi.org/10.4103/joco.joco_153_20.
12. Fernandes M, Sangwan VS, Bansal AK, et al. Outcome of pterygium surgery: analysis over 14 years. Eye (Lond). 2005;19(11):1182–90. https://doi.org/10.1038/sj.eye.6701728.
13. Yong WWD, Shen L, Manotosh R, Tan WTAM, Chai HCC. Impact of fibrin glue versus suture closure on double-headed pterygia in Asian eyes—a 7-year study in a tertiary institution. Ann Med. 2021;53(1):448–55.
14. Ela-Dalman N, Velez FG, Rosenbaum AL. Incomitant esotropia following pterygium excision surgery. Arch Ophthalmol. 2007;125(3):369–73. https://doi.org/10.1001/archopht.125.3.369.
15. Kodavoor SK, Ramamurthy D, Tiwari NN, Ramamurthy S. Double-head pterygium excision with modified vertically split-conjunctival autograft: six-year long-term retrospective analysis. Indian J Ophthalmol. 2017;65(8):700–4. https://doi.org/10.4103/ijo.IJO_284_17.

16. Röck T, Bartz-Schmidt KU, Röck D. Management of double-head pterygium with conjunctival autograft and primary closure. Int Med Case Rep J. 2020;13:111–5. Published 2020 Apr 1. https://doi.org/10.2147/IMCRJ.S203897.
17. Yeung SN, Rubenstein D, Price AJ, Elbaz U, Zhang AQ, Côté E, Slomovic AR. Sequential pterygium excision with conjunctival autograft in the management of primary double-headed pterygia. Can J Ophthalmol. 2013;48(6):521–3. ISSN 0008-4182.
18. Vidal FS, Cronemberger S, Massote JA. Superior conjunctival healing after autografting used in pterygium excision: pre and postoperative outcomes. Invest Ophthalmol Vis Sci. 2019;60(9):6264.

Part II

Infectious Keratitis

Viral Keratitis

7

Shravika Chennupati, Jennifer Lindsey, and Christine Shieh

7.1 Introduction

Viral keratitis is a leading cause of visual impairment and remains responsible for a sizable portion of blindness worldwide. Therefore, proper recognition and treatment are critical to improving clinical outcomes. Herpes simplex virus (HSV) is a herpesvirus with two subtypes, HSV-1 and HSV-2, both of which produce a variety of clinical manifestations. HSV can induce widespread ocular inflammation, leading to complications such as irreversible corneal stromal scarring and vision loss. Varicella zoster virus (VZV) infection can lead to similar findings. This chapter focuses on the ocular manifestations of common causes of viral keratitis such as HSV and VZV and serve as a guide for diagnosing and managing these entities.

7.2 Epidemiology and Pathogenesis

HSV and VZV are double-stranded DNA viruses that infect sensory ganglia during primary infection; they may sporadically reactivate and travel down the ophthalmic division of the trigeminal nerve (V1) to produce recurrent corneal disease [1]. HSV-1 and HSV-2 have a ubiquitous worldwide distribution with seropositivity in more than 90% of adults by the fifth decade of life [2]. Of the 1.5 million new cases of HSV keratitis reported yearly, approximately 6% develop clinical symptoms and

S. Chennupati · C. Shieh (✉)
Vanderbilt Eye Institute, Nashville, TN, USA
e-mail: shravika.chennupati@vumc.org; christine.shieh@vumc.org

J. Lindsey
Massachusetts Eye and Ear, Boston, MA, USA
e-mail: jllindsey@meei.harvard.edu

F. A. Woreta, R. B. Singh (eds.), *Cornea Casebook*, Current Practices in Ophthalmology, https://doi.org/10.1007/978-981-96-0495-1_7

40,000 cases result in severe visual impairment [3]. Studies estimate the overall incidence of zoster in the United States at one million annually, with 10–20% of cases resulting in herpes zoster ophthalmicus (HZO) [4, 5].

7.3 Ocular Herpes Simplex Keratitis

7.3.1 Overview

Ocular herpes simplex virus (ocular HSV) is due to infection of the ocular and/or periorbital structures with HSV-1/2. Manifestations of ocular HSV include blepharoconjunctivitis, epithelial keratitis, stromal keratitis, endotheliitis, keratouveitis, and retinal necrosis. Viral keratitis can involve the retina, and clinicians should have a low threshold for performing a dilated fundus exam. Herpetic keratitis is bilateral in 3% of individuals with ocular HSV, with rates higher among children and atopic or immunocompromised individuals [6]. Primary infection with ocular HSV is often asymptomatic and occurs via direct contact with, or inhalation of respiratory droplets from, an individual with active HSV. Recurrent disease may occur with reactivation of the virus and subsequent involvement of the ophthalmic division of the trigeminal nerve (V1). Treatment with antivirals and other topical interventions may be used to shorten the disease course and reduce long-term complications of ocular HSV.

7.3.2 Eyelid, Conjunctival, and Scleral Involvement

Ocular HSV often produces vesicular lesions on the eyelid and surrounding skin and may also infect the conjunctiva to produce an follicular conjunctivitis and/or blepharoconjunctivitis. Rarely, dendritiform lesions may also be present upon the conjunctiva [7]. In primary ocular HSV, it is more common for patients to present with a self-limiting blepharoconjunctivitis than with corneal involvement. It is estimated that at least 5% of cases of acute conjunctivitis may be attributable to HSV [8]. Care should be taken to evaluate all patients with acute conjunctivitis for additional signs and symptoms of ocular HSV.

7.3.3 Infectious Epithelial Keratitis

The earliest sign of epithelial disease is the transient presence of corneal vesicles or punctate keratopathy (PK). These findings may spontaneously resolve or may form a precursor to the classic HSV keratitis dendritic ulcer. Dendritic ulcers arise when corneal vesicles coalesce into raised plaques and desquamate to form a linear branching ulcer with characteristic terminal buds. These epithelial defects stain with fluorescein dye, while peripheral cells lining the ulcer borders typically stain with rose bengal or lissamine green [9]. Dendritic ulcers may coalesce to form geographic ulcers with scalloped borders that lack a branched appearance. Marginal ulcers may also occur, located alongside the limbus and in some cases accompanied by superficial neovascularization. Recurrent cases of HSV keratitis may result in neurotrophic keratitis, which is characterized by corneal degeneration and desensitization. Damage to corneal sensory nerves leads to an impairment in epithelial cell vitality and disruption of the lacrimation reflex, leading to stromal inflammation and poor tear secretion [10]. Neurotrophic ulcers typically present as oval ulcers with smooth borders. The severity of neurotrophic keratitis has historically been staged using the Mackie classification system. Stage 1 is characterized by epithelial changes such as punctate keratopathy, but without an epithelial defect. Stage 2 is defined by a persistent epithelial defect but without stromal thinning. Stage 3 is the most severe stage with stromal involvement (cornea ulcer or melt) that may progress to corneal perforation [10].

7.3.4 Herpes Stromal Keratitis

Herpes stromal keratitis (HSK) has historically been classified into two categories: necrotizing stromal keratitis (NSK) or immune stromal keratitis (ISK). NSK refers to live virus infection of the cornea stroma and is characterized by an epithelial defect and stromal infiltration. This condition can worsen if left untreated and lead to corneal thinning, necrosis, and even perforation. On exam, NSK can present with single or multiple yellow-white necrotic infiltrations within the corneal stroma [6]. In contrast, immune stromal keratitis (ISK) is thought to occur due to an immune-mediated reaction to viral antigens within the stroma. ISK may be characterized by grainy punctate stromal opacities beneath an intact epithelium [6]. ISK classically presents with cells within the anterior chamber and may be accompanied by ciliary flush, stromal edema, neovascularization, and stromal scarring. An immune ring may also be seen in the mid-stroma or central/paracentral cornea due to the immune response to foreign antigens [6].

7.3.5 HSV Endotheliitis

Viral- or immune-mediated damage of endothelial cells may result in endothelial dysfunction and stromal edema without stromal infiltrate. This phenomenon, termed HSV endotheliitis, is classically categorized into three forms: disciform, diffuse, and linear. Disciform endotheliitis presents as a round disc-like area of stromal edema with underlying well-defined keratic precipitates (KP). This may be accompanied by mild iritis, limbal injection, and elevation of the intraocular pressure (IOP) [11]. Secondary neovascularization and scarring may also rarely occur. Diffuse endotheliitis presents as diffuse "limbus-to-limbus" stromal edema with scattered KP. Iritis may be present in the company of a hypopyon and/or retrocorneal plaque. Linear endotheliitis presents with a linear progression of KP from the limbus to the center of the cornea, with peripheral stromal edema between the KP and the limbus. Microcystic edema may be seen in severe cases of HSV endotheliitis. If left untreated, endotheliitis can result in the permanent loss of endothelial cells and intractable corneal edema [6].

7.3.6 HSV Keratouveitis

Keratouveitis may be associated with HSV, either as its own entity, or in combination with epithelial, stromal, or endothelial disease. Patients may present with ciliary flush, photophobia, visual blurring, and/or pain. This may be accompanied on slit lamp exam with fine or large KP, diffuse corneal edema, posterior synechiae, hyphema, and iris nodules (such as Koeppe nodules) [12]. Segmental iris atrophy and transillumination defects may also occur following ischemic necrosis of the iris stroma. Acute trabeculitis can occur and result in elevation of IOP. Chronic inflammation and obstruction of aqueous outflow may lead to glaucoma.

7.3.7 Laboratory Diagnosis

While viral keratitis is generally diagnosed clinically, laboratory testing may be used to confirm the diagnosis in cases of ambiguous disease. Viral specimens may be obtained from swabs or scrapings of the cornea, conjunctiva, or periorbital skin lesions. The aqueous humor may also be sampled by an anterior chamber tap or paracentesis. These specimens can be subsequently analyzed via qualitative or quantitative polymerase chain reaction (PCR), cytology, or culture to confirm the presence or absence of HSV. Serologic testing for IgG or IgM titers may also be performed to identify primary disease but may produce a false negative result if performed early in the disease course and may be unreliable when attempting to diagnose recurrent disease. While response to treatment is generally gauged by symptomatic improvement, where available, quantitative PCR has been used in some cases to assess changes in aqueous viral load [13].

7.3.8 Treatment

The general mainstay of treatment for HSV viral keratitis is the use of oral antiviral therapy in the form of acyclovir, valacyclovir, or famciclovir. The Herpetic Eye Disease Study (HEDS) II showed that prophylactic oral acyclovir decreases the recurrence of any stromal HSV keratitis by approximately 50% [14]. Valacyclovir, the prodrug of acyclovir, is often the clinician's drug of choice due to its high bioavailability, ease of dosing, and low cost. As these oral antivirals have also been associated with nephrotoxicity, bloodwork should be obtained and followed. Dose reduction may be necessary in patients with kidney disease, and it can be helpful to consult with the patient's nephrologist and primary care doctor. The aforementioned three antivirals are activated by viral thymidine kinase and are therefore less effective against viruses with mutations in the thymidine kinase (TK) gene. Infection with a resistant strain of HSV may be treated in rare cases with epithelial debridement or foscarnet. Topical ganciclovir 0.15% is approved for treatment of acute herpetic keratitis in the United States and is typically dosed five times a day until resolution of the corneal ulcer, followed by prophylactic dosing at the discretion of the clinician [15].

While corticosteroids are generally avoided when treating infectious epithelial keratitis and may lead to worsening, they are widely used in treating viral stromal keratitis and endotheliitis. Treatment of stromal keratitis involves topical corticosteroids and oral antivirals and has been shown by the Herpetic Eye Disease Study (HEDS) I to provide significant benefit in stromal keratitis [14, 16]. In the presence of active epithelial ulceration, aggressive antiviral therapy is pursued, and steroid eye-drops are reduced to a minimum. Notably, some viral keratitis patients may experience recurrence of disease with steroid taper. A slow steroid taper is generally recommended. In cases where it may not be possible to entirely taper off topical steroids clinicians should seek to taper the steroid to the lowest strength and frequency possible (minimum effective dose). Corticosteroid therapy is also the treatment of choice for HSV endotheliitis and keratouveitis, with gradual tapering [17, 18]. Trabeculitis responds to topical corticosteroids, but IOP needs to be monitored and the addition of IOP-lowering drops may be necessary [19, 20]. In neurotrophic keratopathy, treatment may include preservative-free artificial tears, bandage contact lenses, serum tears, cenegermin, amniotic membrane transplantation, and/or tarsorrhaphy [21].

Various surgical treatments may also be employed. Keratoplasty is best reserved for cases of stable or inactive disease, such as old scarring from stromal keratitis. Viral keratitis is a risk factor for reduced transplant survival. Deep anterior lamellar keratoplasty (DALK) may be performed in patients with significant stromal scarring in which the endothelium remains viable. Endothelial keratoplasty is an option for patients who have persistent cornea edema but clear cornea stroma. In patients with profound neurotrophic keratopathy, corneal neurotization has shown potential in restoring corneal sensation [22–24].

7.4 Case 1: A 7-Year-Old Female Presents with Left Eye Pain and Photophobia (Fig. 7.1)

- The patient had a past ocular history significant for HSV interstitial keratitis in the right eye and was maintained on oral acyclovir 400 mg BID.
- A slit-lamp exam revealed a new large central cornea ulcer (Fig. 7.1) in the left eye. Bacteria and fungal cultures were sent, along with viral PCR testing. A diagnosis of active HSV epithelial keratitis complicated by a central corneal ulcer OS was made.

(continued)

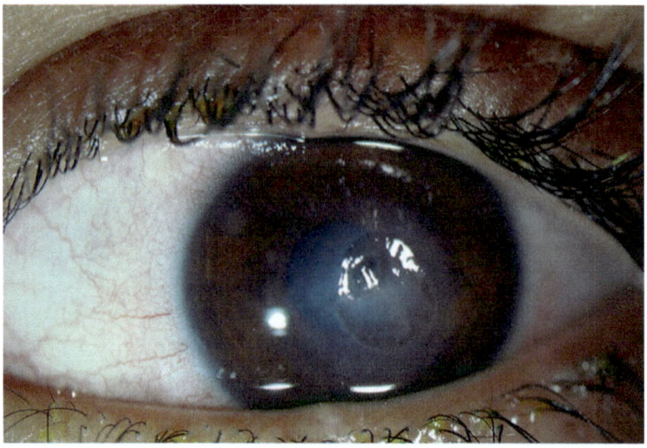

Fig. 7.1 Herpes simplex virus-associated central corneal ulcer with thinning

- Patient's oral acyclovir was raised to therapeutic dosing, and she was started on ganciclovir ophthalmic ointment 5×/day. The patient ultimately required amniotic membrane transplantation to help heal the epithelium.
- Subsequent thymidine kinase mutation panel testing did not reveal a thymidine kinase deficiency. The patient was referred to infectious disease for a consultation, and mutation panel testing ruled out thymidine kinase deficiency. She was switched to liquid oral valacyclovir due to difficulty swallowing pills and has been recurrence-free for 2 years on this regimen.

7.5 Herpes Zoster Keratitis

7.5.1 Overview

HZO is due to the reactivation of latent VZV along the V1 division of the trigeminal nerve and involvement of the orbital and/or periorbital structures. Manifestations of HZO include blepharoconjunctivitis, acute and chronic/relapsing keratitis, endotheliitis, keratouveitis, and neuropathic pain. The diagnosis is generally made clinically, but laboratory testing may be pursued to aid in narrowing the differential diagnosis, especially in cases where adult patients do not recall having childhood chickenpox. Antivirals and other topical interventions may be used to shorten the disease course and reduce long-term complications.

7.5.2 Eyelid, Conjunctival, and Scleral Involvement

HZO classically involves the periorbital structures to produce a painful vesicular rash in the V1 dermatomal distribution. These vesicles may eventually rupture before crusting over and dissipating after approximately 2–3 weeks [6]. Vesicles found at the tip of the nose are known as Hutchinson's sign. As an indicator of nasociliary nerve involvement, Hutchinson's sign is a strong predictor of ocular involvement; however ocular involvement may occur even in the absence of Hutchinson's sign [25]. While uncommon, ocular complications of HZO may occur even when no vesicular rash is visible ("zoster sine herpete") [5]. Other findings may also be noted with HZO, such as blepharitis, secondary ptosis, and extraocular muscle/cranial nerve palsies [26–28]. Significant dermal involvement of the lid may also lead to cicatricial contracture, entropion or ectropion, and lid margin notching. HZO may also produce follicular conjunctivitis, anterior/posterior scleritis, and episcleritis.

7.5.3 Acute Keratitis

The earliest corneal manifestation of acute HZO is a punctate epithelial keratitis that presents shortly after the initial skin rash. This is characterized on exam by swollen epithelial lesions that stain with rose bengal or lissamine green. These edematous, raised epithelial cells coalesce to form pseudodendrites, which appear stellate or dendritic in shape, have tapered ends, and lack central ulceration. Pseudodendrites appear similar to the dendrites of HSK but can be distinguished from dendrites by their minimal staining with fluorescein dye and lack of terminal bulbs or central ulceration.

Following the development of pseudodendrites, anterior stromal keratitis may develop due to either an immune-mediated response to VZV or direct viral cytotoxicity. Nummular keratitis is characterized by the presence of round, coin-shaped granules in the superficial stroma that often underlie areas of previous epithelial keratitis. Limbal vascular keratitis may also be seen during the acute phase of disease due to the extension of preexisting scleritis onto the cornea. Sclerokeratitis can manifest as a crescent-shaped corneal infiltrate adjacent to the area of scleritis [6].

Keratouveitis and endotheliitis may be seen early in the disease course and are typically accompanied by Descemet folds with overlying stromal/epithelial edema [29]. The inflammation may be granulomatous or nongranulomatous, and extensive underlying KP is often visualized. Zoster iritis may occur following ischemic vasculitis, resulting in segmental iris distortion and atrophy. Trabeculitis may occur due to viral invasion or obstruction of the trabecular meshwork by inflammatory cells and debris. Intraocular inflammation may also result in the formation of posterior synechiae and a hypopyon.

7.5.4 Chronic Keratitis

As in ocular herpes, HZO can recur long after the acute phase of the disease has resolved. Dendritiform plaques may arise several months after the initial presentation in a near-quiescent eye and present as elevated gray branching lesions that lack terminal bulbs. In addition, these plaques are migratory in nature and may alter their position upon the corneal epithelium.

Weeks to months after acute keratitis, disciform keratitis (similar to that of HSV keratitis) may arise. This presents with a deep disc-shaped region of stromal edema with minimal infiltrate and an intact overlying epithelium. An immune ring may also develop in the mid-stroma or central/peripheral cornea as a result of the ongoing immune response [6]. Posterior stromal keratitis may also occur months after the onset of disease and can present with corneal edema that is frequently associated with anterior uveitis [30]. A complication of chronic HZO, like HSV, is interstitial keratitis, which may lead to significant corneal scarring and neovascularization. This keratitis can involve deep stromal vessels, and these vessels may exude large amounts of lipid, producing lipid keratopathy [31]. Chronic VZV-related keratitis may also present as a persistent smoldering corneal haze with overlying epithelial irregularity. Without proper identification and treatment, this can lead to progressive visually significant scarring. In patients with chronic or recurrent endotheliitis, sufficient damage to the corneal endothelium may produce permanent corneal edema even in the absence of scarring [6].

As with HSV keratitis, chronic and recurrent disease may result in the development of neurotrophic ulcers. These typically arise months after initial presentation with HZO and are characterized by corneal epithelial breakdown and desensitization leading to poor lubrication and exposure keratopathy. Complications such as scarring, superinfection, corneal thinning, and perforation can occur without proper care.

7.5.5 Laboratory Diagnosis

Diagnosis of VZV keratitis is generally clinical but can be aided by laboratory techniques. Tzank smears of corneal scrapings or samples from the base of a vesicle may demonstrate multinucleated giant cells and acidophilic intranuclear inclusions; however, the sensitivity of this testing is low and cannot distinguish between morphologically-similar viruses such as HSV and VZV. PCR testing and ELISA using lesion samples may also be used to make a diagnosis with high sensitivity. Definitive diagnosis can be made by viral culture using skin or corneal samples but is often challenging to perform in a timely manner. Alternatively, in the case of zoster sine herpete where vesicles are absent, serologic testing may be pursued to look for antibodies against VZV.

7.5.6 Treatment

Treatment of acute VZV keratitis is directed at accelerating healing, treating symptoms, and reducing complications using antiviral medication. Antiviral oral VZV treatment is similar to HSV keratitis, but the dosing for oral VZV keratitis is double that of HSV keratitis: this is true for both therapeutic and prophylactic oral antiviral dosing. As with treatment of HSV keratitis, oral antiviral dose adjustments must be made in patients with renal insufficiency. Oral acyclovir has been shown to reduce the incidence of VZV pseudodendritic keratopathy, stromal keratitis, and iritis [32]. Valacyclovir remains a popular clinician choice in the treatment of VZV keratitis, and its use is being examined in the Zoster Eye Disease Study. Other medications, such as foscarnet and cidofovir, may be used to treat acyclovir-resistant strains of VZV as they do not depend on a viral-specific thymidine kinase for their antiviral activity.

7.6 Case 2: A 59-Year-Old Woman Presents with Blurred Vision and Photosensitivity (Fig. 7.2)

- The patient reported a 1-week history of right eye epiphora with increasing tenderness, blurred vision, and photosensitivity. The patient was treated with an antibiotic ointment at an outside clinic but did not experience any improvement.
- She reported a past medical history of shingles 1 month prior to presentation that was treated with 2 weeks of valacyclovir.
- On presentation, visual acuity was 20/150 OD, and IOP was elevated. A slit lamp exam was performed which revealed corneal edema, diffuse pigmented KP, iritis, and subtle Descemet folds OD. A diagnosis of active viral keratouveitis was made based on history and exam findings.
- The patient was started on valacyclovir 1 g TID, timolol 1 drop BID, and prednisolone 1 drop 8×/day with subsequent clinical improvement.

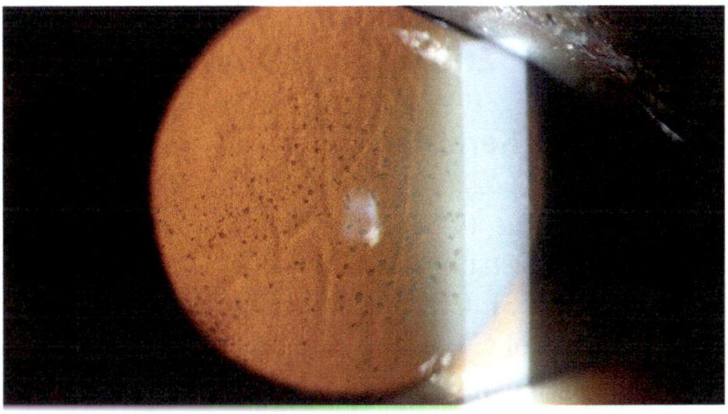

Fig. 7.2 Descemet folds and diffuse pigmented KP associated with herpes zoster keratitis

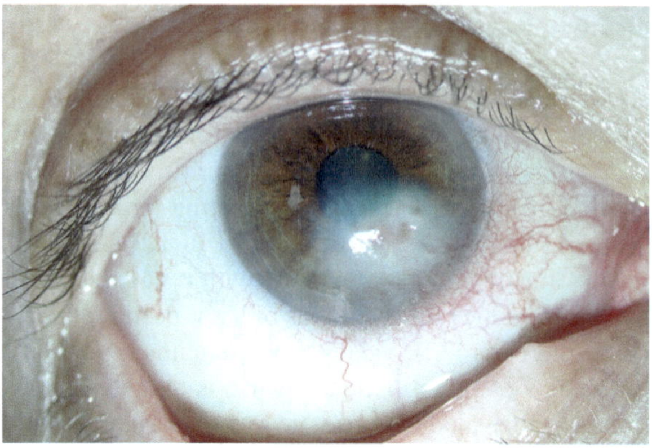

Fig. 7.3 Viral stromal keratitis resulting in cornea scarring and neovascularization

7.7 Case 3: A 66-Year-Old Woman Presents with Worsening Visual Acuity in the Right Eye (Fig. 7.3)

- The patient reported a history of similar issues in the right eye about 20 years ago, with some recurrent issues 2 years prior to presentation: all episodes were successfully treated with oral antivirals.
- A slit-lamp exam was performed which revealed a large inferonasal area of corneal neovascularization and opacification with an associated geographic ulcer. The diagnosis of necrotizing stromal keratitis was made based on history and exam findings.
- The patient ultimately required valacyclovir 1 gram TID PO and ganciclovir ophthalmic ointment to heal the ulcer. Oral valacyclovir was then subsequently decreased to prophylactic dosing and prednisolone eye drops were utilized to decrease the severity of the cornea inflammation.
- At the patient's most recent visit, her condition was stable on oral valacyclovir QD and prednisolone QD. Some residual cornea scarring and neovascularization was noted.

7.8 Other Etiologies of Viral Keratitis

7.8.1 CMV Keratitis

Cytomegalovirus (CMV) is a ubiquitous herpesvirus that may cause keratitis. Corneal manifestations of CMV infection include epitheliitis, stromal keratitis, or endotheliitis [33]. CMV endotheliitis is perhaps the most commonly encountered manifestation of CMV infection and may produce corneal edema, linear and coin-shaped KP, and inflammation within the anterior chamber [6, 33]. As a result, patients may develop anterior uveitis and ocular hypertension that characteristically fails to respond to steroid treatment [33]. Diagnosis of ocular CMV disease is typically made by positive CMV PCR analysis of aqueous fluid. CMV endotheliitis has been shown to respond to treatment with topical ganciclovir, systemic ganciclovir or valganciclovir, or a combination of topical and systemic therapy [6]. However, despite treatment, it has been reported that as many as 40% of patients may fail to retain corneal clarity, further underscoring the importance of early intervention [33].

7.8.2 EBV Keratitis

The Epstein–Barr virus (EBV) is associated with numerous ocular conditions, including unilateral transient follicular conjunctivitis and bilateral stromal keratitis. Corneal exam findings have been reported to include stellate microdendrites, ring-shaped opacities within the anterior stroma, pleomorphic multifocal infiltrates within the peripheral cornea, and subepithelial infiltrates [34]. Diagnosis of ocular EBV disease is generally serologic and can be made by measuring antibody levels against Viral Capsid Antigen (VCA) and EBV Nuclear Antigen (EBNA). Treatment of EBV keratitis is not well-described in the literature; however, topical corticosteroids have been shown to improve the ocular manifestations of EBV interstitial keratitis [35].

7.8.3 Adenovirus Keratitis

Ocular infection with adenovirus is a common cause of viral conjunctivitis and may manifest as epithelial keratitis with subepithelial/anterior stromal infiltrates [36]. Adenovirus-associated keratitis begins with nonstaining epithelial microcysts that progress to a positively-staining focal punctate epithelial keratopathy. Diagnosis is largely clinical but can be confirmed by conjunctival swab culture or utilization of rapid detection immunoassays or PCR. As adenovirus is self-limited, treatment is aimed at relieving symptoms using artificial tears and cold compresses. Topical corticosteroids may be prescribed during the acute phase of disease in severe cases for symptomatic relief but may increase the duration of disease [36]. Stromal infiltrates may develop after a few weeks. These infiltrates are often responsive to steroids but may require a slow steroid taper to prevent recurrence of disease.

References

1. Kinchington PR, Leger AJS, Guedon J-MG, Hendricks RL. Herpes simplex virus and varicella zoster virus, the house guests who never leave. Herpesviridae. 2012;3(1):1–13. https://doi.org/10.1186/2042-4280-3-5.
2. Bennett JE, Dolin R, Blaser MJ. Mandell, Douglas and Bennett's infectious disease essentials. Published online 2017.
3. Farooq AV, Shukla D. Herpes simplex epithelial and stromal keratitis: an epidemiologic update. Surv Ophthalmol. 2012;57(5):448–62. https://doi.org/10.1016/J.SURVOPHTHAL.2012.01.005.

4. Kong CL, Thompson RR, Porco TC, Kim E, Acharya NR. Incidence rate of herpes zoster ophthalmicus: a retrospective cohort study from 1994 through 2018. Ophthalmology. 2020;127(3):324–30. https://doi.org/10.1016/J.OPHTHA.2019.10.001.
5. Johnson RW, Alvarez-Pasquin M-J, Bijl M, et al. Herpes zoster epidemiology, management, and disease and economic burden in Europe: a multidisciplinary perspective. Ther Adv Vaccines. 2015;3(4):109. https://doi.org/10.1177/2051013615599151.
6. Mannis MJ, Holland EJ. Cornea: fundamentals, diagnosis, and management. 5th ed. New York: Elsevier; 2022.
7. Sridhar U, Bansal Y, Choudhury S, Gupta AK. Conjunctival dendrite in a case of primary herpes simplex infection. Br J Ophthalmol. 2004;88(4):590. https://doi.org/10.1136/BJO.2003.028654.
8. Solano D, Fu L, Czyz CN. Viral conjunctivitis. Jpn J Clin Ophthalmol. 2022;70(11):164–9. https://doi.org/10.1016/b978-0-7506-4063-3.50014-8.
9. Shah A, Joshi P, Bhusal B, Subedi P. Clinical pattern and visual impairment associated with herpes simplex keratitis. Clin Ophthalmol. 2019;13:2211–5. https://doi.org/10.2147/OPTH.S219184.
10. Feroze KB, Patel BC. Neurotrophic keratitis. StatPearls. 2022;24. Published online May. https://www.ncbi.nlm.nih.gov/books/NBK431106/. Accessed 16 Aug 2022.
11. Silverstein BE, Chandler D, Neger R, Margolis TP. Disciform keratitis: a case of herpes zoster sine herpete. Am J Ophthalmol. 1997;123(2):254–5. https://doi.org/10.1016/S0002-9394(14)71044-X.
12. Babu K, Konana V, Ganesh S, et al. Viral anterior uveitis. Indian J Ophthalmol. 2020;68(9):1764. https://doi.org/10.4103/IJO.IJO_928_20.
13. Inoue T, Ohashi Y. Utility of real-time PCR analysis for appropriate diagnosis for keratitis. Cornea. 2013;32 Suppl 1(11 SUPPL):S71. https://doi.org/10.1097/ICO.0B013E3182A2C79F.
14. Kalezic T, Mazen M, Kuklinski E, Asbell P. Herpetic eye disease study: lessons learned. Curr Opin Ophthalmol. 2018;29(4):340–6. https://doi.org/10.1097/ICU.0000000000000482.
15. Sahin A, Hamrah P. Acute herpetic keratitis: what is the role for ganciclovir ophthalmic gel? Ophthalmol Eye Dis. 2012;4:23. https://doi.org/10.4137/OED.S7267.
16. Beck RW, Kip KE, Wilhelmus KR. Predictors of recurrent herpes simplex virus keratitis. Herpetic Eye Disease Study Group. Cornea. 2001;20(2):123–8. https://doi.org/10.1097/00003226-200103000-00001.
17. Rowe AM, St. Leger AJ, Jeon S, Dhaliwal DK, Knickelbein JE, Hendricks RL. Herpes keratitis. Prog Retin Eye Res. 2013;32(1):88–101. https://doi.org/10.1016/J.PRETEYERES.2012.08.002.
18. Carter SB, Cohen EJ. Development of herpes simplex virus infectious epithelial keratitis during Oral acyclovir therapy and response to topical antivirals. Cornea. 2016;35(5):692–5. https://doi.org/10.1097/ICO.0000000000000806.
19. Valerio GS, Lin CC. Ocular manifestations of herpes simplex virus. Curr Opin Ophthalmol. 2019;30(6):525. https://doi.org/10.1097/ICU.0000000000000618.
20. Welder JD, Kitzmann AS, Wagoner MD. Herpes simplex keratitis. eyerounds.org. 2012;31. Published December. https://eyerounds.org/cases/160-HSV.htm. Accessed 16 Aug 2022.
21. Labetoulle M, Boutolleau D, Burrel S, Haigh O, Rousseau A. Herpes simplex virus, varicella-zoster virus and cytomegalovirus keratitis: facts for the clinician. Ocul Surf. 2021;28:336. https://doi.org/10.1016/J.JTOS.2021.07.002. Published online.
22. Kim JS, Rafailov L, Leyngold IM. Corneal neurotization for postherpetic neurotrophic keratopathy: initial experience and clinical outcomes. Ophthal Plast Reconstr Surg. 2021;37:42–50. https://doi.org/10.1097/IOP.0000000000001676. Published online.
23. Versura P, Giannaccare G, Pellegrini M, Sebastiani S, Campos EC. Neurotrophic keratitis: current challenges and future prospects. Eye Brain. 2018;10:37. https://doi.org/10.2147/EB.S117261.
24. Adams BS, Patel AR. Cenegermin. StatPearls. Published online May 6, 2022. https://www.ncbi.nlm.nih.gov/books/NBK573069/. Accessed 17 Aug 2022.

25. Zaal MJW, Völker-Dieben HJ, D'Amaro J. Prognostic value of Hutchinson's sign in acute herpes zoster ophthalmicus. Graefes Arch Clin Exp Ophthalmol. 2003;241(3):187–91. https://doi.org/10.1007/S00417-002-0609-1/TABLES/2.
26. Harthan JS, Borgman CJ. Herpes zoster ophthalmicus-induced oculomotor nerve palsy. J Optom. 2013;6(1):60. https://doi.org/10.1016/J.OPTOM.2012.08.005.
27. Park KC, Yoon SS, Yoon JE, Rhee HY. A case of herpes zoster ophthalmicus with isolated trochlear nerve involvement. J Clin Neurol. 2011;7(1):47. https://doi.org/10.3988/JCN.2011.7.1.47.
28. Chaker N, Bouladi M, Chebil A, Jemmeli M, Mghaieth F, El Matri L. Herpes zoster ophthalmicus associated with abducens palsy. J Neurosci Rural Pract. 2014;5(2):180. https://doi.org/10.4103/0976-3147.131673.
29. Li JY. Herpes zoster ophthalmicus: acute keratitis. Curr Opin Ophthalmol. 2018;29(4):328–33. https://doi.org/10.1097/ICU.0000000000000491.
30. Meduri A, Grenga PL, Kaufman SC. Herpes zoster ophthalmicus. Expert Rev Ophthalmol. 2021;4(5):537–45. https://doi.org/10.1586/eop.09.45.
31. Cortina MS, Azar DT. Corneal angiogenesis. Encycl Eye. 2010:408–15. https://doi.org/10.1016/B978-0-12-374203-2.00145-7. Published online
32. Cobo LMMD. Corneal complications of herpes zoster ophthalmicus: prevention and treatment. Cornea. 1988;7(1):50–6. https://journals.lww.com/corneajrnl/Abstract/1988/01000/Corneal_Complications_of_Herpes_Zoster.7.aspx. Accessed 17 Aug 2022.
33. Faith SC, Durrani AF, Jhanji V. Cytomegalovirus keratitis. Curr Opin Ophthalmol. 2018;29(4):373–7. https://doi.org/10.1097/ICU.0000000000000481.
34. Wong KW, Hedges TR, D'amico DJ, Kenyon KR, Soong HK, Schooley RT. Ocular involvement associated with chronic Epstein-Barr virus disease. Arch Ophthalmol (Chicago, Ill 1960). 1987;105(6):788–92. https://doi.org/10.1001/ARCHOPHT.1987.01060060074036.
35. Carl P, Ethan T, Zhenyang Z, Yusra S. An analysis of interstitial keratitis secondary to Epstein-Barr virus. Int J Ophthalmol Clin Res. 2020;7(3) https://doi.org/10.23937/2378-346X/1410118.
36. Omari AA, Mian SI. Adenoviral keratitis: a review of the epidemiology, pathophysiology, clinical features, diagnosis, and management. Curr Opin Ophthalmol. 2018;29(4):365–72. https://doi.org/10.1097/ICU.0000000000000485.

Bacterial Keratitis

8

Shweta Sandhu, Shivani Joshi, Prabhakar Singh,
and Radhika Tandon

Keratitis, an inflammation of the cornea, can result from alterations in corneal anatomy, weakened immunity, or impaired defense mechanisms. The causative agent of bacterial keratitis, which can be either Gram-positive or Gram-negative organisms, determine the nature of the infection. The severity and progression of bacterial keratitis hinge on the virulence of the infecting microorganism and various host factors, such as preexisting ocular surface disorders, ocular surgery, eye injuries, compromised immunity, and systemic diseases.

These cases underscore the importance of tailored treatment strategies, prompt diagnosis, and close follow-up in managing bacterial keratitis, especially in cases with unique medical histories and complex conditions.

8.1 Pediatric Corneal Ulcers

8.1.1 Summary

- A 2-year-old child with congenital hereditary endothelial dystrophy (CHED).
- Infected broken suturepost keratoplasty.
- Removal of infected suture and prompt treatment.

S. Sandhu
Advanced Eye Center, Postgraduate Institute of Medical Education and Research,
Chandigarh, India

S. Joshi · R. Tandon (✉)
Dr. Rajendra Prasad Centre for Ophthalmic Sciences, All India Institute of Medical Sciences,
New Delhi, India

P. Singh
Department of Ophthalmology, All India Institute of Medical Sciences,
Kalyani, West Bengal, India

F. A. Woreta, R. B. Singh (eds.), *Cornea Casebook*, Current Practices in
Ophthalmology, https://doi.org/10.1007/978-981-96-0495-1_8

8.1.2 Clinical Presentation

A 2-year-old child known case of CHED with glaucoma. In the first month of life, surgical trabeculectomy was performed in both eyes for glaucoma. Subsequently, at the age of 1 year, the child underwent optical penetrating keratoplasty in the right eye. Parents presented with distressing symptoms observed almost 1 week postoperatively to penetrating keratoplasty, which included excessive crying, watering redness, and frequent rubbing of the eyes. There was no reported history of ocular trauma.

8.1.3 Diagnosis

The child was taken up for examination under anesthesia (EUA) with corneal scrapings. A bacterial corneal ulcer was diagnosed and etiology was later established as *pseudomonas infection* after microbiological cultures sensitive to moxifloxacin and tobramycin.

8.1.4 Examination

EUA showed a few broken sutures with their ends protruding and 2 × 2.5 mm localised infiltrate. The broken sutures were removed. The infected broken sutures served as a nidus for microbial growth, leading to an corneal graft infection [1–3].

8.1.5 Treatment

While awaiting the culture results, he was empirically started on topical moxifloxacin hydrochloride 0.5%. The antibiotic was prescribed hourly for the first 24 h, then every 2 h for 48 h (round the clock), and subsequently tapered to every 4 h for 1 week, then every 6 h for a week.

8.1.6 Follow-Up and Outcome

The infiltrate resolved with treatment on follow-up EUA. The signs of resolution were observed as healing of epithelial defect, decreasing size and density of infiltrate, decreasing conjunctival injection, and reduced surrounding corneal edema.

Prompt diagnosis and appropriate treatment, including the removal of the infected suture and targeted antibiotic therapy, were crucial in managing this case and thus preserving the child's ambulatory vision [4].

8.2 Bacterial Secondary to Viral Keratitis

8.2.1 Summary

1. Young adult with bilateral chronic viral keratitis.
2. Diagnosed with secondary *Staphylococcus aureus* infection.
3. Improved response in one eye with medical management; therapeutic keratoplasty required in the other eye.
4. Vision improved after 3 weeks of close follow-up care.

8.2.2 Symptoms

A young adult male with a known history of recurrent viral keratitis in the past 2 years, presented with complaints of persistent redness, pain, and watering for last 2 weeks. He had no history of systemic disease, ocular surgery, contact lens use, or drugs/medications use. He was started on antiviral and antibiotic treatment for suspected bacterial infection secondary to viral keratitis [5].

8.2.3 Examination

Visual assessment showed hand motions in right eye and finger counting at 1 m in left eye. Clinical examination showed conjunctival congestion and discharge in both eyes. The cornea unveiled epithelial defect in both eyes (10 × 10 mm in right eye and 3 × 3 mm in left eye), with patchy infiltrates, superior Descemet's folds, and presence of a hypopyon of 1.5 mm in the right eye (Figs. 8.1 and 8.2). Corneal sensations were decreased in both eyes.

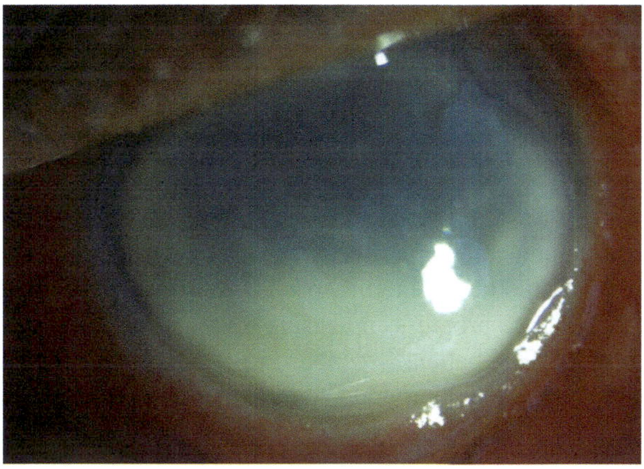

Fig. 8.1 Diffuse clinical picture of right eye shows a large epithelial defect 10 × 10 mm with patchy infiltrates and keratic precipitates, hypopyon of 1.5 mm inferiorly in anterior chamber

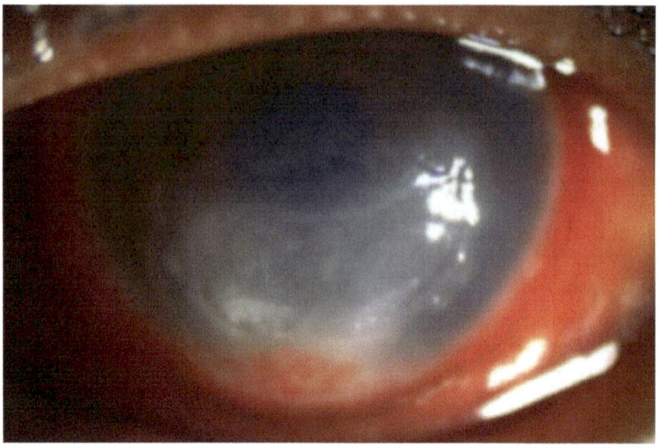

Fig. 8.2 Diffuse clinical picture of left eye showing corneal haze inferiorly with Descemet membrane folds, and an epithelial defect of 3 × 3 mm

8.2.4 Diagnostic Tests

Corneal scraping was performed and inoculated culture plates were sent for microbiological evaluation. The corneal smear showed gram-positive cocci and the culture subsequently grew *Staphylococcus aureus*.

8.2.5 Treatment

The patient's treatment plan involved the commencement of fortified eye drops containing vancomycin 5% and tobramycin 1.3%, administered hourly during the initial 2 days, homatropine 2%, and topical timolol and brimonidine to control the intraocular pressure. Oral ciprofloxacin 500 mg twice a day and with tablet vitamin C 500 mg OD was prescribed. Additionally oral acylovir 400 mg 5 times a day followed by tapered dose (twice daily) and acylovir 3% ophthalmic ointment 5 times a day was also started. The patient responded to therapy with reduced inflammation. The left eye healed on medical therapy alone, while the right eye required therapeutic penetrating keratoplasty (Fig. 8.3).

8.2.6 Follow Up

Patient was followed up daily in outpatient department and after 3 weeks visual acuity demonsrated improvement (Right eye showed finger counting and left eye showed 6/60 Snellen's). Close and consistent follow-up care is crucial to monitor the patient's progress and ensure that the corneal ulcer responds to treatment appropriately. The patient's response to the treatment regimen will guide any necessary adjustments to their medication and overall management.

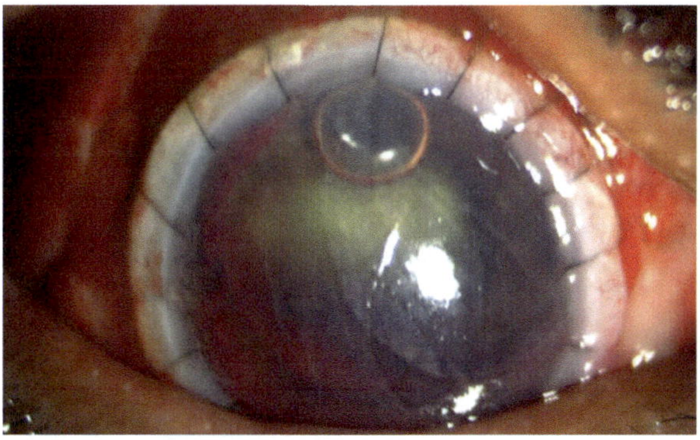

Fig. 8.3 Diffuse clinical picture of right eye post keratoplasty on postoperative day 1 showing a clear graft with a well formed stable anterior chamber, dispersed hyphemac and a small residual air bubble superiorly

8.3 Fulminant Pseudomonal Keratitis

8.3.1 Summary

- Middle-aged male, diagnosed with healed viral keratitis.
- Corneal transplant (optical penetrating keratoplasty) performed in the right eye.
- Post-surgery keratitis, identified as fulminant growth of *Pseudomonal* infection (Fig. 8.4) requiring a regraft (Fig. 8.5).

8.3.2 Symptoms

Middle-aged male, known case of a bilateral healed viral keratitis, had presented to outpatient department of ophthalmology with complaints of diminution of vision in both eyes over the past 2 years. He had no history of contact lens use, any medication use, trauma, or ocular surgery. He had no systemic issues as well.

8.3.3 Examination

Patient had presented with visual acuity of hand motions in right eye and 6/24 Snellen's in the left eye. The patient was diagnosed as bilateral healed viral keratitis with corneal scarring and underwent penetrating keratoplasty (PK) in the right eye. The surgery was uneventful, but on the first postoperative day (POD1), there was evidence of graft infection with whitish infiltrates along the graft-host junction spanning almost 180° with severe anterior chamber inflammation. Corneal scrapings were sent for microbiology. Epithelial defect, altered immune system, vernal keratoconjunctivitis, recurrent herpetic keratitis are common predisposing factors, and when presenting so early as in this case, there was a strong possibility of donor contamination [6, 7].

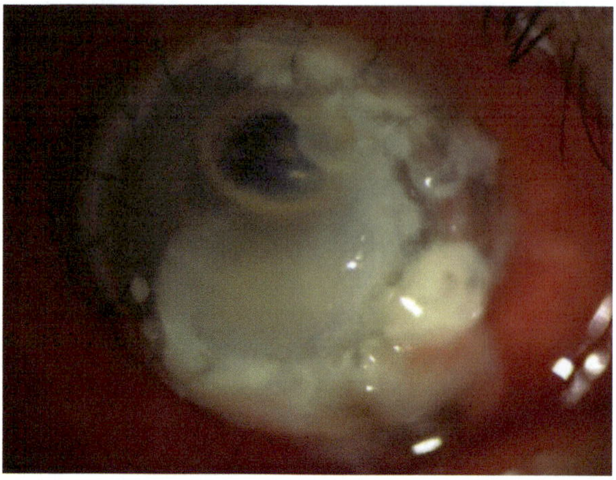

Fig. 8.4 Diffuse clinical picture of POD1 of right-side keratoplasty with infiltrates along the entire graft host junction and hypopyon

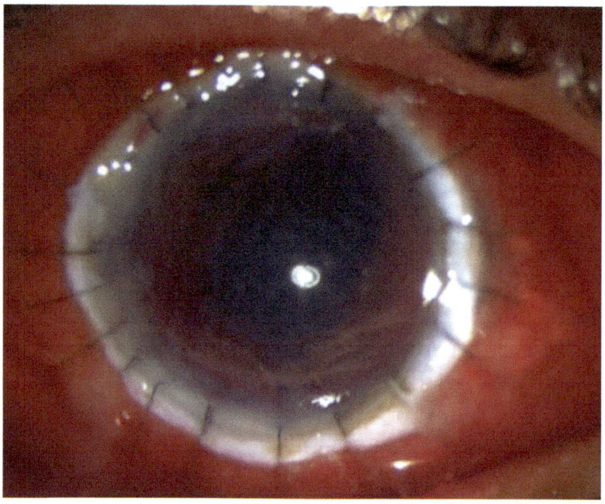

Fig. 8.5 Diffuse clinical picture of POD1 of repeat keratoplasty and PPV (Pars plana vitrectomy) showing large sized graft with scleral rim, graft clarity of grade 2 with all sutures in situ intact, buried, and healthy, AC is formed

8.3.4 Diagnostic Tests

Corneal scraping was performed and inoculated culture plates were sent for microbiological evaluation. The corneal smear showed gram-negative bacilli and the culture subsequently grew *Pseudomonas aeruginosa*.

8.3.5 Treatment

Topical steroids were withheld and topical fortified tobramycin (1.4%) and fortified vancomycin (5%) were started hourly during day and two hourly at night. Report of the corneal scrapings and corneal button, both revealed pseudomonas resistant to cefazolin, amikacin, vancomycin, ceftazidime, ofloxacin, ciprofloxacin, moxifloxacin, cefixime, chloramphenicol, tetracycline, gentamicin, and cefalexin [8]. It was sensitive to imipenem, tigecycline, and partially sensitive to gatifloxacin. Imipenem (5 mg/ml) drops were started hourly during day and two hourly at night. Despite this, the infiltration extended toward center of graft and hypopyon persisted with few vitreous exudates more in the anterior vitreous. Four days later, a repeat PK with pars plana vitrectomy was carried out to reduce microbial load. The next day, the graft was clear without infiltrates or hypopyon. Imipenem was continued. Gatifloxacin drops was added every half hourly. Five days later, prednisolone drops 1% four times a day were added.

In our case, keratitis was seen right on the first POD, suggesting either intraoperative field or donor cornea may be implicated in the infection.

8.4 Diabetes Mellitus, Moraxella Catarrhalis

8.4.1 Summary

- Diabetic patient
- Self-administered steroids
- Moraxella catarrhalis was identified as the cause of keratitis
- Vascularized corneal opacity as sequelae

8.4.2 Symptoms

A 53-year-old diabetic male presented to the ophthalmology outpatient department with complaints of severe pain, redness, photophobia, and decreased vision in the right eye for 10 days duration following history of a fall of dust particles into his eye. There patient had a history of self-medication with topical steroids. The patient consulted a tertiary eyecare facility. He did not give any prior history of such episodes, contact lens wear, or any other ocular or systemic disease.

8.4.3 Examination

Patient presented with visual acuity of hand motions close to the face with accurate projection of rays. On ocular examination, the right eye showed lid edema with conjunctival chemosis. Corneal examination showed a 6 × 5.5 mm corneal infiltrate with an overlying epithelial defect and extensive stromal collagenolysis with central pseudocornea and a flat anterior chamber (Fig. 8.6). The patient underwent tissue adhesive (n-butyl Cyanoacrylate) application with anterior chamber reformation (Fig. 8.7) [9, 10].

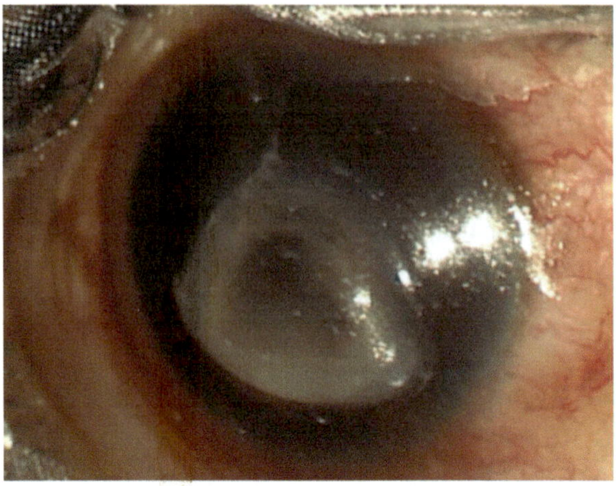

Fig. 8.6 A large (5.5 × 6 mm) corneal infiltrate with overlying epithelial defect and extensive collagenolysis with pseudocornea and flat anterior chamber

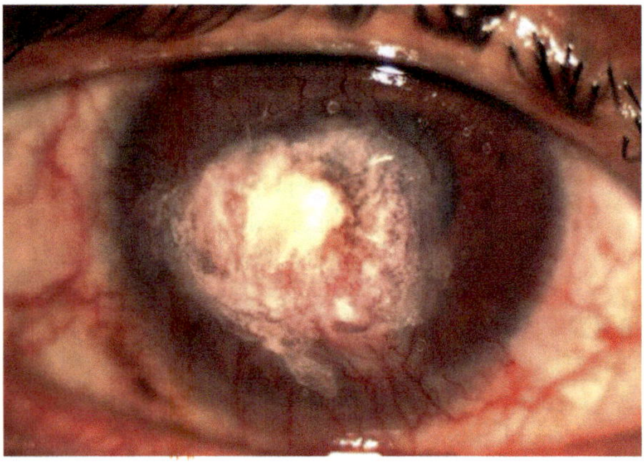

Fig. 8.7 At 1-month status post cyanoacrylate glue application

8.4.4 Diagnostic Tests

Intraoperatively, corneal scraping was performed and inoculated culture plates were sent for microbiological evaluation. The corneal smear showed gram-negative diplococci and the culture subsequently grew Moraxella catarrhalis [11, 12].

8.4.5 Treatment

The patient was started empirically on fortified tobramycin (1.4%) and fortified vancomycin (5%) along with cycloplegic and an oral fluoroquinolone antibiotic (Ciprofloxacin 500 mg BD). Following tissue adhesive application, the anterior chamber was formed and over 2 months the surface healed completely, and the tissue adhesive dislodged on its own (Fig. 8.8). Though the corneal infiltrate resolved with stable ocular surface and a vascularized corneal opacity.

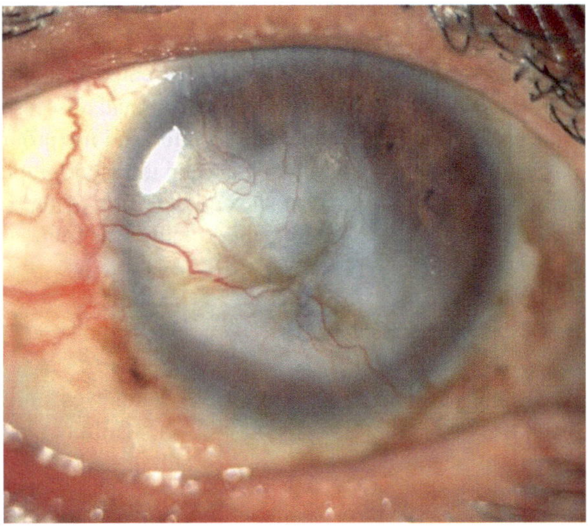

Fig. 8.8 A vascularized corneal scar at the end of 2 months

This case underscores the importance of educating patients, especially those with underlying conditions like diabetes, about the risks of using topical steroids, the need for prompt medical attention for eye problems, and the potential consequences of delayed treatment.

8.5 Post Snake Bite Keratoplasty

8.5.1 Summary

- Male patient with history of snake bite.
- Acute chemical injury causing corneal melting.
- Caution against the use of traditional remedies without medical supervision.

8.5.2 Symptoms

A 38-year-old male presented to emergency hospital with pain, redness, and diminution of vision 10 days after a snake bite on his right foot. History of presenting illness revealed that during treatment for snake bite at a local village health care facility, a traditional eye medicine in the form of a whitish flaky powder was instilled into both his eyes on the advice of a snake charmer. Two days later, the patient developed pain, redness, and diminution of vision in both eyes which was diagnosed elsewhere as bilateral corneal ulcers and subsequently referred to tertiary eye hospital for management [13–15].

8.5.3 Examination

At presentation, ocular examination revealed visual acuity of light perception in both eyes without projection. Bilateral corneal abscesses involving the entire cornea were seen, along with corneal perforation and iris prolapse OD (Figs. 8.9 and 8.10). Posterior segment evaluation on B-scan ultrasonography was unremarkable in both eyes. Systemic examination showed cellulitis of the right foot around the area of snake bite. No other systemic abnormality was found [16, 17].

8.5.4 Diagnostic Tests

A corneal scraping was taken from both eyes and smear preparation showed the presence of gram-positive cocci. Culture growth was consistent with coagulase-negative *Staphylococcus aureus*. Blood coagulation profile and renal

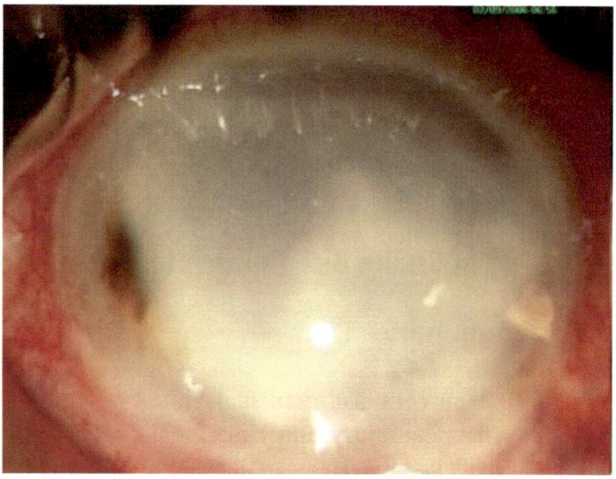

Fig. 8.9 Corneal abscess with perforation in the right eye at presentation

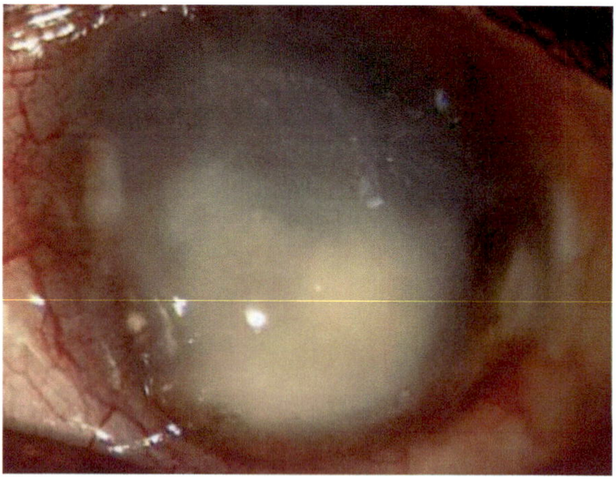

Fig. 8.10 Corneal abscess in the left eye at presentation

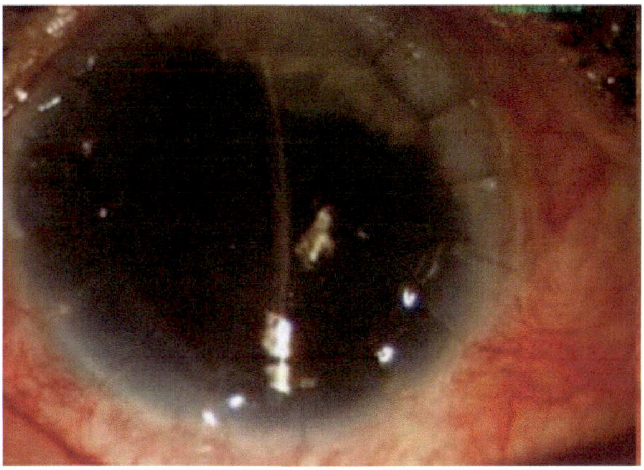

Fig. 8.11 Clear graft in the right eye of after penetrating keratoplasty

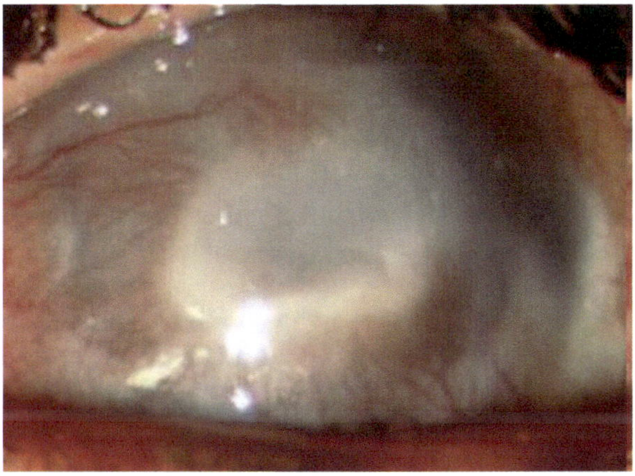

Fig. 8.12 Adherent leucoma in the left eye after medical management

and liver function tests were normal. Chemical analysis of the powder revealed potassium nitrite.

8.5.5 Treatment

The patient was advised to use concentrated 5% cefazolin eye drops at hourly intervals, 0.3% gatifloxacin eye drops every hour, and 2% homatropine eye drops four times a day. Systemic cloxacillin 500 mg QID for 1 week was given for the treatment of foot cellulitis. The right eye continued to worsen and a penetrating keratoplasty with lens aspiration was performed 2 weeks later. The corneal abscess in the left eye responded to medical management with intensive topical antibiotics. Four months later, the graft in the right eye was clear with BCVA of 20/80 (Fig. 8.11). The left eye showed an adherent leucoma with a visual acuity of light perception without projection (Fig. 8.12). Further surgical intervention in the left eye was deferred in view of poor visual prognosis.

8.6 Post Radial Keratotomy Bacterial Keratitis

8.6.1 Summary

- A 45-year-old female with a history of bilateral RK surgery developed keratitis.
- Culture reported positive for Methicillin-Resistant Staphylococcus epidermidis (MRS) keratitis.
- Initial treatment with topical antibiotics was ineffective, necessitating the addition of oral antibiotics for a better response.
- This case underscores the importance of long-term follow-up after RK surgery and the potential for serious complications even decades later.

8.6.2 Symptoms

A 45-year-old female who had undergone bilateral RK (12 corneal incisions per eye) 20 years previously presented with complaints of pain and visual loss in her right eye. Post RK, she had not undergone any long-term follow-up examinations due to the good surgical outcome and the postoperative course being stable and satisfactory for 20 years [18–20]. Although she had been diagnosed with bacterial keratitis by her primary care physician, she was not prescribed any medication and was referred to tertiary eye care hospital for management.

8.6.3 Examination

Patient had no remarkable systemic medical history, and no history of any ocular trauma or contact lens use. Initial examination of her right eye revealed a best-corrected visual acuity (VA) of finger counting close to face. Moreover, we observed a small-sized focus area of epithelial defects with inflammatory infiltrate (5 × 4.5 mm) and endothelial plaque in the deep site in the radial incisions inferotemporally meridian, conjunctival injection, and inflammatory cells in AC (Figs. 8.13 and 8.14) with negative siedel.

8.6.4 Diagnostic Tests

Corneal scrapings were sent for microbiological investigations: Gram stain, Giemsa stain, calcofluor white stain, KOH mount, bacterial culture on blood agar, fungal culture on Sabouraud dextrose agar and thioglycolate broth, and drug sensitivity testing. Culture sensitivity showed Gram-positive cocci arranged in grape-like clusters and appeared on agar as white 1–2 mm colonies suggestive of catalase-positive, coagulase-negative (novobiocin sensitive), facultative anaerobic bacterium suggestive of *Staph epidermidis*.

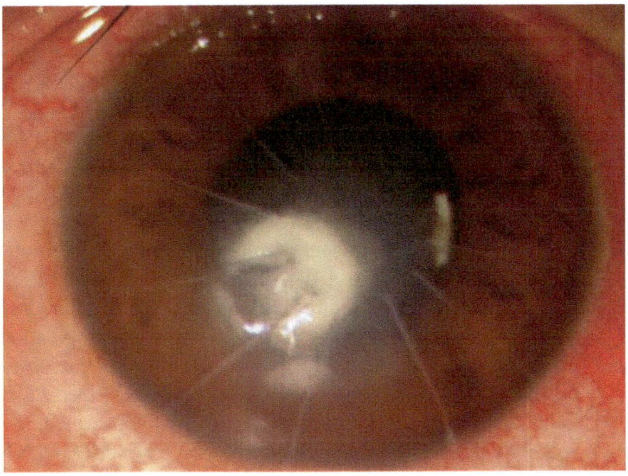

Fig. 8.13 Twelve incisions radial keratotomy with 5 × 4.5 mm focus area of corneal edema with inflammatory infiltrate

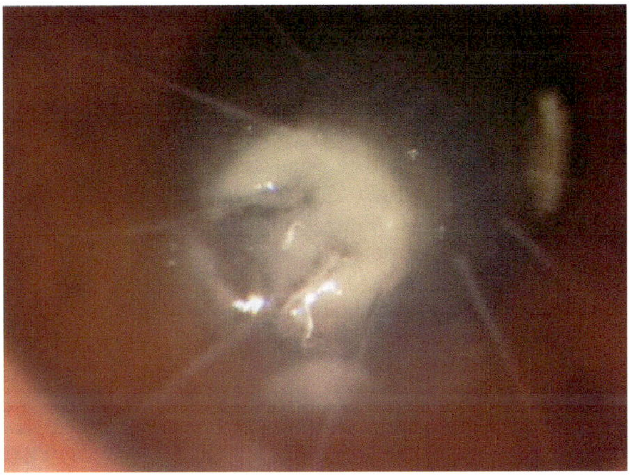

Fig. 8.14 Endothelial plaque in the deep site in the radial incisions at 7 O′ clock infero-temporal meridian

8.6.5 Treatment

Thus, we initiated treatment with an hourly topical administration of 1.5% levofloxacin and 0.5% vancomycin 5% eye drops. However, despite the treatment with broad-spectrum antibiotics, the ocular findings on the following day revealed that the conjunctival injectio and, infiltrate were worsening. Oral Ciprofloxacin (500 mg BD for 1 week) was added to the treatment regimen, leading to better response and resolution of the infection. Superficial stromal infiltrations, minimal melting, and minimal stromal scarring are characteristic of MRSA (Methicillin Resistant Staph Aureus) keratitis. Topical vancomyin is effective in the treatment of MRSA keratitis.

In this case, although early detection and treatment resulted in an good postoperative outcome with no visual dysfunction, our findings reveal that long-term follow-up is necessary post RK since infection may occur many years after surgery [21, 22].

References

1. Davila JR, Mian SI. Infectious keratitis after keratoplasty. Curr Opin Ophthalmol. 2016;27(4):358–66. https://doi.org/10.1097/ICU.0000000000000269. PMID: 27054815.
2. Hood CT, Lee BJ, Jeng BH. Incidence, occurrence rate, and characteristics of suture-related corneal infections after penetrating keratoplasty. Cornea. 2011;30(6):624–8. https://doi.org/10.1097/ICO.0b013e3182041755. PMID: 21282987.
3. Moorthy S, Graue E, Jhanji V, Constantinou M, Vajpayee RB. Microbial keratitis after penetrating keratoplasty: impact of sutures. Am J Ophthalmol. 2011;152(2):189–194.e2. https://doi.org/10.1016/j.ajo.2011.01.038. Epub 2011 May 31. PMID: 21624557.
4. Di Zazzo A, Rajan M, Dureja R, Antonini M, Kanduri V, Madduri B, Mohan N, Mohamed A, Fernandes M. Pediatric microbial keratitis: identification of clinical biomarkers for prognosis and outcome of 218 cases from 2009 to 2019. Cornea. 2022;41(9):1103–9. https://doi.org/10.1097/ICO.0000000000002957. Epub 2021 Dec 22. PMID: 34935663.
5. Yang Z, Yu S, Zhang C, Agrawal R, Feng Y. Nonsurgical management of severe viral keratitis with hypopyon and retrocorneal plaques: a case series. Ophthalmol Ther. 2023;12(1):599–611. https://doi.org/10.1007/s40123-022-00592-x. Epub 2022 Oct 21. PMID: 36269489; PMCID: PMC9834490.
6. Fernandes M, Vira D, Medikonda R, Kumar N. Extensively and pan-drug resistant Pseudomonas aeruginosa keratitis: clinical features, risk factors, and outcome. Graefes Arch Clin Exp Ophthalmol. 2016;254(2):315–22. https://doi.org/10.1007/s00417-015-3208-7. Epub 2015 Nov 4. PMID: 26537122.
7. Vazirani J, Wurity S, Ali MH. Multidrug-resistant Pseudomonas aeruginosa keratitis: risk factors, clinical characteristics, and outcomes. Ophthalmology. 2015;122(10):2110–4. https://doi.org/10.1016/j.ophtha.2015.06.007. Epub 2015 Jul 15. PMID: 26189185.
8. Jain R, Murthy SI, Motukupally SR. Clinical outcomes of corneal graft infections caused by multi-drug resistant Pseudomonas aeruginosa. Cornea. 2014;33(1):22–6. https://doi.org/10.1097/ICO.0000000000000011. PMID: 24240490.
9. Kenny SE, Puig M, Salinas R, Johnson DA, Kheirkhah A. Moraxella keratitis: a case series. Eye Contact Lens. 2021;47(12):674–6. https://doi.org/10.1097/ICL.0000000000000839. PMID: 34520409.
10. Das S, Constantinou M, Daniell M, Taylor HR. Moraxella keratitis: predisposing factors and clinical review of 95 cases. Br J Ophthalmol. 2006;90(10):1236–8. https://doi.org/10.1136/bjo.2006.095182. Epub 2006 Jul 6. PMID: 16825274; PMCID: PMC1857441.
11. Hoarau G, Merabet L, Brignole-Baudouin F, Mizrahi A, Borderie V, Bouheraoua N. Moraxella keratitis: epidemiology and outcomes. Eur J Clin Microbiol Infect Dis. 2020;39(12):2317–25. https://doi.org/10.1007/s10096-020-03985-7. Epub 2020 Jul 9. PMID: 32648113.
12. McSwiney TJ, Knowles SJ, Murphy CC. Clinical and microbiological characteristics of Moraxella keratitis. Br J Ophthalmol. 2019;103(12):1704–9. https://doi.org/10.1136/bjophthalmol-2018-313557. Epub 2019 Feb 1. PMID: 30709811.
13. Price FW. Price's text book of the practice of medicine. Ed. Sir Ronald Bodley: Scott; 1976.
14. Takeshita T, Yamada K, Hanada M, Oda-Ueda N. Case report: extraocular muscle paresis caused by snakebite. Kobe J Med Sci. 2003;49:11–5.
15. Ghosh AK, Bhaduri G, Sarkar AD, Mondal LK, Maiti A, Kishore V, Datta A, Chanda S. Unilateral loss of vision following snakebite. J Indian Med Assoc. 2006;104:404–5.
16. Chen CC, Yang CM, Hu FR, Lee YC. Penetrating ocular injury caused by venomous snakebite. Am J Ophthalmol. 2005;140:544–6.
17. Rojas L, Ortiz G, Gutierrez M, Corredor S. Ghost cell glaucoma related to snake poisoning. Arch Ophthalmol. 2001;119:1212–3.
18. Kawasaki M, Fukuoka H, Kawabata M, Sotozono C. A rare case of infectious keratitis that developed 27-years after radial keratotomy. Am J Ophthalmol Case Rep. 2021;25:101240. https://doi.org/10.1016/j.ajoc.2021.101240. PMID: 34917857; PMCID: PMC8665298.

19. Matoba AY, Torres J, Wilhelmus KR, Hamill MB, Jones DB. Bacterial keratitis after radial keratotomy. Ophthalmology. 1989;96(8):1171–5. https://doi.org/10.1016/s0161-6420(89)32761-8. PMID: 2677887.
20. Procope JA. Delayed-onset pseudomonas keratitis after radial keratotomy. J Cataract Refract Surg. 1997;23(8):1271–2. https://doi.org/10.1016/s0886-3350(97)80327-6. PMID: 9368176.
21. Heidemann DG, Dunn SP, Chow CY. Early- versus late-onset infectious keratitis after radial and astigmatic keratotomy: clinical spectrum in a referral practice. J Cataract Refract Surg. 1999;25(12):1615–9. https://doi.org/10.1016/s0886-3350(99)00285-0. PMID: 10609205.
22. Beldavs RA, al-Ghamdi S, Wilson LA, Waring GO 3rd. Bilateral microbial keratitis after radial keratotomy. Arch Ophthalmol. 1993;111(4):440. https://doi.org/10.1001/archopht.1993.01090040030019. PMID: 8470970.

Fungal Keratitis

9

Savitri Sharma, Aravind Roy, Sujata Das,
and Bhupesh Bagga

9.1 Introduction

Fungal infections of the eye including keratitis can have devastating consequences. Untreated fungal keratitis may progress to endophthalmitis and loss of the eye. Fungal keratitis is relatively rare in the United States except in the southern states. However, contact lens-associated fungal keratitis caused by *Fusarium* species was reported in at least 130 patients from 26 states [1]. In South Asia, Africa, and other tropical climates, fungal keratitis occurs more commonly. Reports from India show that as much as 44% of microbial keratitis could be caused by fungi [2]. *Candida* species and filamentous fungi, such as *Fusarium* species, are the most frequent fungal isolates associated with keratitis in patients treated at the Bascom Palmer Eye Institute in the United States [3]. Of the 421 corneal isolates identified, *Fusarium* species were the most frequent fungal pathogen (49.4%), followed by *Curvularia* (8.1%), *Aspergillus* (7.1%), and *Paecilomyces* species (5%). Other studies have also

S. Sharma (✉)
Laboratory Services, KAR Campus, L V Prasad Eye Institute, Hyderabad, Telangana, India
e-mail: savitri@lvpei.org

A. Roy
Cornea and Anterior Segment Services, KVC campus, L V Prasad Eye Institute, Vijaywada, Andhra Pradesh, India
e-mail: aravindroy@lvpei.org

S. Das
Shantilal Shanghvi Cornea Institute, MTC Campus, L V Prasad Eye Institute, Bhubaneswar, Odisha, India
e-mail: sujatadas@lvpei.org

B. Bagga
Ramoji Foundation Centre of Ocular Infections, Shantilal Shanghvi Cornea Institute, KAR Campus, L V Prasad Eye Institute, Hyderabad, Telangana, India
e-mail: Bhupesh@lvpei.org

F. A. Woreta, R. B. Singh (eds.), *Cornea Casebook*, Current Practices in Ophthalmology, https://doi.org/10.1007/978-981-96-0495-1_9

reported *Fusarium* species as the commonest cause of fungal keratitis [4]. Fungal keratitis is a significant cause of corneal blindness, particularly in developing countries, in tropical and subtropical regions where approximately half of the world's fungal keratitis cases occur [5], and the contribution of fungal keratitis, as one of the major causes of visual loss, cannot be ignored [6].

Clinical features to determine the causative agent of fungal keratitis have been reported to be not more than 70% by experienced clinicians [7]. In the clinic, in vivo method such as confocal microscopy is helpful to the clinicians to make the clinical diagnosis with greater confidence, especially for *Acanthamoeba* and fungal keratitis [8]. However, confirmation by direct microscopic examination and culture of the corneal samples remains the gold standard for the etiological diagnosis. Currently, very high sensitivity and specificity are being reported in the diagnosis of fungal keratitis by using molecular methods such as polymerase chain reaction (PCR) and PCR-based DNA sequencing.

Current treatment protocols for mycotic infections of the cornea are far from optimal owing to a combination of factors such as delayed diagnosis, scarcity of effective antifungal agents, and poor tissue penetration of the currently available antifungal agents. Topical natamycin, a polyene, is the only FDA-approved and commercially available topical antifungal for the eye. It has good efficacy against filamentous fungi but does not penetrate well into the cornea. Additionally, it forms precipitates upon instillation and degrades easily, requiring storage in a dark container. Topical amphotericin B is often used in the management of fungal keratitis; however, it requires preparation by a compounding pharmacy. The fungal keratitis cases discussed in this chapter bring out the possibility of mixed infection, a variety of methods for diagnosis, and the modification of the treatment strategies for achieving optimum results.

9.2 Case 1

A 68-year-old male presented to the cornea clinic with complaints of blurring vision and watering of left eye of 15 days duration. He had a history of injury with a paddy leaf 15 days ago. He was using topical moxifloxacin 0.5% prior to presentation. Visual acuity was 20/20p in left eye. There was no history of any systemic diseases. Slit-lamp examination showed mild conjunctival congestion with minimal infiltrate mimicking a dendrite near temporal limbus (Fig. 9.1a). Corneal scrapings were submitted for microbiological evaluation. Direct microscopy of corneal scraping using Gram stain and 10% potassium hydroxide with 0.1% calcofluor white (KOH + CFW) wet mount (examined by fluorescence microscope) did not reveal any organism. While the culture reports were awaited, basis clinical suspicion the patient was started on topical natamycin 5% hourly, homatropine 2% thrice daily, and oral paracetamol 650 mg and asked to review after 3 days. On the next visit, the patient complained of increased pain and visual acuity reduced to 20/40 in the left eye. The clinical picture was unchanged. Microscopy of repeat corneal scrapings revealed septate fungal filaments in both Gram stain (Fig. 9.1b) and KOH + CFW mount.

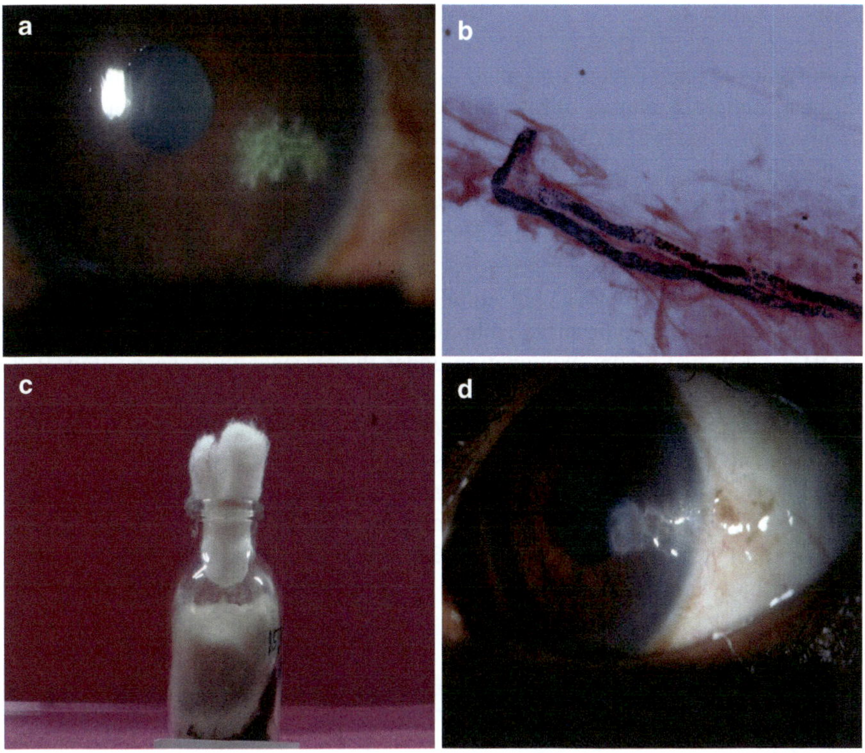

Fig. 9.1 (**a**) Slit-lamp picture of left eye in diffuse illumination showing mild conjunctival congestion and superficial infiltrate arranged in a dendritic pattern, (**b**) septate fungal filaments in microscopy of corneal scraping (Gram stain, ×1000 total magnification), (**c**) fluffy fungal growth, pinkish below and cream colored above (unidentified hyaline fungus, potato dextrose agar), (**d**) slit-lamp picture showing resolved keratitis with corneal scar

Meanwhile, significant fungal growth was noted on blood agar and potato dextrose agar (Fig. 9.1c) from the primary corneal scraping taken on the first visit. The fungus grown was nonpigmented and remained unidentified due to lack of sporulation. The patient was continued on the same treatment regimen. After 1 month of presentation, the corneal infiltrate had scarred and the patient had responded well to medication (Fig. 9.1d).

Learning Points

1. Early fungal keratitis may mimic dendrite of viral keratitis.
2. Repeat corneal scraping needs to be considered in case of negative results in microbiology at the first attempt.
3. Direct microscopy of corneal scrapings is helpful in the rapid diagnosis of fungal keratitis.

9.3 Case 2

A 66-year-old male patient presented to the cornea clinic with complaints of pain, redness, and photophobia in his right eye since 2 weeks. There was a history of injury with a paddy leaf. There was history of any other systemic disease. He was using topical natamycin 5% two hourly and topical gatifloxacin 0.5% 8 times per day at presentation. His visual acuity was perception of light with projection of rays. Left eye visual acuity was 20/30. Slit lamp examination showed conjunctival congestion and full thickness infiltrate of 7 mm × 5 mm with tentacle-like edges with guttering from 7 to 9 o'clock paracentral cornea (Fig. 9.2a). There was hypopyon of 2.8 mm. Corneal scraping revealed broad, sparsely septate, branching filaments in KOH + CFW wet mount examination under fluorescence microscope (Fig. 9.2b) and in Gomori methenamine silver stain (Fig. 9.2c). The filaments resembled zygomycete fungal filaments. To rule out *Pythium* and to differentiate from mucorales, corneal scraping was subjected to potassium iodide-sulfuric acid (IKI-H_2SO) stain which was positive and confirmed *Pythium* (Fig. 9.2d). Patient was started on topical linezolid (2%) hourly and systemic azithromycin (500 mg) BD. Despite intensive medical therapy, the condition worsened to corneal perforation after 1 month of presentation (Fig. 9.2e), and required tissue adhesive application and bandage

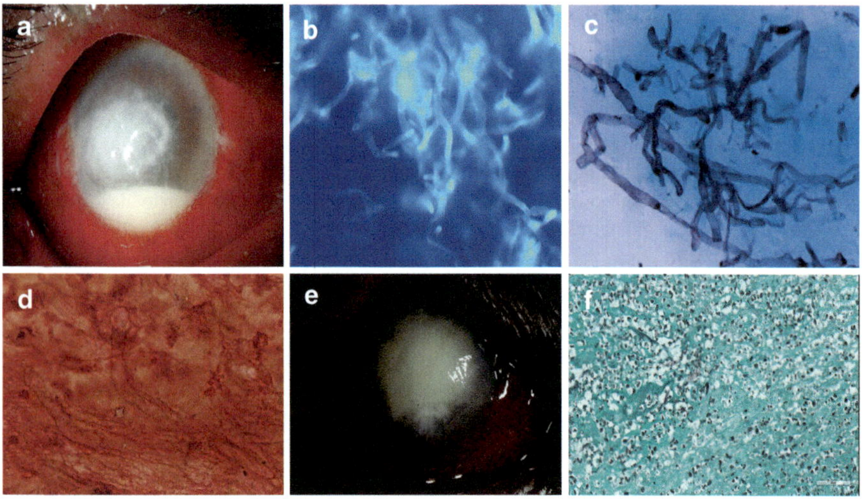

Fig. 9.2 (**a**) Slit-lamp picture of right eye showing conjunctival congestion and corneal infiltrate with guttering from 7 to 9 o'clock, (**b**) direct fluorescence microscopy of corneal scraping showing broad, aseptate, branching hyphae with ribbon-like folds (potassium hydroxide with calcofluor white wet mount, ×400 total magnification), (**c**) direct microscopy of corneal scraping showing black, broad, aseptate, branching hyphae with ribbon-like folds (Gomori methenamine silver stain, ×400 total magnification), (**d**) corneal scraping showing bluish broad hyphal fragments (potassium iodide-sulfuric acid stain, x400 total magnification), (**e**) slit-lamp picture of the cornea showing total corneal infiltrate, (**f**) histopathology picture showing black, broad, aseptate hyphal fragments (Gomori methenamine silver stain, ×400 total magnification)

contact lens followed by therapeutic penetrating keratoplasty. Histopathology of corneal tissue further confirmed the presence of *Pythium* in corneal tissue as well as in anterior chamber exudate (Fig. 9.2f).

Learning Points

1. *Pythium* keratitis needs to be differentiated from fungal keratitis since treatment of both entities is completely different.
2. Potassium iodide-sulfuric acid (IKI-H_2SO_4) stain is a sensitive diagnostic test to confirm *Pythium* species in corneal tissue.
3. Despite specific therapy, an advanced *Pythium* keratitis may not respond favorably to medical therapy and require surgical intervention.

9.4 Case 3

A 50-year-old controlled diabetic and hypertensive man presented with 5-month history of pain, watering, and redness in the left eye with history of vegetative injury sustained 5 years ago. He was empirically treated with topical voriconazole 1% hourly a few months ago. Presenting unaided visual acuity of the left eye was 20/60. Slit lamp examination showed deep stromal supero-nasal corneal scar with multiple stromal infiltrates (Fig. 9.3a), edema, localized keratic precipitates, cells in anterior chamber (AC), and intraocular pressure (IOP) 12 mm of Hg. Etiology was presumed to be non-necrotizing HSV deep stromal keratitis based on clinical signs. He was advised topical prednisolone acetate 1% 6 times per day, atropine 1% three times per day, and oral acyclovir 400 mg 5 times a day. After 2 weeks of therapy, there was worsening of stromal infiltrate with large mutton fat-like exudates on endothelium and hypopyon. Corticosteroids were stopped; corneal biopsy and diagnostic AC tap for quantitative real-time PCR (qPCR) was performed for HSV-1 DNA. Corneal scrapings from deeper cornea were submitted for mirobiological evaluation. Gram-stained smear showed septate fungal filaments on microscopy (Fig. 9.3b) and no growth in culture media (5% sheep blood agar, chocolate agar, Sabouraud dextrose agar). qPCR of AC tap for HSV 1 showed 438 copy numbers per milliliter. Corneal biopsy specimen on histopathologic evaluation showed fungal filaments in Gomori methenamine silver (GMS) stain. The patient was started on treatment with topical natamycin 5%, atropine 1% eye drops, and oral ketoconazole 200 mg twice daily. He continued to worsen with active infiltrates approaching limbus (Fig. 9.3c) and underwent therapeutic penetrating keratoplasty. Histopathology of corneal button showed fungal filaments in the posterior corneal stroma in Gomori methenamine silver (GMS) stain (Fig. 9.3d). Culture of corneal button was negative for bacteria and fungus. Topical prednisolone acetate 1% 8 times a day and prophylactic oral acyclovir 400 mg 2 times a day were started after 2 weeks of antifungal therapy. Postoperative course was uneventful without recurrence after 4 months of follow-up.

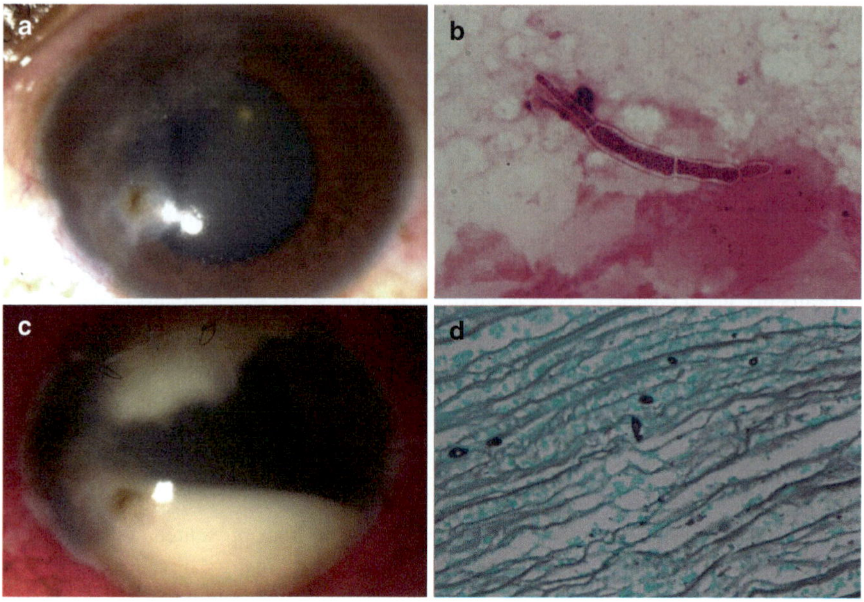

Fig. 9.3 (**a**) Slit-lamp picture of the cornea showing superonasal scar and multiple mid-stromal infiltrates, (**b**) direct microscopy of the corneal biopsy from the superior cornea showing septate fungal filaments (Gram stain, ×1000 total magnification), (**c**) slit-lamp picture showing worsened corneal infiltrates with active infiltrates approaching the limbus at 12 o'clock, (**d**) histopathology of the corneal tissue shows black fungal filaments in the corneal stroma (Gomori methenamine silver stain, ×400 total magnification)

Learning Points

1. Corneal biopsy is a useful investigation for diagnosis of deep-seated corneal infection.
2. Real-time PCR is a reliable investigation to establish diagnosis of viral keratitis including HSV 1.
3. Co-infection of HSV 1 stromal keratitis with fungi is a possibility in a hot and humid tropical climate.
4. Fungi can remain dormant in corneal tissues for a long time and may get reactivated after treatment with corticosteroids.
5. Topical corticosteroids with long-term oral acyclovir prophylaxis are necessary to control HSV 1-associated inflammation.

9.5 Case 4

A 55-year-old uncontrolled diabetic man presented with 20-day history of pain, redness, and defective vision in the left eye. There was no antecedent history of trauma and no other significant ocular or systemic history. His visual acuity was hand motions in left eye. There was a large paracentral corneal stromal infiltrate 8 mm × 6 mm with feathery margins extending up to the posterior stroma and approaching 5 o'clock limbus. Inferior cornea showed thinning with iris incarceration. Anterior chamber was formed and had 3 mm hypopyon with exudates on the endothelium. The lens and posterior segment were not visualized. The left eye B scan ultrasonography was normal. The right eye was essentially normal. Corneal scraping from the lesion was negative for bacteria and fungus in smear and culture. The patient was advised tissue adhesives and application of bandage contact lenses (TA + BCL) and topical broad-spectrum antibiotics (fortified vancomycin 5% + ciprofloxacin 0.5%) were administered hourly along with atropine 1% eye drops thrice daily. The infiltrates worsened with increase in endoexudates after 1 week of treatment (Fig. 9.4a). Blood sugar was under control. Following the same treatment for another week, the infiltrates decreased with corneal scarring and vascularization and persistence of deep stromal endoexudates. The patient was advised AC wash and corneal biopsy and subjected to microbiologic evaluation (Fig. 9.4b). AC wash on microbiologic evaluation showed septate fungal filaments in 1% acid-fast stain, while Gram stain and KOH + CFW wet mount was negative, culture showed no growth of organisms. AC wash was subjected to PCR analysis for fungus and HSV 1 DNA. ITS-based panfungal PCR was positive for fungal DNA and real-time PCR for HSV 1 DNA showed 8239 copies/ml. Corneal biopsy from an area of stromal infiltrate was subjected to histopathology and was found to be negative. On the basis of visualization of fungal filaments and high copy numbers of HSV 1 DNA in AC wash sample, the patient was advised a therapeutic dose of oral acyclovir 400 mg five times a day and topical natamycin 5% hourly for 8 weeks. This led to resolution of the infiltrates with scarring and vascularization. Following this, the frequency of acyclovir 400 mg was reduced to twice daily and prednisolone 1% eye drops 8 times a day with weekly taper for 8 weeks. The prophylactic dose of acyclovir 400 mg twice daily was continued and at the last follow-up at 15 months, the left eye cornea was scarred and vascularized (Fig. 9.4c).

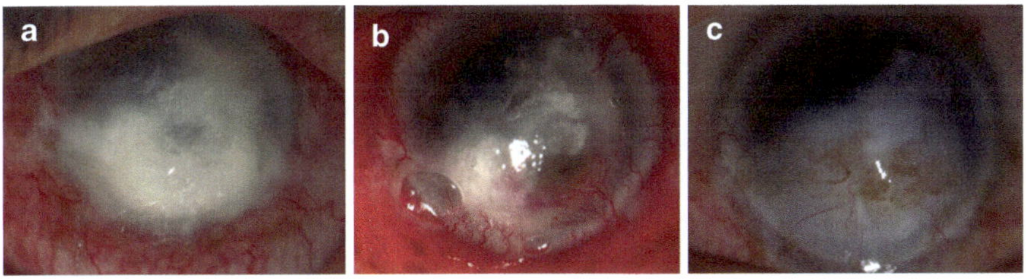

Fig. 9.4 (**a**) Slit-lamp biomicroscopy shows corneal infiltrates with ill-defined margins approaching limbus at 5 o'clock with inferior corneal thinning and iris incarceration, (**b**) tissue adhesive and bandage contact lens application done, (**c**) vascularized and scarred cornea seen with healing of microbial keratitis after 15 months follow-up

Learning Points

1. Herpes simplex keratitis is primarily a clinical diagnosis, but the existence of clinical HSV keratitis should be supported by demonstration of HSV 1 DNA in PCR.
2. Realtime PCR with high copy numbers of HSV-1 DNA is suggestive of active viral replication and needs therapy with antivirals.
3. Co-infection of the cornea with HSV 1 and fungus is rarely reported and needs combination antifungal and antiviral therapy.

9.6 Case 5

A 65-year-old woman presented to the cornea clinic with decreased vision along with redness and pain in her left eye since 2 months. She had a previous history of uneventful cataract surgery of her left eye 2 months prior to presentation and achieved the best corrected visual acuity of 20/20 after 6 weeks duration. However, she developed sudden onset of pain and redness along with evidence of anterior chamber inflammation. She had undergone a diagnostic anterior chamber tap which did not reveal any organism and topical corticosteroids were given. On follow-up, she worsened with the increase in redness and pain and decreased vision and was referred to our institute.

At presentation, the vision was 20/500 in the affected eye while the right eye was essentially within normal limits. On slit-lamp examination of the cornea of the left eye, there were multiple pin point stromal infiltrates diffusely spread across the entire stroma (Fig. 9.5a). As the epithelium was intact, we scraped off the epithelium to get material from the anterior stromal infiltrate and sent for complete microbiological examination. Posterior segment examination was found to be normal by ultrasonic examination.

No organisms were demonstrated in the microscopic examination of the corneal scrapings stained with KOH + CFW and Gram stain. Corticosteroids were discontinued while the patient was started on combination of antibiotics including hourly fortified vancomycin 5% and ciprofloxacin 0.5% topically. With no clue to the etiological diagnosis, we performed confocal microscopy which revealed multiple double-walled filamentous structures (Fig. 9.5b) with branches extending from anterior to posterior stroma. These findings were suggestive of fungal filaments. The diagnosis was confirmed by repeat corneal scraping performed on the next follow-up which showed septate filaments in KOH + CFW wet mount (Fig. 9.5c) and GMS stain. The patient was started on hourly topical 5% natamycin along with oral ketoconazole (200 mg twice a day) and followed-up daily. On follow-up, there was increase in the size and density of the infiltrate. As there was significant worsening of the corneal infiltrates (Fig. 9.5d), the patient was subjected to therapeutic penetrating keratoplasty. The culture from the excised corneal button grew *Aspergillus flavus* (Fig. 9.5e). On histopathology examination of the corneal button, septate

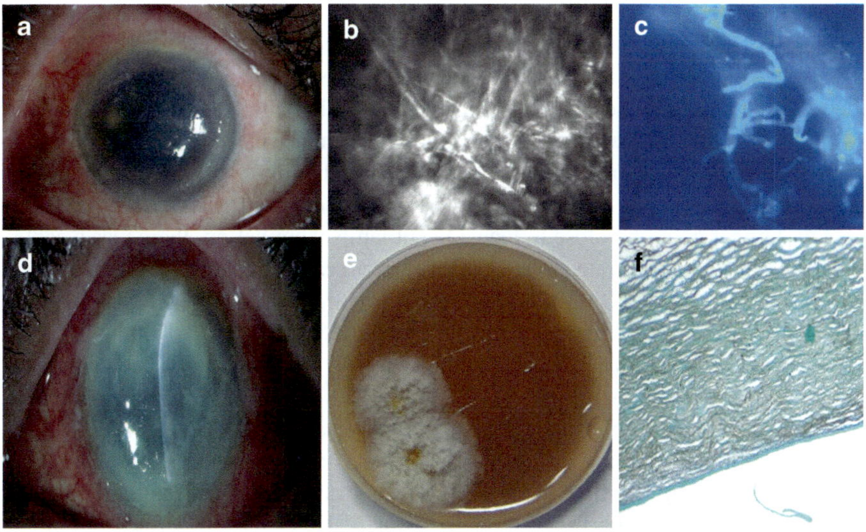

Fig. 9.5 (**a**) Slit-lamp photograph at the time of presentation showing small pin head lesions diffusely arranged in the entire corneal stroma, (**b**) confocal microscopy image shows double walled linear structures with branches suggestive of fungal filaments, (**c**) direct fluorescence microscopy of repeat sample of corneal scraping (potassium hydroxide with calcofluor white mount, ×400 total magnification) shows septate branching filaments suggestive of fungus, (**d**) slit-lamp photograph showing increased size and density of infiltrate over 1 week time, (**e**) culture of excised corneal tissue shows white fluffy fungal colony with yellow pigment in the center on chocolate agar suggestive of *Aspergillus flavus*, (**f**) histopathology of the excised corneal button shows multiple inflammatory cells in the anterior stroma with black fungal fragments primarily in mid stroma (Gomori methenamine silver stain, ×100 total magnification)

fungal filaments could be identified extending till the posterior stroma (Fig. 9.5f). On regular follow-up the graft was clear and there was no recurrence. After 3 weeks, while the patient was still on topical and oral antifungals, corticosteroids were started topically. At this point of time, the retina examination revealed a normal and attached retina with 0.6 C:D ratio of the disc. On regular follow-up until 2 years the best corrected visual acuity improved to 20/30 and the graft was clear.

Learning Points

1. This case report highlights the importance of confocal microscopy in the diagnosis of fungus in cases of deep stromal involvement.
2. Fungal keratitis after cataract surgery is uncommon, however, should be included in the differential diagnosis when dealing with increased delayed anterior chamber inflammation after cataract surgery.
3. Corticosteroids should be withheld in patients with microbial keratitis until the etiology is determined by microbiological investigation or confocal microscopy.

9.7 Case 6

A 31-year-old female patient presented with redness, pain, and watering along with decrease in vision in her left eye since 1 week following trauma with leaf while working in the agriculture field. At the time of presentation, she was using combination of antibiotics and antifungals both topically and orally. On examination, her left eye was essentially within normal limits. The best corrected visual acuity in the left eye was finger counting close to face. On slit lamp examination, there was a central raised plaque-like infiltrate (Fig. 9.6a) in the cornea with hyphate extensions. The size of the infiltrate was 4 mm × 4.5 mm. The depth of involvement, as assessed by slit-lamp, was mid stromal which was observed in AS-OCT to be 300 μm (Fig. 9.6b). There were two satellite infiltrates (2 mm in size) supero-nasally and temporally along with hypopyon of 1.5 mm.

After documentation of the clinical findings, as a standard protocol of the management, corneal scrapings were collected under topical anesthesia for microbiological evaluation. This included direct smear examination and culture. Multiple fungal filaments were observed in microscopy of KOH + CFW mount and Gram-stained smear (Fig. 9.6c). Culture confirmed significant growth of fungus that was identified as *Fusarium solani* (Fig. 9.6d). After microbiological confirmation of fungal filaments on smears, the patient was started on hourly topical natamycin 5% and oral ketoconazole 200 mg twice a day. Along with the continuation of medical treatment the patient was also subjected to photodynamic antimicrobial therapy (PDAT) with rose bengal. This was performed by applying Rose Bengal (0.1%) to the de-epithelialized cornea for 30 min, followed by irradiation with a 6 mW/cm^2 custom-made green LED source for 15 min (5.4 J/cm^2). Irradiation was performed using a green LED array (Fig. 9.6e) with peak wavelength of 518 nm in a dark room. Rose Bengal concentration on the eye was maintained with soak and sponge. The above protocol of Rose Bengal-assisted photodynamic therapy was done according to the protocol used previously at Bascom Palmer Eye Institute, USA [9, 10]. On serial follow-up, there was an improvement in the clinical signs of infection with complete resolution of infection in 25 days with resultant corneal scar formation (Fig. 9.6f) with visual acuity of 20/25.

Learning Points

1. This case report highlights the importance of PDAT with RB as an adjuvant treatment in fungal keratitis.
2. Medical therapy coupled with PDAT + RB can result in successful resolution of severe *Fusarium* keratitis.

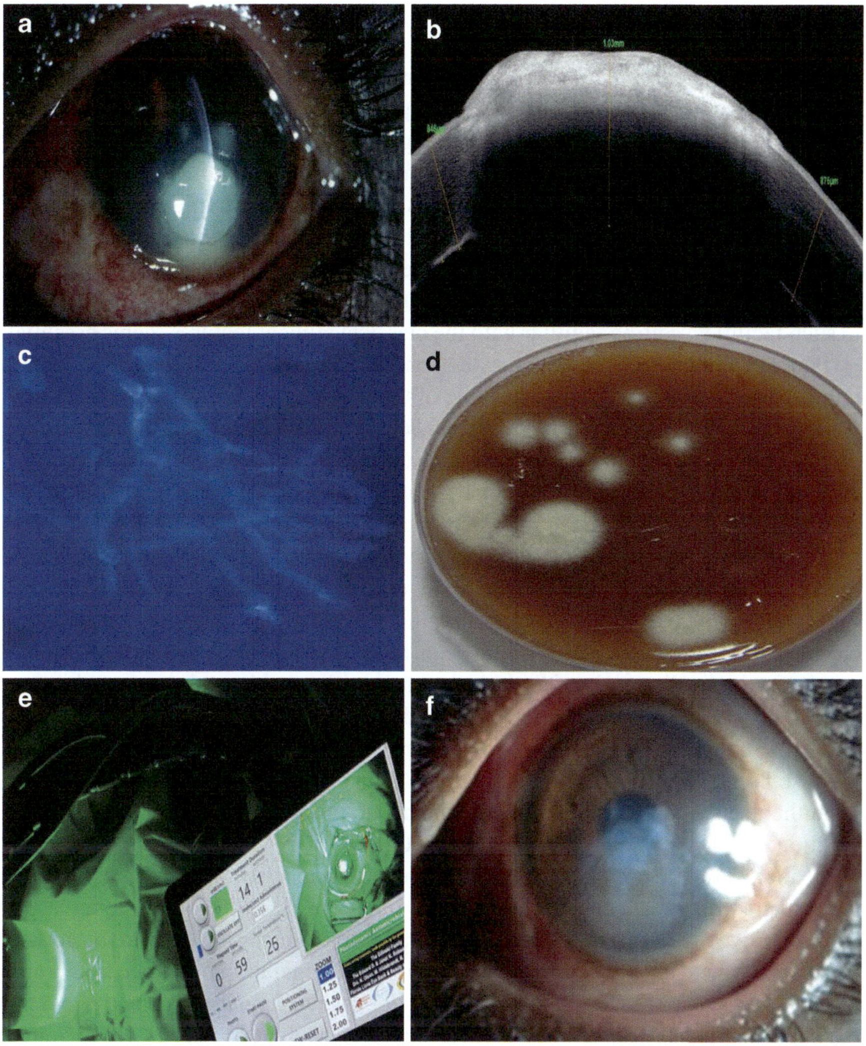

Fig. 9.6 (**a**) Slit-lamp photograph depicting a plaque-like raised corneal infiltrate with associated endoexudates along with two satellite infiltrates and hypopyon, (**b**) anterior OCT image of the corneal infiltrate at the time of presentation showing the depth of involvement till the anterior to mid stroma and raised thick plaque like infiltrate, (**c**) direct fluorescence microscopy of corneal scraping showing septate branching filaments (potassium hydroxide with calcofluor white, ×400 total magnification), (**d**) multiple, creamy-white, feathery fungal colonies on the inoculum marks on chocolate agar suggestive of *Fusarium* species, (**e**) green LED system used as the light source for photosensitizer in photodynamic therapy, (**f**) slit-lamp photograph showing complete clinical resolution with evident corneal scarring

9.8 Discussion

The onset of fungal infection of cornea is mostly insidious. Classical clinical features of fungal keratitis may vary widely. A prospective study looking at the characteristic clinical features as an aid to the diagnosis concluded that no single clinical feature can be considered as absolutely pathognomonic of a particular type of etiological agent [11]. The traditional academic approach for the initial diagnosis and management of microbial keratitis considers diagnostic scraping of corneal ulcers mandatory. However, this requires a well-equipped laboratory with trained manpower to process minute samples. Since many ophthalmologists do not have access to such facilities, getting familiar with the classical clinical features seems essential.

Fungal keratitis in early stage may be confused as dendritic ulcer as noted in case number 1. Close observation at the edge of the lesion and history help to differentiate. It is noted in case number 2 that *Pythium* keratitis, an emerging new entity, closely resembles fungal keratitis clinically, microbiologically, and histopathologically. Among the various clinical manifestations of *Pythium* keratitis, the common distinguishing features are the presence of central/paracentral dense grey infiltrate, multiple mid stromal "tentacle-like-infiltrates", peripheral guttering, classical subepithelial or superficial stromal infiltrate arranged in reticular pattern [12–14]. Fluorescence microscopy of corneal scraping stained with potassium hydroxide and calcofluor white (KOH+ CFW) has been reported to be of good sensitivity and specificity in the diagnosis of *Pythium* keratitis with good interobserver and intraobserver concordance [15, 16]. Potassium iodide with sulphuric acid (IKI-H2SO4) is another simple cost effective sensitive and specific stain for diagnosis [17].

Case numbers 3 and 4 demonstrated the utility of corneal biopsy and scrapings from the deeper corneal lamellae as a diagnostic modality for detecting fungus. In addition, qPCR showed high copy numbers of HSV1 DNA suggestive of active viral replication. Previous published reports have recommended >50 copies/ml to be a confirmatory diagnostic test for active HSV keratitis [18, 19]. While histopathology was definitive for fungal diagnosis in case 3, lack of fungal growth from the corneal button could be due to inactivation upon prior antifungal therapy or decreased load of the organisms in the half corneal button. For case 4, fungal filaments were demonstrated in smear from deeper corneal lamellae, and panfungal PCR for fungal DNA was positive from AC exudates, though there was no growth of fungus either due to lack of viable organisms or reduced fungal load. Absence of growth of fungus from both samples was suggestive of a chronic indolent infection that was deep seated with reduced load of organisms. Vemuganti et al. [20] in an analysis of corneal buttons suggested possible fungal etiology in deep stromal corneal lesions with anterior chamber exudates. In absence of confocal microscopy corneal biopsy in deep stromal corneal lesions has been reported to improve the diagnostic accuracy of causative organisms [21, 22].

The role of confocal microscopy in diagnosis of deep-seated fungal keratitis is well demonstrated in case 5. The noninvasive technique of confocal microscopy has been very effective in providing correct and precise diagnosis in many of the corneal infections especially fungal and *Acanthamoeba* keratitis [23]. The sensitivity of confocal microscope in expert hands can be as high as 90% in the detection of these organisms [8, 24]. However, stand-alone use of confocal microscopy for the diagnosis of microbial keratitis is not recommended [25].

Case 6 in this series of fungal keratitis has been treated with a realtively recent adjuvant therapy of photodynamic therapy with Rose Bengal (PDAT+RB) with promising results. In the last decade, photoactivated chromophore for keratitis-collagen cross-linking (PACK-CXL) has been introduced for the management of microbial keratitis. Discrepancy of in vitro susceptibility of microorganisms to PACK-CXL and clinical effect on patients with keratitis has been reported [26]. Adding other photosensitizers have been recent advancements in these techniques [27–30]. PDAT with Rose Bengal is reported to have better in vitro efficacy as compared to riboflavin and has been found to be useful in refractory cases of microbial keratitis lowering the rate of therapeutic keratoplasty [9]. In a pilot trial, we treated seven cases of fungal keratitis with antifungal medication along with PDAT+RB as adjuvant therapy. We also tested the in vitro effect of PDAT+RB on the corresponding fungal isolates. *Fusarium* species were susceptible in vitro to PDAT+RB and the patients with *Fusarium* keratitis responded well [15, 16] to this novel therapy. Case 6 re-iterates our earlier experience with this promising therapy.

This chapter describes six cases of fungal keratitis that were challenging to diagnose and treat. The repertoire for diagnosis must include a combination of clinical acumen and microbiological methods including molecular techniques. Similarly, a multipronged approach is called for in the treatment of fungal keratitis that may or may not have mixed infection. Cognizance of systemic diseases such as diabetes is also an important consideration in the course of the management of fungal keratitis.

References

1. Centers for Disease Control (CDC). Update: *Fusarium* keratitis—United States, 2005–2006. Morbidity and Mortality Weekly Report (MMWR). 2006;55:563–4.
2. Sharma S, Srinivasan M, George C. The current status of *Fusarium* species in mycotic keratitis in South India. J Med Microbiol. 1993;11:140–7.
3. Marangon FB, Miller D, Giaconi JA, Alfonso EC. In vitro investigation of voriconazole susceptibility for keratitis and endophthalmitis fungal pathogens. Am J Ophthalmol. 2004;137:820–5.
4. Gopinathan U, Sharma S, Garg P, Rao GN. Review of epidemiological features, microbiological diagnosis and treatment outcome of microbial keratitis: experience of over a decade. Indian J Ophthalmol. 2009;57:273–9.
5. Thomas P, Kaliamurthy J. Mycotic keratitis: epidemiology, diagnosis and management. Clin Microbiol Infect. 2013;19:210–20.
6. Garg P, Roy A, Roy S. Update on fungal keratitis. Curr Opin Ophthalmol. 2016;27:333–9.
7. Rautaraya B, Sharma S, Kar S, Das S, Sahu SK. Diagnosis and treatment outcome of mycotic keratitis at a tertiary eye care centre in Eastern India. BMC Ophthalmol. 2011;11:39.
8. Vaddavalli PK, Garg P, Sharma S, Sangwan VS, Rao GN, Thomas R. Role of confocal microscopy in the diagnosis of fungal and *Acanthamoeba* keratitis. Ophthalmology. 2011;118:29–35.

9. Naranjo A, Arboleda A, Martinez JD, Durkee H, Aguilar MC, Relhan N, et al. Rose Bengal photodynamic antimicrobial therapy for patients with progressive infectious keratitis: a pilot clinical study. Am J Ophthalmol. 2019;208:387–96.
10. Martinez JD, Arrieta E, Naranjo A, Monsalve P, Mintz KJ, Peterson J, et al. Rose Bengal photodynamic antimicrobial therapy: a pilot safety study. Cornea. 2021;40:1036–43.
11. Thomas PA, Leck AK, Myatt M. Characteristic clinical features as an aid to the diagnosis of suppurative keratitis caused by filamentous fungi. Br J Ophthalmol. 2005;89:1554–8.
12. Sharma S, Balne PK, Motukupally SR, Das S, Garg P, Sahu SK, Arunasri K, Manjulatha K, Mishra DK, Shivaji S. Pythium insidiosum keratitis: clinical profile and role of DNA sequencing and zoospore formation in diagnosis. Cornea. 2015;34:438–42.
13. Hasika R, Lalitha P, Radhakrishnan N, Rameshkumar G, Prajna NV, Srinivasan M. Pythium keratitis in South India: incidence, clinical profile, management, and treatment recommendation. Indian J Ophthalmol. 2019;67:42–7.
14. Agarwal S, Iyer G, Srinivasan B, Agarwal M, Panchalam Sampath Kumar S, Therese LK. Clinical profile of pythium keratitis: perioperative measures to reduce risk of recurrence. Br J Ophthalmol. 2018;102:153–7.
15. Bagga B, Vishwakarma P, Sharma S, Jospeh J, Mitra S, Mohamed A. Sensitivity and specificity of potassium hydroxide and calcofluor white stain to differentiate between fungal and *Pythium* filaments in corneal scrapings from patients of *Pythium* keratitis. Indian J Ophthalmol. 2022a;70:542–5.
16. Bagga B, Sharma S, Ahirwar LK, Sheba E, Vaddavalli PK, Mishra DK. Clinical outcomes of Rose Bengal mediated photodynamic antimicrobial therapy on fungal keratitis with their microbiological and pathological correlation. Curr Eye Res. 2022b;47:987–94.
17. Mittal R, Jena SK, Desai A, Agarwal S. *Pythium insidiosum* keratitis: histopathology and rapid novel diagnostic staining technique. Cornea. 2017;36:1124–32.
18. Guda SM, Sontam B, Bagga B, Ranjith K, Sharma S, Joseph J. Evaluation of multiplex real-time polymerase chain reaction for the detection of herpes simplex virus-1 and 2 and varicella-zoster virus in corneal cells from normal subjects and patients with keratitis in India. Indian J Ophthalmol. 2019;67:1040–6.
19. Kaye SB, Baker K, Bonshek R, Maseruka H, Grinfeld E, Tullo A, et al. Human herpesviruses in the cornea. Br J Ophthalmol. 2000;84:563–71.
20. Vemuganti GK, Garg P, Gopinathan U, Naduvilath TJ, John RK, Buddi R, et al. Evaluation of agent and host factors in progression of mycotic keratitis: a histologic and microbiologic study of 167 corneal buttons. Ophthalmology. 2002;109:1538–46.
21. Lee P, Green WR. Corneal biopsy. Indications, techniques, and a report of a series of 87 cases. Ophthalmology. 1990;97:718–21.
22. Hudson J, Al-Khersan H, Carletti P, Miller D, Dubovy SR, Amescua G. Role of corneal biopsy in the management of infectious keratitis. Curr Opin Ophthalmol. 2022;33:290–5.
23. Chidambaram JD, Prajna NV, Larke NL, Palepu S, Lanjewar S, Shah M, et al. Prospective study of the diagnostic accuracy of the in vivo laser scanning confocal microscope for severe microbial keratitis. Ophthalmology. 2016;123:2285–93.
24. Kumar RL, Cruzat A, Hamrah P. Current state of in vivo confocal microscopy in management of microbial keratitis. Semin Ophthalmol. 2010;25:166–70.
25. Hau SC, Dart JKG, Vesaluoma M, et al. Diagnostic accuracy of microbial keratitis with in vivo scanning laser confocal microscopy. Br J Ophthalmol. 2010;94:982–7.
26. Martinez JD, Naranjo A, Amescua G, Dubovy SR, Arboleda A, Durkee H, Aguilar MC, Flynn HW, Miller D, Parel JM. Human corneal changes after Rose Bengal photodynamic antimicrobial therapy for treatment of fungal keratitis. Cornea. 2018 Oct;37:e46–8.
27. Kasetsuwan N, Reinprayoon U, Satitpitakul V. Photoactivated chromophore for moderate to severe infectious keratitis as an adjunct therapy: a randomized controlled trial. Am J Ophthalmol. 2016;165:94–9.

28. Bilgihan K, Kalkanci A, Ozdemir HB, Yazar R, Karakurt F, Yuksel E, Otag F, Karabicak N, Arikan-Akdagli S. Evaluation of antifungal efficacy of 0.1% and 0.25% riboflavin with UVA: a comparative in vitro study. Curr Eye Res. 2016;41:1050–6.
29. Kling S, Hufschmid FS, Torres-Netto EA, Randleman JB, Willcox M, Zbinden R, Hafezi F. High fluence increases the antibacterial efficacy of PACK cross-linking. Cornea. 2020;39:1020–6.
30. Amescua G, Arboleda A, Nikpoor N, Durkee H, Relhan N, Aguilar MC, Flynn HW, Miller D, Parel JM. Rose Bengal photodynamic antimicrobial therapy: a novel treatment for resistant Fusarium keratitis. Cornea. 2017;36:1141–4.

10 Parasitic Keratitis

Sujata Das, Aravind Roy,
and Smrutirekha Priyadarshini

10.1 Introduction

Parasitic infections of the eye may be a manifestation of generalized systemic disease or a localized phenomenon. Infection of the cornea due to various etiological agents is a leading cause of corneal blindness worldwide. The etiological agents vary significantly according to geographic location. Although corneal infection due to parasites constitutes a relatively small proportion of microbial keratitis, treatment poses a challenge for ophthalmologists. In this chapter, we discuss microsporidia and acanthamoeba keratitis as these are more common in the practice.

Microsporidia are small, obligate, spore-forming, intracellular living eukaryotes that infect a broad range of vertebrates and invertebrates [1]. Microsporidial keratitis mostly occurs in two forms: (i) superficial keratoconjunctivitis, and (ii) deep stromal keratitis. Ocular infections due to microsporidia have received considerable importance in recent years. Earlier considered to be a disease of immunocompromised patients, superficial keratoconjunctivitis is now known as a common infection in immunocompetent patients [2, 3].

Acanthamoeba is one of the most common free-living amoebae found in the environment. It has two forms: (i) asexually reproducing trophozoite form, and (ii) dormant double-walled cyst form. Keratitis due to *Acanthamoeba* has been recognized in almost all parts of the world [4–7]. Contact lens is a common risk factor in western world. Cases reported from India have found previous injury with muddy

S. Das (✉) · S. Priyadarshini
Cornea and Anterior Segment Service, L V Prasad Eye Institute, Bhubaneswar, Odisha, India
e-mail: sujatadas@lvpei.org; smruti@lvpei.org

A. Roy
Cornea and Anterior Segment Service, L V Prasad Eye Institute,
Vijayawada, Andhra Pradesh, India
e-mail: aravind@lvpei.org

F. A. Woreta, R. B. Singh (eds.), *Cornea Casebook*, Current Practices in Ophthalmology, https://doi.org/10.1007/978-981-96-0495-1_10

water and or associated vegetative trauma rather than contact lens use is a risk factor. If not diagnosed early and treated aggressively, extensive ocular damage can occur.

The cases discussed here highlight natural course, alternative method of diagnosis, and differential diagnosis of keratitis due to two common parasites, i.e., *Acanthamoeba* and Microsporidia.

10.2 Case 1

A 43-year-old male presented to us with complaints of redness, pain, watering, and foreign body sensation of 1-week duration in his right eye. He had a vague history of some particle going inside the eye while riding a bike. His visual acuity was 20/30p. Slit-lamp examination revealed mild conjunctival congestion, multiple epithelial lesions involving cornea (Fig. 10.1a, b). Direct smear examination from the cornea scraping revealed microsporidial spores in Gram and 10% Potassium Hydroxide with 0.1% Calcoflour White (KOH + CFW) stain. He was prescribed Carboxymethyl cellulose (0.5%) and asked to review after 2 weeks. Patient was symptomatically better when patient visited after 2 weeks. His vision improved to 20/20p. There were multiple fresh keratic precipitates (KPs) (Fig. 10.1c, d). Anterior chamber was quiet. There was no congestion. While ocular lubricants were continued for 2 weeks, Loteprednol etabonate (0.5%) was started four times a day with a

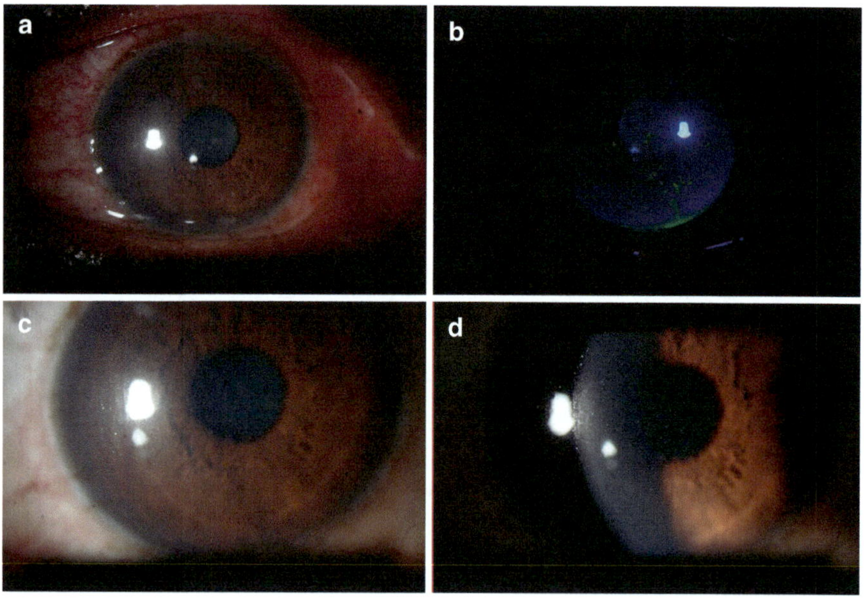

Fig. 10.1 (**a**) Diffuse slit-lamp examination showing conjunctival congestion, multiple epithelial lesions. (**b**) Fluorescein positive lesions in cobalt blue filter. (**c**) Multiple keratic precipitates on endothelium during follow-up in diffuse illumination. (**d**) Slit view

weekly tapering dosage over 4 weeks. The keratoconjunctivitis resolved completely without any residual corneal scarring.

Learning Points

(a) Clinical and direct smear examination helps in establishing the diagnosis.
(b) Ocular lubricants help in symptomatic relief in keratoconjunctivitis patients. There is no role of antibiotic or antiparasitic medication.
(c) Keratic precipitates are seen in some cases of keratoconjuntivitis patients after 1–2 weeks of onset of disease.

10.3 Case 2

A 48-year-old male, who was a manual labourer by occupation, presented to cornea clinic with complaints of blurring vision and pain in right eye of 12 days duration. He had a history of injury with an unknown object. He was using topical homatropine eyedrops 2% prior to presentation. Visual acuity was 20/125 in the right eye. There was no history of systemic disease. Slit-lamp examination showed mild conjunctival congestion with a foreign body embedded (hair-like structure) with two midstromal infiltrates (one large and one small), endoexudate paracentrally near temporal limbus along with diffusely present mutton fat KPs (Fig. 10.2a). Endoscraping and foreign body removal were planned. Sample did not reveal

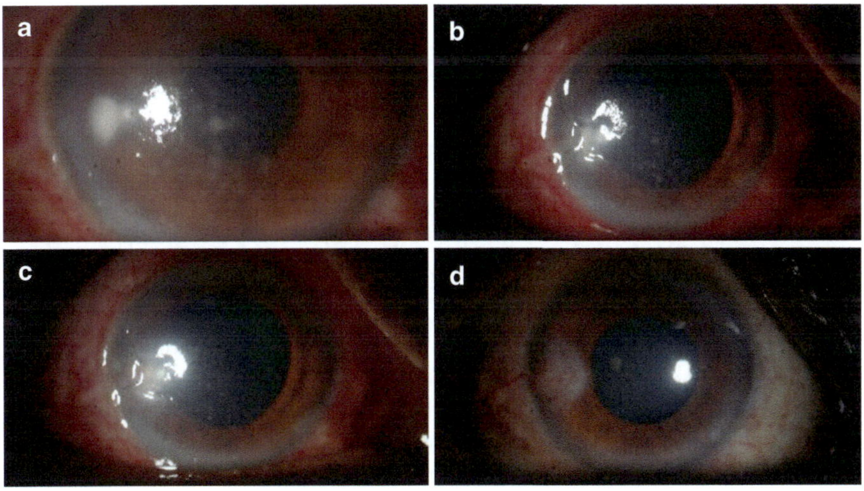

Fig. 10.2 (**a**) Diffuse slit-lamp examination showing mid-stromal infiltrates, endoexudate and mutton fat KPs. (**b**) Following corneal biopsy, the lamellar flap was apposed with two interrupted 10-0 nylon sutures. (**c**) Onset of resolution with appearance of superficial vascularisation and decreased density of KPs. (**d**) Complete resolution of infection with corneal scarring, superficial vascularisation and few pigments on endothelium

presence of any organism. Thus, based on clinical suspicion, Voriconazole 1% eyedrop along with atropine sulfate 1% eyedrops were started. Foreign body plated on blood agar media also did not show any growth of microorganism. After 10 days, the two infiltrates were still present and the presence of large KPs adjacent to the corneal lesions warranted a Corneal biopsy. A lamellar flap was made and material scraped from bed of the flap (Fig. 10.2b). Corneal scrapings were submitted for microbiological evaluation. Direct microscopy of corneal scraping using KOH + CFW wet mount showed the presence of microsporidial spores. Culture reports did not reveal any growth of organism. Due to the scanty sample amount, histopathological evaluation was not possible. The patient was started on topical polyhexamethylene biguanide (PHMB) 0.02% hourly and atropine 1% thrice daily. At 2 weeks visit, there was presence of superficial new lesions at 9 o'clock, density of KPs had reduced and vascularisation started. His vision had improved to 20/60 and he was symptomatically better (Fig. 10.2c). At about 2 months from the date of biopsy and starting of PHMB, the biopsied site had healed completely with intensive vascularisation and scarring, and few pigments persisted on the endothelium. His vision had improved to 20/40p improving to 20/25 with pinhole (Fig. 10.2d).

Learning Points

(a) History of trauma should be elicited in all cases of corneal ulcer.
(b) Direct microscopy of corneal scrapings is the most feasible method for diagnosing microsporidial stromal keratitis apart from PCR.
(c) Corneal biopsy can be considered in the case of deep-seated ulcers.
(d) Medical management with PHMB 0.02% can at times be helpful in microsporidial stromal keratitis and defer the need of therapeutic penetrating keratoplasty.

10.4 Case 3

A 55-year-old male presented to our cornea clinic with complaints of redness, watering, and diminution of vision in her right eye for past 6 months. There was no history of any ocular trauma. He had diabetes and hypertension for past 7 and 3 years, respectively. He was already on topical antibiotic eyedrops (Tobramycin) and antivirals (acyclovir eye ointment) at the time of presentation without any improvement. The visual acuity was 20/40 in the affected eye. Slit-lamp examination showed the presence of an intact epithelium, multifocal areas of fluffy greyish-white stromal infiltrate, stromal edema, and KPs adjacent to the lesion (Fig. 10.3a). The fellow eye was unremarkable on examination. A clinical differential of Herpes simplex virus (HSV) endotheliitis and microsporidial stromal keratitis was made and systemic acyclovir (Tab. Acivir 400 mg, 5 times/day) along with topical Prednisolone acetate 1% eyedrop 8 times/day was started. After 1-week, the infiltrate had consolidated. At this visit, corneal scrapings revealed presence of microsporidial spores (Gram stain and KOH mount). Hence, topical steroids were stopped

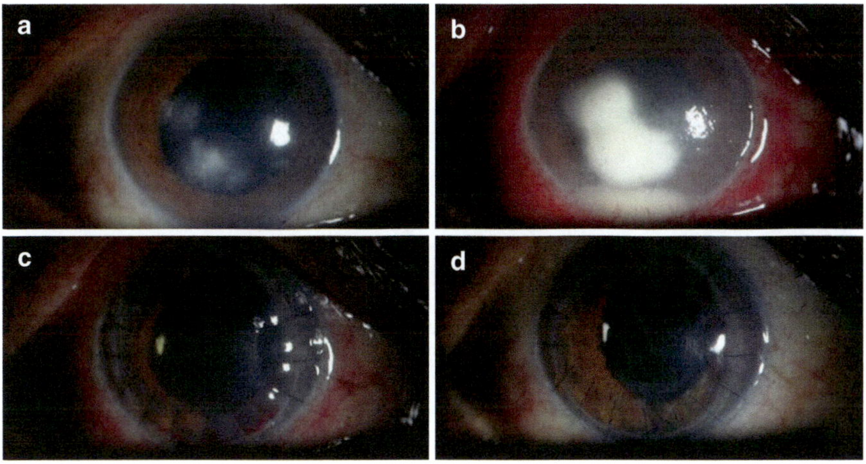

Fig. 10.3 (**a**) At presentation, (**b**) worsening of ulcer with medical management, (**c**) 1 week following therapeutic keratoplasty, (**d**) 4 months post keratoplasty

and he was started on topical polyhexamethylene biguanide hydrochloride 0.02% (PHMB). At 1 week follow-up, he had worsening of the infiltrate along with appearance of hypopyon for which Voriconazole 1% eyedrop was added to the treatment regimen (Fig. 10.3b). Later, in view of worsening of the infection, he underwent a therapeutic penetrating keratoplasty with a large 9.5 mm donor graft. Histopathological examination of the corneal button revealed the presence of Gram-positive spores. Furthermore, Kinyoun stain (1% Acid fast stain) highlighted the presence of microsporidial spores. Postoperatively he was continued with PHMB 0.02% eyedrops hourly (Fig. 10.3c). After 1 week, prednisolone acetate 1% eyedrops 8 times/day was added to PHMB and closely observed for recurrence. At 4 months follow-up, he had a vision of 20/60 with clear graft (Fig. 10.3d).

Learning Points

(a) HSV endotheliitis can mimic microsporidia stromal keratitis clinically. A basic microbiologic workup (Gram stain) can help in confirming the diagnosis and guiding treatment.
(b) Microsporidial stromal keratitis unresponsive to medical treatment warrants therapeutic keratoplasty for resolution of infection.

10.5 Case 4

A 22-year-old male presented with complaints of redness, watering, diminution of vision of right eye of 3 months duration. His visual acuity was 20/160. He gave an history of fall of insect. He has lid edema associated with diffuse conjunctival congestion. He had localized greyish-white irregular epithelium in central cornea

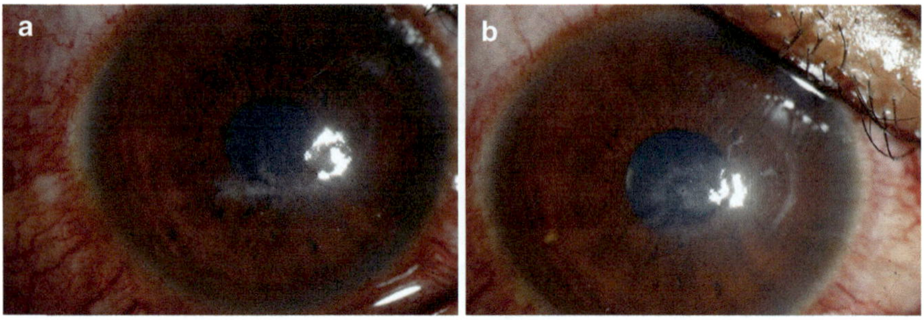

Fig. 10.4 (**a**) Slit-lamp examination showing conjunctival congestion associated with irregular hazy epithelium in the central cornea during presentation, (**b**) decreased congestion with scarring of cornea following 3 weeks of treatment

(Fig. 10.4a). He was on multiple medication including traditional eye drops. There was suspicion of toxic keratitis. He was asked to discontinue all medication and asked to come after 1 week. Though patient felt marginally better, clinical picture was status quo. He was continued lubricants for 2 weeks. Since there was no improvement clinically, corneal scraping was performed. Cornea scraping revealed cysts of *Acanthamoeba* in KOH + CFW, which later grew *Acanthamoeba* in Non-Nutrient Agar with *E. coli*. He was started with 0.02% PHMB. Patient visited 3 weeks after starting medication. His visual acuity improved to 20/100. Congestion has reduced and corneal finding was better than presentation (Fig. 10.4b). He was lost to follow-up after 3 weeks.

Learning Points

(a) Irregular greyish epithelium should raise suspicion of *Acanthamoeba* keratitis.
(b) Disproportionate pain may not be typical feature of *Acanthamoeba* keratitis always.

10.6 Case 5

A 49-year-old male presented with a 50-day history of blurring of vision, watering, pain, and redness in his left eye. He was on a cocktail of topical antibiotics. At presentation, his visual acuity was finger counting 1 m and the cornea showed a 6.5 × 5.5 mm corneal infiltrate with diffuse margins restricted to anterior half of the corneal stroma. The anterior chamber showed a 1 mm hypopyon. The fellow eye was essentially normal. The systemic and ocular history was unremarkable. Corneal scraping was negative for any organism. Therefore, empirical treatment with 0.5% ciprofloxacin and 5% fortified vancomycin was started hourly with 1% atropine three times for 3 weeks. The lesion was status quo and a viral etiology was suspected, he was started on topical 1% prednisolone 6 times and 3% acyclovir ointment 5 times. After 2 weeks, the lesion worsened with appearance of ring infiltrate.

Over the next 8 weeks, the patient had waxing and waning clinical course. Repeat scraping and drug holiday was negative. A second trial with topical 1% prednisolone acetate 8 times/day with 1% atropine thrice and 3% acyclovir was administered for 3 weeks leading to worsening of lesions. Third scraping taken after 13 weeks of presentation with a limbal nodule showed of acanthamoeba cysts in 10% KOH + CFW wet mount. The culture was negative after 14 days of incubation. The patient was started on 0.02% Chlorhexidine and 0.02% PHMB hourly with 1% atropine sulfate. Over the next 1-week multiple limbal nodules were noted (Fig. 10.5a) and the patient was started on oral ketoconazole 100 mg twice daily and oral prednisolone 60 mg once daily for 8 weeks. This led to reduction of the size of limbal nodules, organizing corneal and limbal infiltrates with superficial and deep corneal vascularization. (Fig. 10.5b) after 2 weeks of the same treatment the continued corneal inflammation led to central corneal melt with perforation for which therapeutic keratoplasty(TPK) was performed. Following TPK topical 1% prednisolone acetate 8 times with 0.02% Chlorhexidine and 0.02% PHMB hourly and 1% atropine sulfate was continued for 3 weeks. After this, the anti-acanthamoeba medications were stopped and corticosteroids were continued. The patient was followed up for 8 months post TPK during which the graft failed and at the last follow up the vision was light perception, graft edema, and disorganized anterior segment (Fig. 10.5c). He was advised cosmetic tattooing for the unsightly appearance of eye.

Learning Points

(a) *Acanthamoeba* keratitis (AK) may require multiple corneal scrapings before yielding positive results.
(b) Worsening of microbiology-negative corneal infiltrates after an initial period of improvement and with a provisional diagnosis of viral keratitis is suggestive of acanthamoeba or fungal keratitis.
(c) Limbal nodules are usually a sign of intense anterior segment inflammation and are usually immune mediated, they require oral ketoconazole and immunosuppressants with continued anti-acanthamoeba medications.

10.7 Case 6

A 42-year-old woman, who is an agricultural laborer, presented with right eye redness, pain, and diminution of vision after sustaining an injury with vegetative trauma while working in chilly field 3 weeks earlier. She was treated elsewhere prior to presentation and was using combination moxifloxacin 0.5% with dexamethasone 0.1% topical preparation 2-hourly for 1 week. On examination here her systemic status was within normal limits, uncorrected visual acuity was 20/250 for distance improving to 20/80 with pin hole and <N36 for near with no improvement. The left eye was essentially normal. Her right eye showed minimal conjunctival congestion with ring-shaped dry appearing corneal infiltrate of 7.6 mm × 8.4 mm, the infiltrate was restricted to the anterior half of the corneal stroma (Fig. 10.6a). There were no

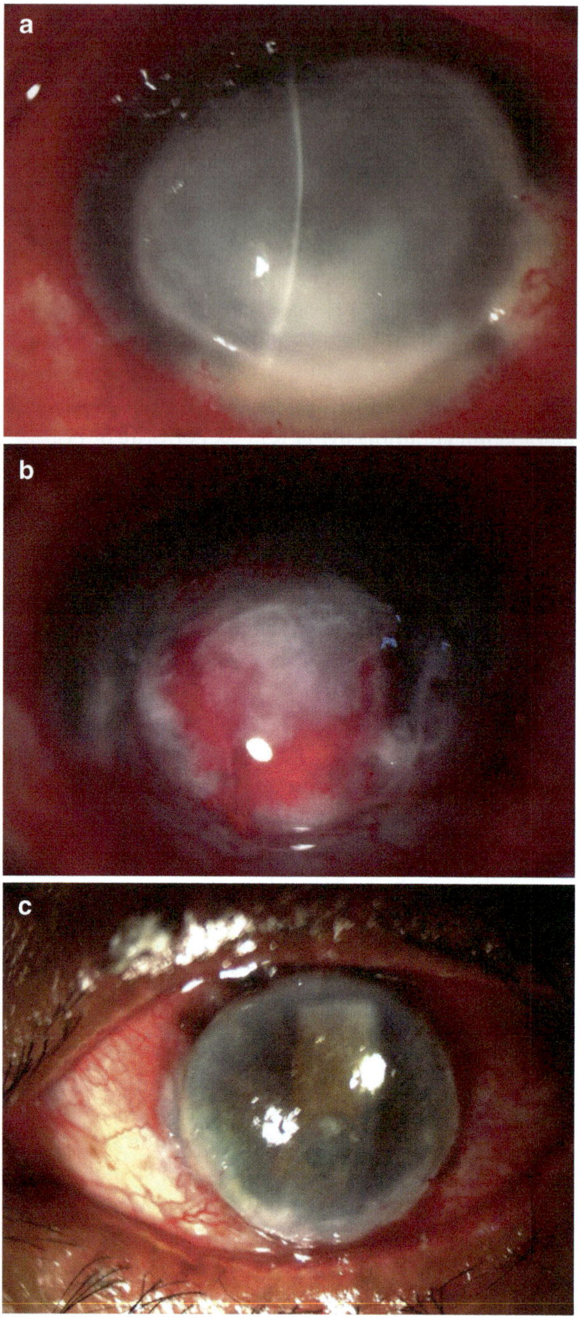

Fig. 10.5 (**a**) Clinical picture at 3 months with limbal nodule at 4 o'clock limbus, (**b**) clinical picture at 5.5 months with central perforation, (**c**) last follow-up at 8 months after therapeutic PKP with failed graft

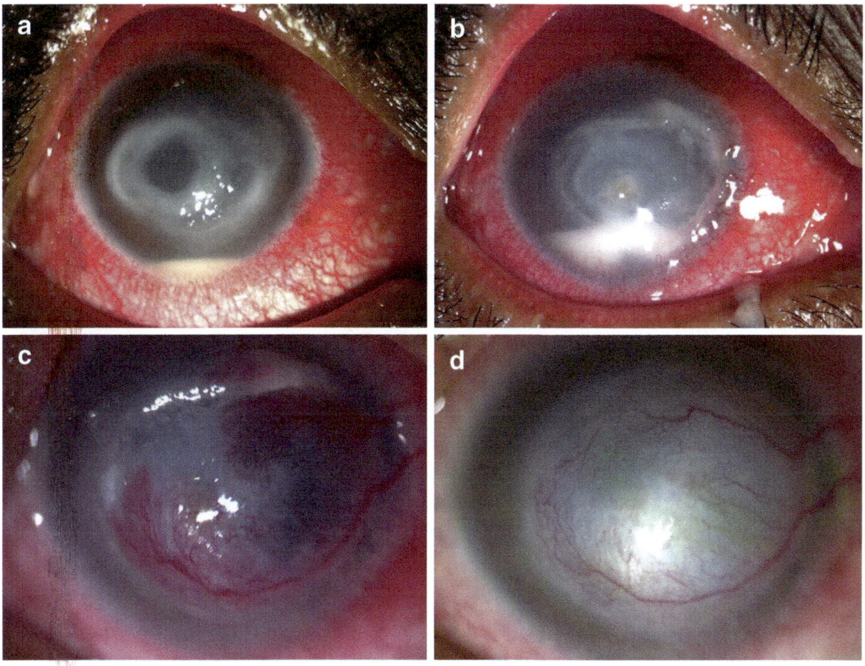

Fig. 10.6 (**a**) Clinical picture of right eye at presentation, (**b**) clinical picture after 8 weeks with central corneal melt and thinning with infiltrate progressing to 2 o'clock limbus, (**c**) clinical picture at 6 weeks after application of tissue adhesive and a bandage contact lens with scarring, superficial and deep vascularization, and small focus of paracentral corneal infiltrate, (**d**) at last follow-up at 21 weeks follow-up with complete resolution, scarring and vascularization

peripheral corneal lesions or superficial/deep vascularization. Scraping of the infiltrate yielded acanthamoeba cysts 0–10 per high power field on 10% KOH + CFW wet mount and on Gram stain. The patient was advised to stop the antibiotic and corticosteroid combination and started on anti-acanthamoeba (AAK) regimen consisting of PHMB 0.02% hourly and Chlorhexidine 0.02% eyedrops with atropine 1% three times and oral aceclofenac 100 mg as needed. The therapy was continued for 8 weeks during which the hypopyon started increasing to 2 mm and there was progressive central corneal melting with peripheral corneal vascularization and corneal infiltrates progressing to the 2o'clock limbus (Fig. 10.6b). Suspecting a secondary infection, a second scraping was performed which was positive for acanthamoeba cysts. Tissue adhesives (TA) with bandage contact lens (BCL) were applied for tectonic support. The anti-acanthamoeba keratitis regimen was continued for another 6 weeks following which there was scarring of paracentral cornea with thinning and vascularization of central cornea with a paracentral focal infiltrate (Fig. 10.6c). Tissue adhesive and bandage contact lens were removed, and AAK regimen was continued for 7 weeks before complete scarring and resolution (Fig. 10.6d).

Learning Points

(a) Agricultural trauma or injury with muddy water could predispose to AK.
(b) Ring infiltrate is suggestive of fungal, gram-negative bacilli, and *Acanthamoeba* keratitis. This needs confirmation on microbiology before initiating AAK regimen.
(c) Intense ocular surface inflammation due to AK and AAK regimen may cause corneal melting and requires TA + BCL application. AAK regimen needs to be continued for at least 2 weeks of scarring for optimum resolution.

10.8 Discussion

Keratoconjunctivitis is the most common ocular involvement resulting from microsporidia. Typical clinical features of microsporidial keratoconjunctivitis include diffuse, multifocal, coarse, raised, punctate, round to oval epithelial lesion in the cornea, with or without anterior chamber reaction [2, 3]. It is usually associated with mild to moderate conjunctival congestion. Central corneal edema, mild secondary uveitis, and fine keratic precipitates are usually seen after few days of initial presentation. Although microsporidial keratoconjunctivitis was believed to occur in immunocompromised patients, it is observed more and more in immunocompetent patients. Case 1 presented with typical clinical features at first visit, and keratic precipitates during second visit. Direct smear examination using different stains such as KOH + CFW, Gram, Giemsa, and Acid-Fast stain is useful in diagnosis [8]. Both topical and systemic treatments have been described in the literature for management of keratoconjunctivitis. Randomized controlled trial established no significant benefit of PHMB compared to placebo suggesting the self-limiting nature of the disease [9].

Clinically microsporidial stromal keratitis could mimic suppurative or nonsuppurative inflammation and vascularization of cornea. The durations of symptoms range from a few months to years. It may present like progressive herpes disciform keratitis with recurrent stromal infiltration and uveitis and should be considered in the differential diagnosis of culture-negative stromal keratitis not responding to standard medical therapy [10]. Case 3 presented with history of 6 months duration and initially treated as HSV keratitis. Although smear examination helps in diagnosis, biopsy may be required in some cases of microsporidial stromal keratitis with deep-seated infiltrate like Case 2. Stromal keratitis is refractory to medical management. Therefore, early surgical intervention is recommended. While Case 2 responded to medical management, Case 3 required keratoplasty.

The earliest signs of *Acanthamoeba* keratitis may be micro-erosion, irregularities, opacities, or micro-cystic edema, often with patchy anterior stromal infiltrate. Radial neuritis is a pathognomonic sign for *Acanthamoeba* keratitis. Ring infiltrate with an overlying epithelial defect is commonly observed. Although, the epithelium is intact in early stages, in long-standing cases, a central defect, which is often associated with stromal thinning. The inflammation may involve sclera [4]. None of three cases described above was clinically suspected earlier to be *Acanthamoeba*. While Case 4 had minimal clinical findings. Case 5 presented with scleral involvement. Neither of these patients had a history of contact lens wear.

Direct smear examination, culture, polymerase chain reaction (PCR), and confocal microscopy have been used to confirm the diagnosis of *Acanthamoeba* keratitis [11]. Though direct smear examination revealed *Acanthamoeba* cyst in all cases, Case 5 required multiple scrapings for confirmation. The diamidine and biguanide are the most effective cysticidal antiamoebics in-vitro [12]. Voriconazole has been used for *Acanthamoeba* stromal keratitis [13].

In advanced cases, keratoplasty may be necessary. There is a high risk of recurrence if the infection is not controlled. Lamellar keratoplastyc can be considered in cases of *Acanthamoeba* keratitis [14, 15]. Antiamoebic therapy should be used prior to surgery and to be continued postoperatively.

References

1. Sharma S, Das S, Joseph J, Vemuganti GK, Murthy S. Microsporidial keratitis: need for increased awareness. Surv Ophthalmol. 2011;56(1):1–22.
2. Das S, Sharma S, Sahu SK, Nayak SS, Kar S. Diagnosis, clinical features and treatment outcome of microsporidial keratoconjunctivitis. Br J Ophthalmol. 2012;96(6):793–5.
3. Loh RS, Chan CM, Ti SE, Lim L, Chan KS, Tan DT. Emerging prevalence of microsporidial keratitis in Singapore: epidemiology, clinical features, and management. Ophthalmology. 2009;116(12):2348–53.
4. Jain R, Garg P, Motukupally SR, Geary MB. Clinico-microbiological review of non-contact-lens-associated acanthamoeba keratitis. Semin Ophthalmol. 2015;30(4):281–8.
5. Woodruff SA, Dart JK. Acanthamoeba keratitis occurring with daily disposable contact lens wear. Br J Ophthalmol. 1999;83(9):1088–9.
6. Stehr-Green JK, Bailey TM, Visvesvara GS. The epidemiology of Acanthamoeba keratitis in the United States. Am J Ophthalmol. 1989;107(4):331–6.
7. Kamel AG, Norazah A. First case of Acanthamoeba keratitis in Malaysia. Trans R Soc Trop Med Hyg. 1995;89(6):652.
8. Joseph J, Murthy S, Garg P, Sharma S. Use of different stains for microscopic evaluation of corneal scrapings for diagnosis of microsporidial keratitis. J Clin Microbiol. 2006;44(2):583–5.
9. Das S, Sahu SK, Sharma S, Nayak SS, Kar S. Clinical trial of 0.02% polyhexamethylene biguanide versus placebo in the treatment of microsporidial keratoconjunctivitis. Am J Ophthalmol. 2010;150(1):110–115.e2.
10. Sabhapandit S, Murthy SI, Garg P, Korwar V, Vemuganti GK, Sharma S. Microsporidial stromal keratitis: clinical features, unique diagnostic criteria, and treatment outcomes in a large case series. Cornea. 2016;35(12):1569–74.
11. Fanselow N, Sirajuddin N, Yin XT, Huang AJW, Stuart PM. *Acanthamoeba* keratitis, pathology, diagnosis and treatment. Pathogens. 2021;10(3):323.
12. Lorenzo-Morales J, Khan NA, Walochnik J. An update on Acanthamoeba keratitis: diagnosis, pathogenesis and treatment. Parasite. 2015;22:10.
13. Bagga B, Sharma S, Gour RPS, Mohamed A, Joseph J, Rathi M, V, Garg P. A randomized masked pilot clinical trial to compare the efficacy of topical 1% voriconazole ophthalmic solution as monotherapy with combination therapy of topical 0.02% polyhexamethylene biguanide and 0.02% chlorhexidine in the treatment of Acanthamoeba keratitis. Eye (Lond). 2021;35(5):1326–33.

14. Sarnicola E, Sarnicola C, Sabatino F, Tosi GM, Perri P, Sarnicola V. Early Deep Anterior Lamellar Keratoplasty (DALK) for Acanthamoeba keratitis poorly responsive to medical treatment. Cornea. 2016;35(1):1–5.
15. Bagga B, Garg P, Joseph J, Mohamed A, Kalra P. Outcome of therapeutic deep anterior lamellar keratoplasty in advanced *Acanthamoeba* keratitis. Indian J Ophthalmol. 2020;68(3):442–6.

Part III

Endothelial Disorders

Fuchs Endothelial Corneal Dystrophy

11

Kyongjin Cho, Muhammad Ali, Albert S. Jun, and Divya Srikumaran

11.1 Introduction

Fuchs endothelial corneal dystrophy (FECD) is the most common primary corneal endothelial dystrophy and the leading indication for corneal transplantation worldwide [1]. FECD is characterized by a progressive decline in the density and function of corneal endothelial cells (CECs) which manifests as polymegathism, pleomorphism, and the formation of guttae. Primary dysfunction of the endothelial cells manifests as corneal swelling. Persistent corneal edema leads to keratocyte death and subepithelial fibrosis [2]. FECD is a complex and heterogeneous genetic disease with the interaction between genetic and environmental factors.

In this chapter, we use a case-based approach to review the clinical characteristics of FECD and the tools available for diagnosis and prognostication. We will also review the current medical and surgical management and discuss emerging therapeutic options.

K. Cho
Wilmer Eye Institute, Johns Hopkins University, Baltimore, MD, USA

Department of Ophthalmology, Dankook University, Cheonan, South Korea

M. Ali · D. Srikumaran (✉)
Wilmer Eye Institute, Johns Hopkins University, Baltimore, MD, USA
e-mail: dsrikum1@jhmi.edu

A. S. Jun
Wilmer Eye Institute, Johns Hopkins University, Baltimore, MD, USA

Department of Ophthalmology, University of Virginia, Charlottesville, VA, USA

F. A. Woreta, R. B. Singh (eds.), *Cornea Casebook*, Current Practices in Ophthalmology, https://doi.org/10.1007/978-981-96-0495-1_11

Table 11.1 Comparison according to FECD classification

Classification	Early onset FECD	Late-onset FECD
Onset time	First decade	Fourth to fifth decade
Female-to-male ratio	1: 1	2.5:1 to 3:1
Causal gene	COL8A2	TCF4, TCF8(ZEB1), AGBL1, LOXHD1, SLC4A11, KANK4, LAMC1, ATP1B1, DMPK

11.2 Classification and Molecular Genetics

The progression of the disease is bilateral but may be asymmetric with four clinical stages over a period of two to three decades. FECD can be divided into two subtypes: the more common late-onset subtype initially presents in the fourth decade or later, and the less common early onset presents within the first decade of life. The exact pathogenesis of FECD continues to be investigated and multiple genes have been implicated (Table 11.1) [3, 4]. Early onset FECD has been linked to a mutation in the gene for the α 2 chain of collagen 8 (COL8A2). The gene locus has not been identified in most patients with late-onset FECD. Less commonly, genetic loci have been identified in some cases of late-onset FECD. The genetic mutations may result in oxidative damage and apoptosis, dysregulation of the mitochondria, unfolded protein response and endoplasmic reticulum (ER) stress, dysregulation of the MicroRNA, and/or induction of a mesenchymal to epithelial transition.

11.3 Clinical Presentation and Diagnosis <Case 1>

Early onset FECD begins as early as 3 years of age with equal sex distribution. Corneal guttae are small and rounded, in a fine patchy distribution, in contrast to the coarse and distinct guttae of late-onset FECD. By age 30 or 40, affected individuals may develop the end-stage disease [5]. Late-onset FECD presents in the fourth decade or later, with a female-to-male ratio ranging from 2.5:1 to 3:1.

In the early stages, forward light scatter caused by corneal guttae may result in visual disturbances, and the area ratio of corneal guttae is correlated with visual acuity, contrast sensitivity, and intraocular straylight [6, 7]. In advanced stages, patients tend to suffer from blurred vision and pain or foreign body sensations caused by corneal edema and epithelial bullae.

COL8A2, α2 chain of collagen 8; TCF4, transcription factor 4; ZEB1, transcription factor Zinc finger E-Box binding homeodomain 1; AGBL1, ATP/GTP binding protein like 1; LOXHD1, lipoxygenase homology domain 1; SLC4A11, solute carrier family 4 member 11; KANK4, KN motif and ankyrin repeat domains 4; LAMC1, laminin subunit gamma 1; ATP1B1, ATPase Na+ /K+ transporting subunit beta 1; DMPK, dystrophia myotonica protein kinase (Fig. 11.1).

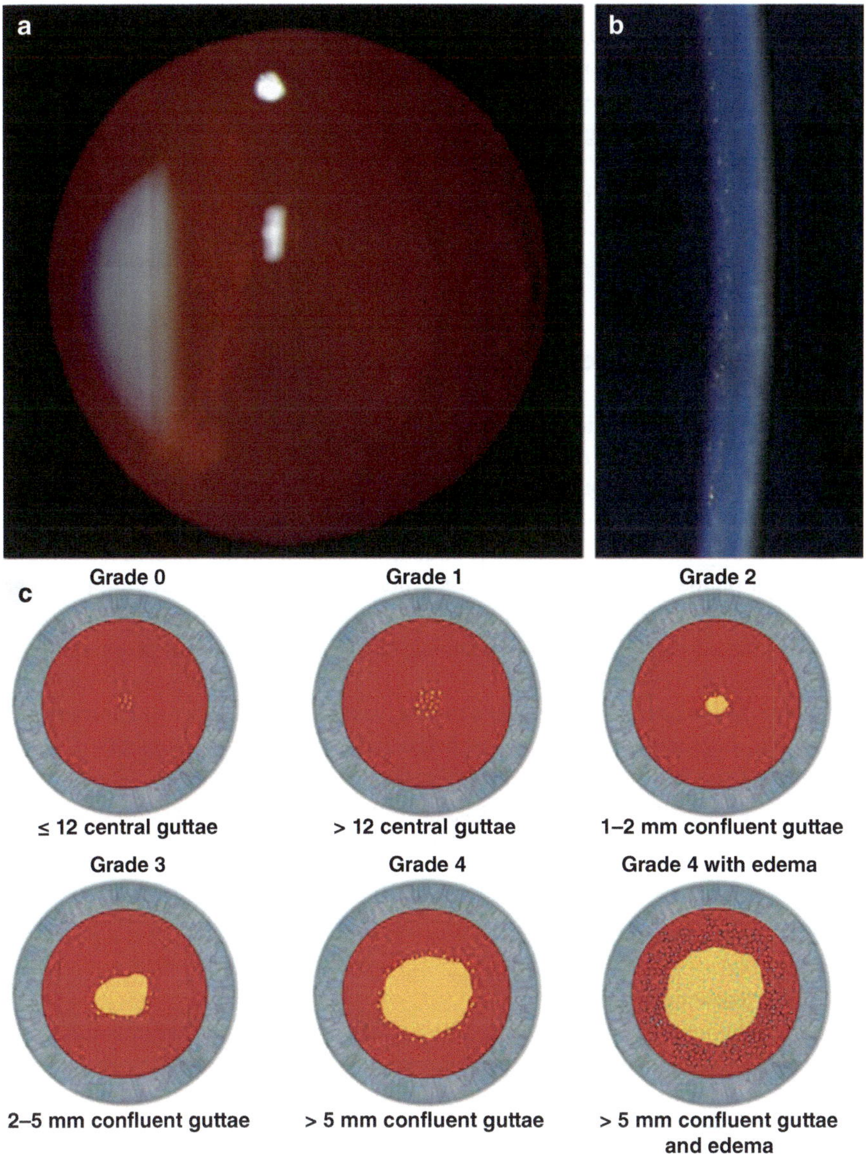

Fig. 11.1 <Case 1> Left eye of a 47-year-old female with cornea guttae of grade 4 severity. Guttae are best visualized using retroillumination on a slit lamp (**a**) or focusing directly on Descemet's membrane (**b**). The cornea reveals large areas with a fine-grained distribution of guttae. FECD classification adapted from Krachmer et al. (1978) [8] (**c**)

Case 1—Guttae in FECD

1. First signs occur mostly in the fourth to fifth decade of life as guttae in the central corneal endothelium.
2. Guttae are best diagnosed using retroillumination on a slit lamp with the pupils dilated.
3. In the next stage, guttae spread peripherally and may coalesce.
4. In advanced FECD, the cornea has with >5 mm diameter of confluent guttae or visible stromal or epithelial edema.

11.3.1 Clinical Course and Staging

Stage 1: Central cornea guttae which appear as dark spots on the posterior corneal surface. Some patients develop guttae but never progress to later stages, whereas others advance to endothelial decompensation and stromal edema.

Stage 2: Endothelial decompensation and stromal edema. The guttae have spread peripherally and may coalesce, producing a beaten-metal appearance with or without pigment dusting. Descemet membrane is thickened, gray, and irregular. Progressive stromal edema results in a ground-glass opacification of the cornea with marked central thickening causing visual reduction, most prominently in the morning.

Stage 3: Stromal edema may progress to involve the epithelium causing intraepithelial and interepithelial edema (epithelial bullae), bullous keratopathy. Corneal surface irregularity and stromal haze further reduce vision.

Stage 4: Subepithelial fibrosis, scarring, and peripheral superficial vascularization from chronic edema occur in long-standing cases.

11.3.2 Associated Diseases

11.3.2.1 Keratoconus

Although the underlying etiology leading to the expression of keratoconus (KC) and FECD in the same patient is unknown, the association between KC and FECD has been reported previously [9]. Oxidative stress, reactive oxygen species (ROS), and mitochondrial dysfunction are known to play a role in the pathogenesis of both diseases [10]. Clinicians should be wary of the possibility of corneal thinning caused by KC and concurrent increase in corneal thickness caused by FECD. This may lead to unexpected postoperative visual outcomes after cataract surgeries. Therefore, routine preoperative topography and specular microscopy would minimize this risk.

Glaucoma

Several studies have proposed an association between FECD and glaucoma. However, in a large retrospective study with 841 patients, higher prevalence of glaucoma or ocular hypertension in FECD patients could not be demonstrated [11]. In a study with 1610 patients in families, glaucoma prevalence of up to 11% compared to 6% in a normal population was found [12]. However, this study may include several undetected PEX keratopathy eyes in the presumed FECD group [13].

Myotonic Dystrophy

Myotonic dystrophy (MD) is the most common inherited muscle disease in adults and has an autosomal dominant inheritance. Some studies suggest that MD patients are at risk for FECD. In a study by Winkler et al., the prevalence of FECD in the cohort of patients with MD was 36% and 46%, which is higher than the general population [14]. Their data suggest a shared pathophysiologic mechanism of RNA toxicity due to CTG repeat expansion between FECD and MD.

Diabetes Mellitus

Some studies have described the association between diabetes and increased central corneal thickness (CCT) in FECD cases and controls [15]. The pathophysiology has been hypothesized to be due to abnormally functioning CECs and reduced ECD. Consistent with this hypothesis is the fact that the recipients with diabetes experienced more endothelial cell loss following DMEK, as compared to those without diabetes [16].

11.3.3 Diagnosis

Because not every case of cornea guttae is progressive and develops into FECD, a thorough examination of family history, symptoms, and signs such as corneal is warranted before diagnosing FECD [17].

11.3.3.1 Corneal Thickness and Tomography <Case 2>

The CCT could be used to determine the grade of disease progression, but this alone might not be accurate because of the interindividual variety of CCT and the difficulty in defining the exact center of the cornea. Corneal tomography such as Anterior segment optical coherence tomography (AS-OCT) or Scheimpflug imaging enables measurement at multiple locations and high repeatability [18].

For the treatment decision of FECD, it is very useful to divide corneal edema into clinically definite corneal edema, subclinical edema, or no edema. However, it is difficult to detect subclinical edema only with slit lamp microscopy and pachymetry. Three Scheimpflug tomography pachymetry map and posterior elevation map patterns are useful for detecting subclinical edema and can predict FECD prognosis independent of CCT [19, 20] (Fig. 11.2).

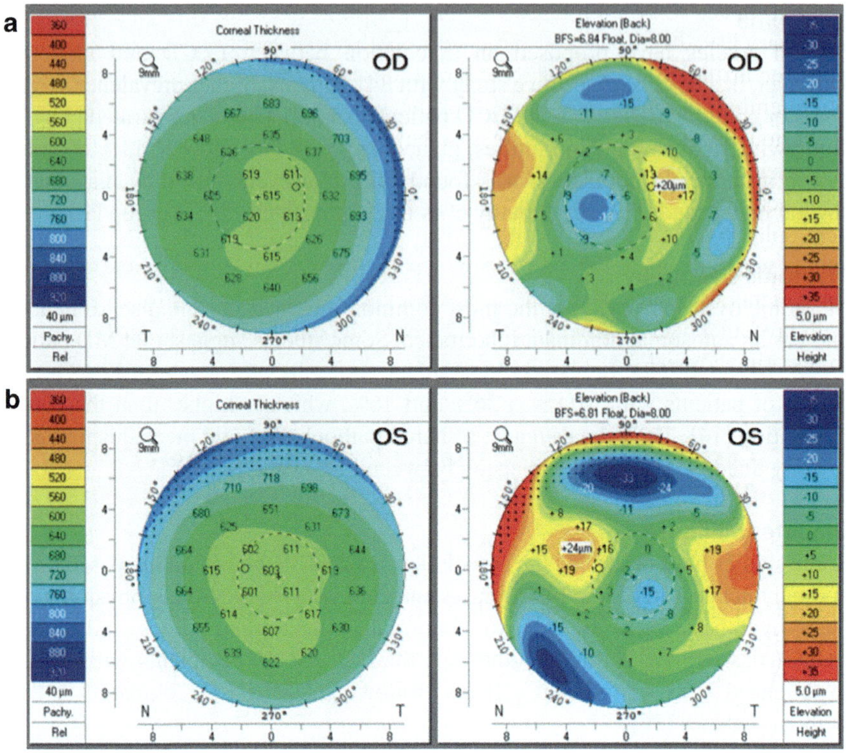

Fig. 11.2 <Case 2> Scheimpflug tomographic features of corneal edema in a 63-year-old female patient with FECD and cataract in both eyes. The tomography maps of the right (**a**) and left (**b**) cornea show loss of parallel and circular/oval isopachs and displacement of the thinnest point of the cornea from its normal inferotemporal location to the nasal in the pachymetry map (*N* nasal, T temporal), and focal posterior depression of the posterior corneal surface (to −18 and −15 relative to the best-fit sphere in right and left, respectively) in the posterior elevation map. She noticed worsening visual acuity and the best corrected visual acuities (BCVA) are 20/30 (right) and 20/40 (left). The measured values of central cornea pachymetry were 634 μm and 612 μm, right and left, respectively. Cataract was grade two nuclear sclerosis in both eyes. The patient underwent a triple procedure (phacoemulsification, intraocular lens insertion, and DMEK)

Case 2—Tomographic Features of Corneal Edema in FECD

1. FECD can be classified as having clinically definite corneal edema, subclinical edema, or no edema.
2. If guttae are present and typically confluent without clinically definite edema, subclinical corneal edema in FECD can be detected by Scheimpflug tomography.
3. Tomographic features of subclinical edema are (1) loss of parallel isopachs, (2) displacement of the thinnest point of the cornea, and (3) focal posterior corneal surface depression.
4. Subclinical edema should be considered when evaluating FECD eyes for cataract surgery or DMEK.

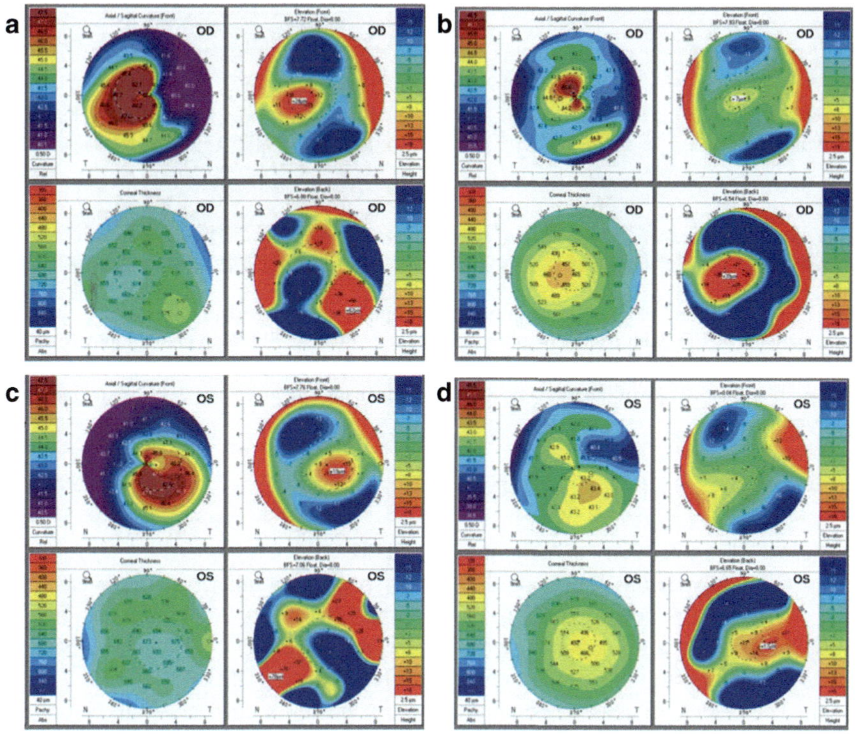

Fig. 11.3 <Case 3> Tomographic features of corneal edema in a 71-year-old male patient with FECD and cataract in both eyes. The tomography maps show high irregular astigmatism in both eyes. Irregularities appear both in the anterior and posterior surfaces of the cornea (**a**. right eye, **c**. left eye). He noticed worsening visual acuity and best corrected visual acuities are 20/60 (right) and 20/125 (left). The measured values of central cornea pachymetry were 615 μm and 622 μm, right and left, respectively. The irregular astigmatism was decreased after triple procedure in both eyes (**b**, **d**)

11.3.3.2 Optical Changes and Corneal Curvature <Case 3>

Early in the course of FECD, anterior and posterior corneal surfaces can be irregular, and both corneal surfaces can backscatter more light than normal. Irregular surfaces and increased backscatter are associated with increased high order aberrations (HOAs) and forward scatter, which in turn decrease visual acuity and increase disability glare. Posterior surface irregularity and backscatter might also be caused by guttae [21].

Corneal edema in FECD changes the normal ellipsoid posterior profile to a more spherical shape, effectively inducing less negative power and loss of normal posterior surface toricity. Similarly, the steep anterior and posterior surface meridians, which are usually oriented vertically in normal corneas, are more often oblique or horizontal in FECD. These changes may partially explain the hyperopic shift after endothelial keratoplasty and might contribute to inaccurate refractive outcomes after cataract surgery [22].

Patients with severe FECD could show larger amount of asymmetry and higher-order irregularity components of the anterior and posterior corneal surfaces [23] (Fig. 11.3).

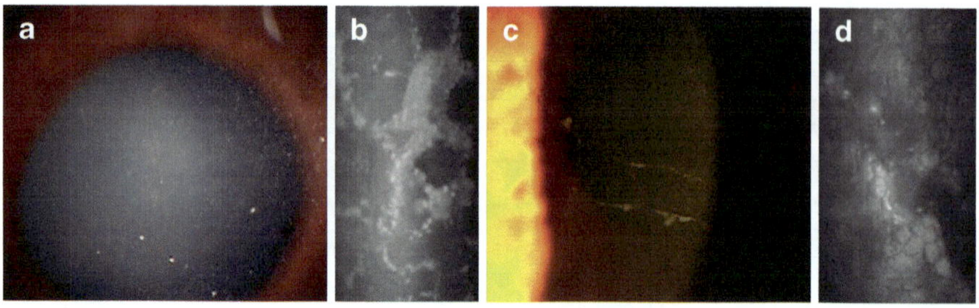

Fig. 11.4 FECD and PPCD. Slit lamp (**a**) and specular microscopy (**b**) images of a 47-year-old male patient (FCED) with confluent guttae and pigment dusting. Slit lamp photography (**c**) of the right of a 33-year-old male (PPCD) showing a railroad-shaped pattern at posterior membrane level; the specular microscopy of the same eye (**d**) shows the bands, reduced cell density, and increased cell size

Case 3—Irregular Corneal Astigmatism in FECD

1. Clinically definite corneal edema may show focal anterior surface elevation corresponding to region of focal posterior surface depression resulting in irregular astigmatism in corneas affected by FECD.
2. Irregular astigmatism may improve or resolve after DMEK.
3. The change of astigmatism and refractive power of cornea should be considered in IOL calculation.
4. Toric intraocular lens (IOL) should be used with caution.

11.3.4 Differential Diagnosis

11.3.4.1 Posterior Polymorphous Corneal Dystrophy

In posterior polymorphous corneal dystrophy (PPCD), the underlying corneal abnormality occurs in the Descemet membrane and the endothelium, with vesicle-like lesions, band lesions, and/or diffuse opacities. A railroad-shaped pattern of the corneal endothelium is a hallmark of PPCD (Fig. 11.4).

Congenital Hereditary Endothelial Dystrophy

Corneal opacification in congenital hereditary endothelial dystrophy (CHED) is full thickness, with milky ground glass appearance but normal corneal thickness. Corneal clouding is usually present at birth. Specular microscopy in parents of CHED patients may show cornea guttae.

Chandler's Syndrome

Chandler's syndrome is a form of Iridocorneal endothelial (ICE) syndrome that presents unilaterally with a hammered silver appearance of the corneal endothelium and shallow anterior chamber with peripheral anterior synechiae. Diagnosis of FECD would be less likely when it presents with such unilateral atypical characteristics.

X-Linked Endothelial Corneal Dystrophy

X-linked endothelial corneal dystrophy (XECD) is congenital, and it affects males much more severely than females. Some males have congenital clouding ranging from a diffuse haze to a milky, ground-glass appearance with moon crater-like changes to the endothelium. In later life, a band keratopathy may develop.

Pseudoexfoliation Keratopathy

FECD could show similarities with PEX keratopathy. The diffuse decompensation pattern on PEX eyes can be distinguished clinically from the corneal edema in FECD, which usually starts centrally and spreads peripherally.

Pseudophakic Bullous Keratopathy

Pseudophakic bullous keratopathy (PBK) is irreversible corneal edema induced by anterior segment surgery most commonly cataract surgery but also glaucoma and other IOL surgeries. This edema can progress to the subepithelial and epithelial layers and results in bullae formation.

11.4 Management

11.4.1 Medical Treatment

In early stages, FECD can be observed. However, many patients will develop visual impairment with progression of the disease. Currently, no medical therapy is available to interfere with the progression of FECD. Hyperosmotic drops may temporarily improve symptoms in earlier stages. However, a recent randomized trial has revealed that the drops might not offer much benefit and might result in more adverse events when compared to a placebo [24].

Rho-associated protein kinase (ROCK) inhibitors are actively being investigated for the treatment of FECD. Netarsudil is a drug known as a rho kinase inhibitor and approved for treatment of glaucoma. In a randomized pilot study, Price and colleagues showed that use of netarsudil was associated with reduction of corneal edema and improvement in scotopic corrected distance vision in FECD patients [25].

11.4.2 Surgical Treatment

11.4.2.1 Keratoplasty

For over a century, penetrating keratoplasty (PK) has remained the main treatment modality for FECD [26]. However, the surgical management has evolved from PK to endothelial keratoplasty including first Deep lamellar endothelial keratoplasty (DLEK) then Descemet Stripping (Automated) Endothelial Keratoplasty (DSEK/DSAEK), and finally Descemet Membrane Endothelial Keratoplasty (DMEK) over the past two decades.

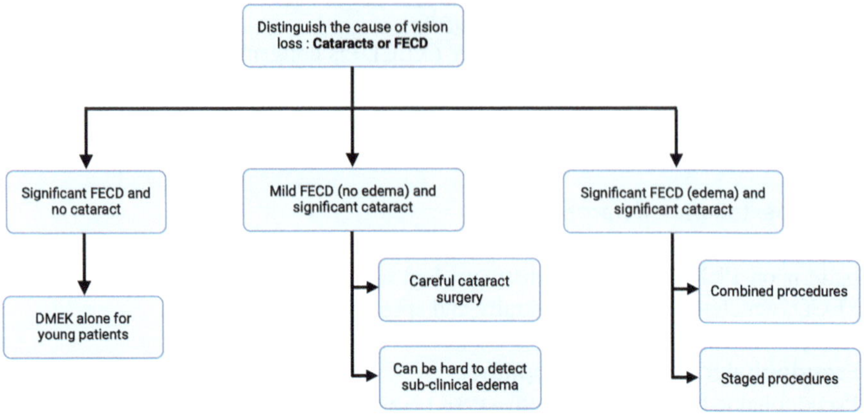

Fig. 11.5 Algorithm describing the approach to Fuchs Endothelial Corneal Dystrophy (FECD) with Cataract. Slit lamp examination is important in assessing the stage and density of the cataract, depth of the anterior chamber, and presence of clinically evident corneal edema. Scheimpflug tomography is useful for detecting subclinical edema of cornea

Cataract Surgery in FECD Patients

When FECD and cataracts coexist, surgeons must decide whether to perform cataract surgery or keratoplasty or both. It is important to determine whether the cause of vision loss is cataract, corneal edema or both in deciding whether to perform combined procedures, cataract surgery, or DMEK alone (Fig. 11.5). Cataracts may be associated with a myopic shift. On the other hand, FECD patients may report blurry vision upon awakening, or foreign body sensation and pain if bullae are present [27]. In addition to careful slit lamp examination, the use of Scheimpflug tomography is helpful in detecting subclinical edema as described above.

The DMEK triple procedure (DMEK combined with phacoemulsification and posterior chamber lens implantation) is a good option to treat patients with both visually significant cataracts and corneal edema, due to rapid visual recovery and the reduced risks relative to two separate surgeries.

Cataract Surgery Alone in FECD <Case 4>

For patients with a visually significant cataract, but without evidence of subclinical corneal edema, cataract surgery alone would be preferred. Moreover, early cataract surgery may be preferred since the increased ultrasound energy is needed to remove a dense cataract. Certain surgical techniques (tri-soft shell technique, Phaco-Chop technique, and low flow irrigation) may help reduce endothelial cell loss in such cases. In terms of IOL selection, hydrophobic IOLs are preferred if a future DMEK is anticipated due to the risk of opacification of hydrophilic IOLs. In a large cohort of Medicare beneficiaries with FECD, the probability of receiving EK after cataract surgery was only 2.3% at 8 years [28]. The use of Scheimpflug tomography can help predict which eyes may progress disease to need keratoplasty after cataract surgery. The 4-year cumulative risk of disease progression and intervention after uncomplicated cataract surgery was 0%, 50%, and 75% when none, 1 or 2, and all 3 pachymetry map and posterior elevation map parameters were present, respectively [20].

Phakic DMEK

For young patients with significant FECD, but without a cataract, phakic DMEK might be the preferred. In a case series of 1000 eyes, Birbal et al. found that the patient's lens status did not influence DMEK outcomes [29]. In addition, recent studies showed that a subsequent cataract extraction was feasible with minimal endothelial cell loss if performed carefully in patients with a DMEK graft [30]. Additionally, the 5-year phacoemulsification rate among FECD patients with no cataract is reported to be just 16.9% [31].

Combined Procedure (Cataract Surgery and DMEK)

For patients with both a visually significant cataract and FECD, a combined procedure should be considered. Visual outcomes, endothelial cell loss, and rebubbling rates remain comparable between combined procedure and staged procedures (DMEK after cataract surgery) [32]. Shahnazaryan et al. reported that while rates of rebubbling remained low with good visual outcomes, the rates of endothelial cell loss at 1 month and 1 year were higher after DMEK triple when compared with DMEK alone [33]. Thus, the mixed results in the literature suggest that the decision to perform a staged versus combined procedure should be based on surgeon experience.

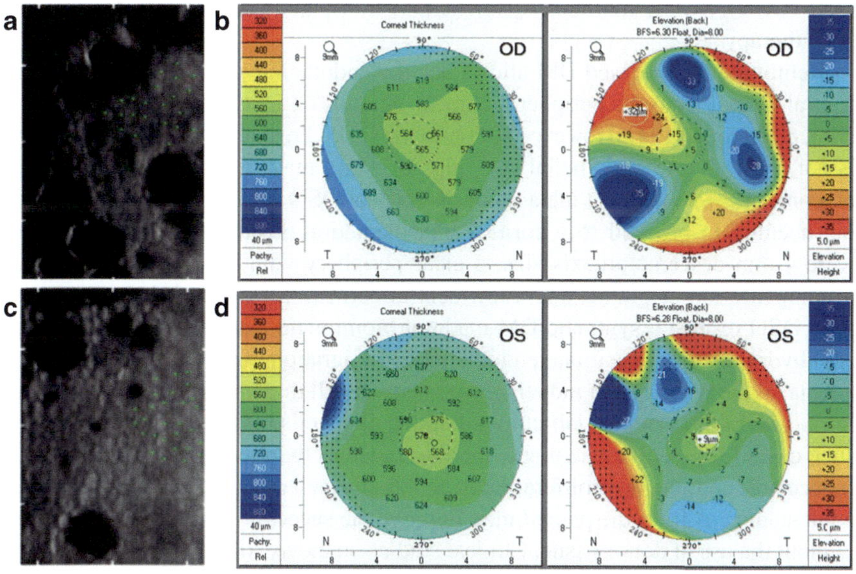

Fig. 11.6 <Case 4> The 66-year-old female patient with FECD and cataract in both eyes. Her best corrected visual acuities are 20/30-1 (right) and 20/40 (left). She noticed difficulty with near vision reading and computer. Her specular microscopy does show guttae in both eyes (**a**. right, **c**. left) and much lower cell counts in right eye. The tomography maps show that the right eye has two features of edema, irregular isopachs and displacement of the thinnest point while in the left eye, there are mildly irregular isopachs (**b**. right, **d**. left). The measured values of central cornea pachymetry were 546 μm and 564 μm, right and left, respectively. We discussed the risk of corneal decompensation but since her left eye has few tomographic features of edema even though central corneal thickness is higher in the left eye the patient underwent cataract surgery alone with DMEK in the future if needed

Surgical modifications when performing a combined procedure include avoiding the use of dilating agents in the irrigation fluid, smaller rhexis that covers the optic edge, careful removal of the viscoelastics before graft insertion, and using cohesive viscoelastics instead of dispersive (Fig. 11.6).

Case 4—Cataract Surgery in FECD Patients

1. Given the high incidence of both FECD and cataracts, patients present with varying stages of both conditions simultaneously.
2. It is important to determine if the cause of vision loss is cataract or the corneal disease.
3. Scheimpflug tomography is useful for discriminating subclinical edema of cornea.
4. Certain surgical techniques are helpful to reduce endothelial cell loss.
5. Hydrophobic IOLs are preferred if a future DMEK is anticipated.

11.4.3 Regenerative and Emerging Treatments <Case 5>

There are newer modalities are emerging therapies including Descemet Stripping Only (DSO), ROCK Inhibitor, synthetic DM transplant, injection cell therapy, and gene therapy.

Removing the diseased DM allows healthy endothelial cells to migrate over the central cornea from the peripheral corneal. Studies on DSO have shown favorable clinical outcomes [34]. However, in some cases, DSO results in an environment that is not conducive to endothelial cell migration and may result in poor or delayed outcomes [35]. In a recent meta-analysis, 85% of DSO cases were successful without needing to proceed to a corneal transplantation. Factors influencing success were 4-mm descemetorhexis size, a clear periphery with no clinical sequelae of decompensation or guttae, and a low central corneal thickness [36]. In cases with poor DSO results, a synthetic DM made of biomimetic materials (e.g., hyaluronic acid hydrogels) may facilitate endothelial cell migration, and resolution of corneal edema, as shown in rabbit models [37]. Injection cell therapy via a cell carrier or an intra-cameral injection of lab-cultured endothelial cells may prove to be helpful in such cases [38]. A pharmacologic approach such as the use of ROCK inhibitors to induce host endothelial proliferation or endothelial cell culture using reprogrammed adult stem cells from the patient may improve the success of this descemetorrhexis without the use of donor tissue. Clinical studies on the use of ROCK inhibitors have shown favorable outcomes [39].

To expand the pool of donor tissue, a new technique has been introduced in which a single donor corneal button is divided into two segments for transplantation in two different patients. This technique, referred to as hemi-DMEK, may not be adopted in the United States because of regulatory, billing, and liability challenges, but it may be more acceptable in areas where there is donor tissue shortage.

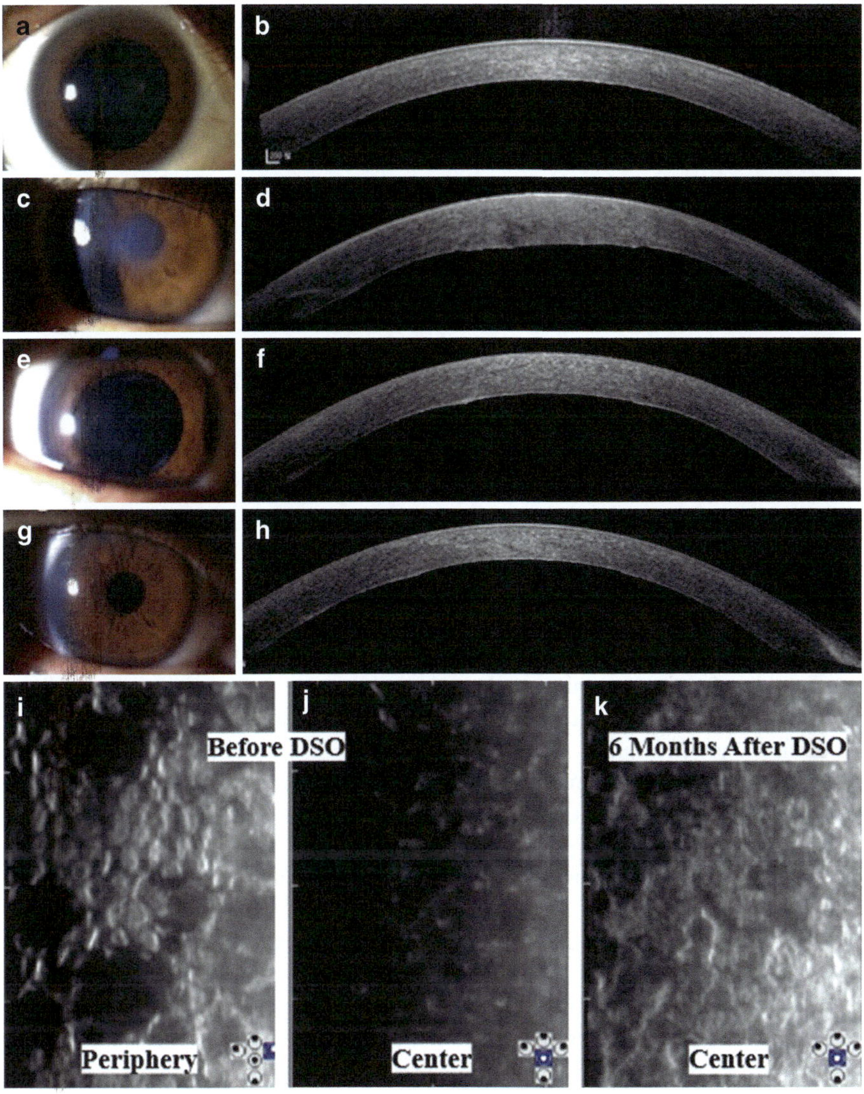

Fig. 11.7 <Case 5> The 62-year-old woman with FECD and cataract in both eyes. Her best corrected visual acuity (BCVA) and central cornea thickness (CCT) are 20/40 and 581 μm, respectively in right eye. She underwent phacoemulsification, intraocular lens insertion, and 4-mm central Descemet stripping only (DSO). The images of slit lamp microscopy and anterior segment optical coherent tomography (OCT) before surgery (**a**, **b**), 7 days (**c**, **d**), 3 months (**e**, **f**), and 6 months (**g**, **h**) after surgery. Immediately after DSO, corneal edema worsened, but over time, a corneal endothelial cell layer was formed, and corneal edema disappeared. Before DSO, endothelial cells and guttae were observed only in the peripheral cornea, not center (specular microscopic images of peripheral (**i**) and central (**j**) cornea). After 6 months of DSO, endothelial cells were observed in the central cornea (**k**). BCVA and CCT measured 6 months after surgery improved to 20/20 and 556 μm, respectively (Photo courtesy of Kim HK)

With increasing understanding of the genes implicated in FECD and the advancement in gene therapy, gene editing tools, e.g., CRISPR-Cas9 for editing genomes, present an opportunity to use gene therapy in the treatment of FECD [40] (Fig. 11.7).

Case 5—Descemet Stripping Only (DSO)

1. DSO involves removing the diseased DM thus allowing healthy endothelial cells to migrate over the central cornea.
2. DSO is a viable treatment option for patients who have localized endothelial disease within the central 5 mm of the cornea and have a clear peripheral endothelial layer.
3. While DMEK remains the gold standard, DSO provides an alternative if donor tissue isn't readily available and graft rejection is a concern.
4. Descemetorhexis size, surgical technique, and patient factors (age, genetic factors, etc.) may influence the rate of corneal clearance.

11.5 Summary Points

1. FECD is the most common primary corneal endothelial dystrophy and the leading indication for corneal transplantation.
2. First signs occur mostly in the fourth to fifth decade of life as guttae in the central corneal endothelium.
3. FECD may be accompanied by keratoconus with corneal ectatic changes.
4. Corneal edema could show irregular astigmatism which may improve or resolve after DMEK.
5. Scheimpflug tomography is useful for discriminating subclinical edema and irregular astigmatism of cornea.
6. It is important to determine if the cause of vision loss is cataract or the corneal disease.
7. In combined procedure (cataract surgery and DMEK), the change of astigmatism and refractive power of cornea should be considered in IOL calculation, and toric intraocular lens (IOL) should be used with caution.
8. DSO is a viable treatment option, however, patient selection and determination of who will be a responder versus nonresponder remains challenging.
9. Advances in minimally invasive surgical techniques such as cell-based approaches, in addition to nonsurgical treatments, may improve therapeutic outcomes in the future.

Acknowledgments Funding Statement: No funding or sponsorship was received for this chapter.

Disclosures Kyongjin Cho, Muhammad Ali and Albert S Jun have no disclosures.

Divya Srikumaran: Eye Bank Association of America: Grant Support; AAO Hoskins Center: Grant Support; National Eye Institute: Grant Support; Johns Hopkins ICTR/NCATS: Grant Support; ABMS-REF: Grant Support; Alcon: Consultant; Expert Testimony: Legal Fees.

Conflict of Interest No conflicting relationship exists for any author.

References

1. Gain P, et al. Global survey of corneal transplantation and eye banking. JAMA Ophthalmol. 2016;134(2):167–73.
2. Hamill CE, Schmedt T, Jurkunas U. Fuchs endothelial cornea dystrophy: a review of the genetics behind disease development. Semin Ophthalmol. 2013;28(5–6):281–6.
3. Matthaei M, et al. Fuchs endothelial corneal dystrophy: clinical, genetic, pathophysiologic, and therapeutic aspects. Annu Rev Vis Sci. 2019;5:151–75.
4. Nanda GG, Alone DP. REVIEW: current understanding of the pathogenesis of Fuchs' endothelial corneal dystrophy. Mol Vis. 2019;25:295–310.
5. Cockerham GC, et al. An immunohistochemical analysis and comparison of posterior polymorphous dystrophy with congenital hereditary endothelial dystrophy. Cornea. 2002;21(8):787–91.
6. Oie Y, Watanabe S, Nishida K. Evaluation of visual quality in patients with Fuchs endothelial corneal dystrophy. Cornea. 2016;35(Suppl 1):S55–s58.
7. Watanabe S, et al. Relationship between corneal Guttae and quality of vision in patients with mild Fuchs' endothelial corneal dystrophy. Ophthalmology. 2015;122(10):2103–9.
8. Krachmer JH, et al. Corneal endothelial dystrophy. A study of 64 families. Arch Ophthalmol. 1978;96(11):2036–9.
9. Jurkunas U, Azar DT. Potential complications of ocular surgery in patients with coexistent keratoconus and Fuchs' endothelial dystrophy. Ophthalmology. 2006;113(12):2187–97.
10. Vallabh NA, Romano V, Willoughby CE. Mitochondrial dysfunction and oxidative stress in corneal disease. Mitochondrion. 2017;36:103–13.
11. Rice GD, Wright K, Silverstein SM. A retrospective study of the association between Fuchs' endothelial dystrophy and glaucoma. Clin Ophthalmol. 2014;8:2155–9.
12. Nagarsheth M, et al. Relationship between Fuchs endothelial corneal dystrophy severity and glaucoma and/or ocular hypertension. Arch Ophthalmol. 2012;130(11):1384–8.
13. Naumann GO, Schlötzer-Schrehardt U. Keratopathy in pseudoexfoliation syndrome as a cause of corneal endothelial decompensation: a clinicopathologic study. Ophthalmology. 2000;107(6):1111–24.
14. Winkler NS, et al. Fuchs' endothelial corneal dystrophy in patients with myotonic dystrophy, type 1. Invest Ophthalmol Vis Sci. 2018;59(7):3053–7.
15. Luo XY, et al. Association of diabetes with central corneal thickness among a multiethnic Asian population. JAMA Netw Open. 2019;2(1):e186647.
16. Price MO, et al. Effect of donor and recipient diabetes status on Descemet membrane endothelial keratoplasty adherence and survival. Cornea. 2017;36(10):1184–8.
17. Vedana G, Villarreal G Jr, Jun AS. Fuchs endothelial corneal dystrophy: current perspectives. Clin Ophthalmol. 2016;10:321–30.
18. Rio-Cristobal A, Martin R. Corneal assessment technologies: current status. Surv Ophthalmol. 2014;59(6):599–614.
19. Sun SY, et al. Determining subclinical edema in Fuchs endothelial corneal dystrophy: revised classification using Scheimpflug tomography for preoperative assessment. Ophthalmology. 2019;126(2):195–204.
20. Patel SV, et al. Predicting the prognosis of Fuchs endothelial corneal dystrophy by using Scheimpflug tomography. Ophthalmology. 2020;127(3):315–23.
21. Wacker K, et al. Corneal high-order aberrations and backscatter in Fuchs' endothelial corneal dystrophy. Ophthalmology. 2015;122(8):1645–52.
22. Wacker K, McLaren JW, Patel SV. Directional posterior corneal profile changes in Fuchs' endothelial corneal dystrophy. Invest Ophthalmol Vis Sci. 2015;56(10):5904–11.
23. Oie Y, et al. Fourier analysis on regular and irregular astigmatism of anterior and posterior corneal surfaces in Fuchs endothelial corneal dystrophy. Am J Ophthalmol. 2021;223:33–41.
24. Zander DB, et al. Hyperosmolar eye drops for diurnal corneal edema in Fuchs' endothelial dystrophy. Ophthalmology (Rochester, Minn.). 2021;128(11):1527–33.

25. Price MO, Price FW Jr. Randomized, double-masked, pilot study of netarsudil 0.02% ophthalmic solution for treatment of corneal edema in Fuchs dystrophy. Am J Ophthalmol. 2021;227:100–5.
26. Güell JL, et al. Historical review and update of surgical treatment for corneal endothelial diseases. Ophthalmol Therapy. 2014;3(1–2):1–15.
27. Fritz M, et al. Diurnal variation in corneal edema in Fuchs endothelial corneal dystrophy. Am J Ophthalmol. 2019;207:351–5.
28. Heckenlaible NJ, et al. Predictors of receiving keratoplasty for Fuchs' endothelial corneal dystrophy among medicare beneficiaries. Ophthalmology. 2022;130:28.
29. Birbal RS, et al. Effect of surgical indication and preoperative lens status on Descemet membrane endothelial keratoplasty outcomes. Am J Ophthalmol. 2020;212:79–87.
30. Gundlach E, et al. DMEK in phakic eyes: targeted therapy or highway to cataract surgery? Graefes Arch Clin Exp Ophthalmol. 2015;253(6):909–14.
31. Birbal RS, et al. Five-year graft survival and clinical outcomes of 500 consecutive cases after Descemet membrane endothelial keratoplasty. Cornea. 2020;39(3):290–7.
32. Tey KY, et al. Effects of combined cataract surgery on outcomes of Descemet's membrane endothelial keratoplasty: a systematic review and meta-analysis. Front Med (Lausanne). 2022;9:857200.
33. Campbell JA, et al. Refractive accuracy in eyes undergoing combined cataract extraction and Descemet membrane endothelial keratoplasty. Br J Ophthalmol. 2022;106(5):623–7.
34. Garcerant D, et al. Descemet"s stripping without endothelial keratoplasty. Curr Opin Ophthalmol. 2019;30(4):275–85.
35. Soh YQ, et al. Predicative factors for corneal endothelial cell migration. Invest Ophthalmol Vis Sci. 2016;57(2):338–48.
36. Din N, et al. Surgical management of Fuchs endothelial corneal dystrophy: a treatment algorithm and individual patient meta-analysis of Descemet stripping only. Cornea. 2022;41(9):1188–95.
37. Bhogal M, et al. Allogeneic Descemet's membrane transplantation enhances corneal endothelial monolayer formation and restores functional integrity following Descemet's stripping. Invest Ophthalmol Vis Sci. 2017;58(10):4249–60.
38. Soh YQ, Peh GSL, Mehta JS. Translational issues for human corneal endothelial tissue engineering. J Tissue Eng Regen Med. 2017;11(9):2425–42.
39. Davies E, Jurkunas U, Pineda R 2nd. Pilot study of corneal clearance with the use of a rho-kinase inhibitor after descemetorhexis without endothelial keratoplasty for Fuchs endothelial corneal dystrophy. Cornea. 2021;40(7):899–902.
40. Richard GF. Shortening trinucleotide repeats using highly specific endonucleases: a possible approach to gene therapy? Trends Genet. 2015;31(4):177–86.

Pseudophakic Bullous Keratopathy

12

Roma B. Pegany, Richard D. Stutzman, Afshan A. Nanji, and Winston D. Chamberlain

12.1 Introduction

Pseudophakic bullous keratopathy (PBK) is irreversible stromal edema in the cornea, resulting from injury to the corneal endothelium, most commonly occurring after intraocular surgery. Aphakic bullous keratopathy (ABK) refers to corneal edema that develops in the absence of an intraocular lens (IOL). While any intraocular surgery can potentially cause endothelial damage, PBK most commonly occurs after cataract surgery [1]. Approximately 26 million cataract surgeries are performed worldwide each year [2]. From 1980 to 2014, PBK or ABK was the leading indication for a penetrating keratoplasty (PKP) in the United States, representing 28% of the cases during this period [3]. While the advancement of modern phacoemulsification techniques, viscoelastic devices, and IOL design have reduced the incidence of PBK since the 1960s, it still remains a significant cause of vision loss [1]. The corneal edema and corneal scarring that develop in PBK compromise the refractive and transparency properties of the cornea, which are critical to the function of the human optical system.

12.2 Pathophysiology of Corneal Edema in Bullous Keratopathy

Corneal transparency is maintained through intact epithelial and endothelial barriers and transport mechanisms. The endothelium lines the posterior surface of the cornea. It is a highly specialized monolayer mosaic of hexagonal cells with a

R. B. Pegany · R. D. Stutzman · A. A. Nanji · W. D. Chamberlain (✉)
Division of Cornea and Refractive Surgery, Casey Eye Institute, Oregon Health & Science University, Portland, OR, USA
e-mail: chamberw@ohsu.edu

F. A. Woreta, R. B. Singh (eds.), *Cornea Casebook*, Current Practices in Ophthalmology, https://doi.org/10.1007/978-981-96-0495-1_12

Na+/K+ ATPase ion transport system that actively pumps fluid out of the corneal stroma into the aqueous humor, keeping the stroma in a relative state of deturgescence (78% water content) [4]. The mechanisms leading to edema and PBK are not fully understood, but exposure to mechanical trauma and other forms of cellular stress during and after intraocular surgery can disrupt this barrier and the metabolic pump. Human corneal endothelial cells have a low proliferation rate and damaged cells are replaced by the enlargement of neighboring cells and their centripetal migration into an injured region [5, 6]. Corneal epithelial cells have tight junctional complexes between cells that normally prevent penetration of fluid from the precorneal tear film into deeper layers of the cornea.

In bullous keratopathy, epithelial Na+/K+ ATPase function may be altered, and there may also be increase aquaporin 3 levels, and abnormal integrin patterns [1]. In advanced bullous keratopathy, aqueous fluid can enter and accumulate under the epithelium from the stroma and form small vesicles (bullae). Eventual epithelial rupture and corneal nerve exposure lead to ocular pain [1]. Bullae may become secondarily infected from surface toxins and microbes, further complicating the condition. Histological studies of PBK reveal bullous separation of the epithelial cell layer from Bowman's membrane, separation of stromal collagen fibrils with increased interstitial fluid, thickening of Descemet's membrane, and decreased endothelial cell number [7].

12.3 Mechanisms of Bullous Keratopathy

12.3.1 Surgical

Surgical trauma is the most common cause of endothelial decompensation in bullous keratopathy. Before the 1980s, PBK was a common complication because of the high rate of intracapsular cataract extraction and anterior chamber IOL placement [8]. Modern, less-traumatic, phacoemulsification techniques and foldable posterior chamber IOLs have resulted in a decline in pseudophakic corneal edema. However, corneal edema following cataract surgery remains a common indication for corneal transplantation in the United States [9, 10]. Endothelial damage can occur from prolonged or high-energy phacoemulsification, which is associated with the production of free radicals that induce oxidative stress [6], as well as from the use of high fluidic parameters and intraocular irrigating solutions [11] or drugs that alter the pH and osmotic balance of the endothelium [1]. Mechanical contact between the endothelium and surgical instruments or lens fragments can also occur, especially in an eye with a shallow anterior chamber or dense cataract. Surgical complications, including a capsular tear or rupture with vitreous prolapse into the anterior chamber or a Descemet's membrane detachment that causes persistent post-operative corneal edema, are also contributors.

Other intraocular surgeries can compromise the endothelium. Long-term use of intraocular silicone oil as a tamponade for repair of complex retinal detachments has been shown to cause corneal edema and keratopathy when the silicone oil contacts the endothelium, particularly in aphakic eyes [12]. Endothelial cytotoxicity has been demonstrated with the use of anti-proliferative drugs such as 5-fluorouracil and mitomycin-C during trabeculectomies [13]. Mechanical trauma from conventional glaucoma drainage devices [14] and intracameral sustained release drug delivery devices for glaucoma (Durysta) are also contributors and have safety concerns [15]. Central endothelial cell loss from the newer and expanding pool of Minimally Invasive Glaucoma Surgery (MIGS) devices could be problematic based on the 5-year results of the COMPASS-XT trial that revealed a significantly greater central endothelial cell loss with the CyPass Micro-Stent combined with phacoemulsification versus phacoemulsification alone. The FDA withdrew this device from the market in 2018 [16]. Long-term studies are needed to determine the mechanisms and impact of other novel devices on corneal endothelial damage.

12.3.2 Other Predispositions

Several patient factors (Fig. 12.1) may increase the risk of corneal decompensation and lead to PBK. These include an abnormally low endothelial cell count, as in Fuch's endothelial corneal dystrophy or from prior surgeries, as well as other endothelial disorders, such as posterior polymorphous corneal dystrophy or iridocorneal endothelial syndromes [17]. Other causes include a history of glaucoma, uveitis, previous eye trauma causing corneal touch with the iris or lens, penetrating foreign

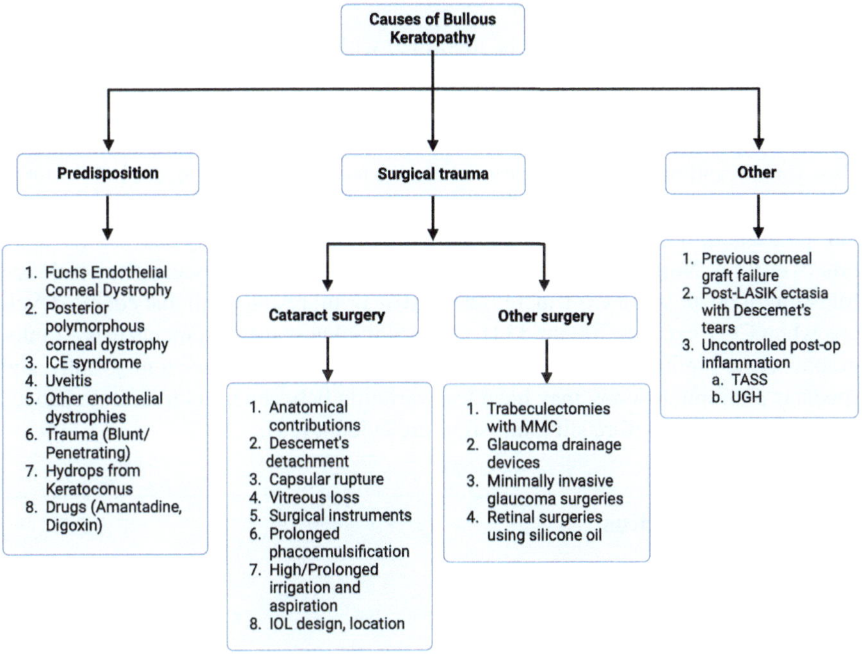

Fig. 12.1 Causes of bullous keratopathy

body, and hydrops developing from corneal ectasias such as keratoconus, pellucid marginal degeneration, and post-LASIK ectasia [1]. Systemic medications should be carefully reviewed as some (amantadine and digoxin) can cause endothelial toxicity [18, 19]. Other causes include uncontrollable postoperative inflammation – such as that seen in toxic anterior segment syndrome (TASS) [20] and uveitis-glaucoma-hyphema (UGH) syndrome (commonly seen after ACIOL placement and with some PCIOL surgeries) [21] as well as secondary graft failure from chronic or acute immunologic rejection [22].

12.4 Clinical Presentation

Patients with pseudophakic bullous keratopathy present with a history of intraocular surgery, which may have been prolonged or complicated. The average time for development of PBK after cataract surgery ranges from 8 months to 7 years [1]. Symptoms include fluctuating vision that is worse in the morning. Corneal edema tends to be more severe upon awakening due to the hypertonic environment and lack of evaporation during the night when the eyes are closed [1]. Chronic edema may lead to the development of corneal haze, scarring, and neovascularization, as well as tearing and pain resulting from ruptured bullae.

12.5 Diagnostic Evaluation

Signs of bullous keratopathy can be identified with a detailed slit lamp examination looking for microcystic epithelial edema, stromal edema, and Descemet's membrane folds. Additionally, signs of anterior chamber inflammation, such as keratic precipitates and anterior segment cell and flare, and the location of the intraocular lens, shunts, and other device positions relative to the endothelium, are important to note. Ultrasound or optical pachymetry measurements of central corneal thickness (CCT) are helpful in assessing corneal hydration and monitoring endothelial function over time. Normal CCT is approximately 540 μm [23]. Descemet's membrane folds might occur when CCT increases by 10% or more and epithelial edema develops when CCT exceeds 700 μm [24]. Corneal thickness measurements using tomographic Scheimpflug imaging, anterior segment optical coherence tomography, and specular photomicroscopy may have less variation between users to detect changes to the endothelium before slit lamp signs are evident [25].

12.6 Case Studies

12.6.1 Case 1

- Pseudophakic Bullous Keratopathy in a patient with uveitic glaucoma and multiple glaucoma surgeries.

- 6 years after the glaucoma surgeries, the patient developed corneal edema and painful epithelial blisters.
- Management included a staged procedure with repositioning of both glaucoma tube implants from the anterior chamber to the sulcus followed by an Ultrathin-DSAEK.

This 36-year-old female has a history of undifferentiated spondyloarthropathy on immunosuppression, idiopathic non-granulomatous anterior uveitis, and well-controlled uveitic glaucoma. The patient had previously undergone multiple uneventful intraocular surgeries, including two Baerveldt glaucoma tube shunts that were placed in the anterior chamber and phacoemulsification with placement of a posterior chamber IOL. Six years later, the patient developed endothelial decompensation manifesting as foggy vision, an increase in corneal pachymetry, and corneal edema with painful ruptured bullae. The exam was notable for stromal swelling, multiple Descemet's membrane folds and striae, and a tube positioned in close proximity to the corneal endothelium. A staged procedure was recommended and involved re-positioning the glaucoma tubes from the anterior chamber to the sulcus followed by endothelial keratoplasty. This was done to correct ongoing intermittent contact of the tubes with the posterior corneal surface and to create space for performing endothelial keratoplasty. Perioperative, intraoperative, and postoperative systemic steroids were given to optimize control of post-surgical inflammation in this patient with a history of uveitis, which is an underlying risk factor for endothelial decompensation. The patient underwent an uncomplicated ultra thin-DSAEK. Postoperatively, the patient developed interface haze (Fig. 12.2d) likely from inflammatory mediators and chronic edema but is clearing over time.

12.6.2 Case 2

- Pseudophakic Bullous Keratopathy in a patient with an anteriorly dislocated intraocular lens (Fig. 12.3).
- The patient had an open globe injury and was left aphakic at the time of repair; 3 years later the patient underwent placement of a secondary IOL with an ACIOL, which did not exhibit phacodynesis.
- A decade later, the patient developed bullous keratopathy (Fig. 12.4) with painful bullae.
- Management included ACIOL explantation, a scleral-sutured IOL, and endothelial keratoplasty.

This 52-year-old patient has a history of an open globe injury with an intraocular metallic foreign body, traumatic cataract, and retinal detachment and underwent repair with removal of the foreign body, lensectomy, and pars plana vitrectomy with a scleral buckle and air-fluid exchange, endolaser, and 20% SF6 gas. Three years later, secondary IOL placement with an ACIOL was performed and the patient did well. However, a decade later, the patient developed cloudy vision,

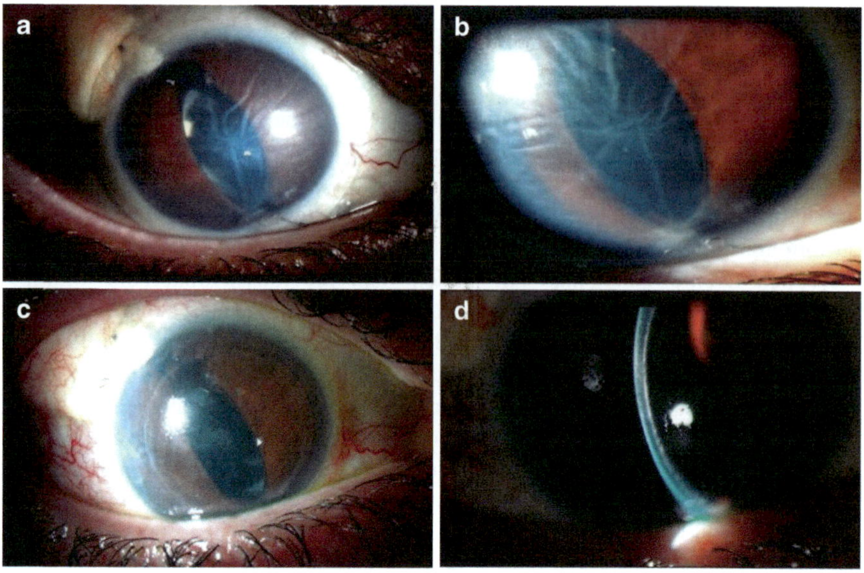

Fig. 12.2 (**a**) Baerveldt superotemporally with sulcus tube visible through a peaked pupil. Patient is wearing a bandage contact lens to alleviate pain from bullae (**b**) Deep corneal stromal edema with star-shaped Descemet's membrane folds. (**c**) and (**d**). The patient's eye after an ultra thin-DSAEK was performed. There is some reticular haze in the interface only. Slit beam showing interface haze

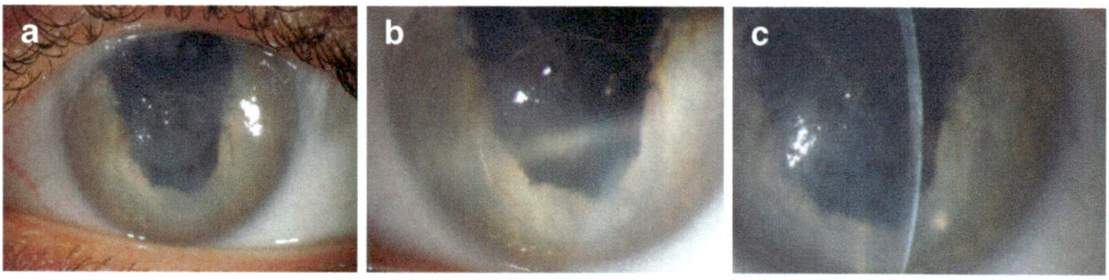

Fig. 12.3 (**a**) Diffuse corneal edema with bullous changes. A large superior iris defect is also present. (**b**) An intraocular lens is visible inferiorly in the anterior chamber and a superior haptic is visible. (**c**) Slit beam showing diffuse corneal edema

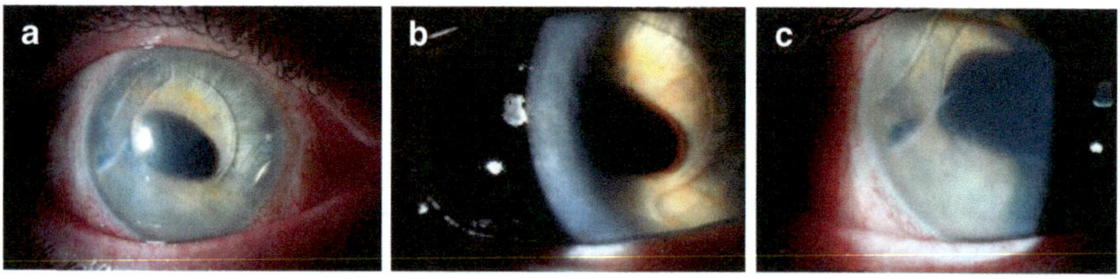

Fig. 12.4 (**a**) Anterior Chamber IOL visible with corneal edema temporally and a surgical, oval pupil. (**b**) Slit beam highlighting diffuse cornea edema with Descemet's membrane folds. (**c**) ACIOL haptic overlying peripheral iridotomy

corneal edema, and pain from epithelial breakdown. Corneal pachymetry measured 798 microns. Management included ACIOL explantation, a scleral-fixated lens, and DSAEK.

12.6.3 Case 3

- Pseudophakic Bullous Keratopathy in a patient with an anteriorly dislocated intraocular lens.
- The patient underwent IOL explantation, penetrating keratoplasty, and was left aphakic.
- Endothelial Keratoplasty was not recommended given an underlying large iris defect and planned aphakia (due to severe amblyopia limiting vision to count fingers), both of which would make air management of the graft difficult.

This 30-year-old patient presented with PBK secondary to anterior dislocation of a posterior chamber IOL. The patient has a history of severe amblyopia, a history of strabismus surgery, medically controlled glaucoma, and a traumatic iris with no superior iris remaining. The mechanism of the traumatic iris was unknown. The patient had received cataract surgery outside of the United States and years later developed diffuse microcystic and stromal corneal edema and pain due to ruptured bullae. The IOL model was unknown but was presumably originally placed posteriorly. On slit lamp exam, two superior haptics were visualized. Ultrasound biomicroscopy showed the haptics extending posterior to the iris with evidence of posterior synechiae from the iris to the haptic inferiorly as well as iris contact with the cornea inferiorly. Corneal pachymetry measured 882 μm. The patient underwent removal of the lens and a penetrating keratoplasty. The patient was left aphakic. Endothelial keratoplasty was not recommended given difficulty of air/gas management in the setting of a large iris defect and aphakia. The patient's graft remained clear for 3 years, but the patient was then lost to follow-up.

12.7 Treatment

12.7.1 Conservative Management

Medical treatment of PBK and ABK is aimed at alleviating patient pain and discomfort. Usually, these treatments are temporizing in preparation for a more definitive treatment. Therapeutic options include the use of topical sodium chloride agents (2% drops and 5% drops or ointment), which form a hypertonic layer that draws water out of the cornea by osmosis. This hypertonic reservoir might be prolonged with the use of a bandage soft contact lens which also reduces pain by preventing rupture of epithelial bullae. Concurrent use of dilating drops has been shown to further reduce pain from the concomitant iritis present in bullous keratopathy [26].

12.7.2 Surgical Management—Corneal Transplantation

12.7.2.1 Penetrating Keratoplasty (PKP)

A PKP is performed by transplanting all five layers of the cornea. Overall graft survival at 5 and 10 years is excellent and demonstrates that PKP is an effective and safe long-term treatment [27]. Graft failure rate at 10 years is significantly lower for PBK eyes undergoing PKP plus an ACIOL exchanged for a PCIOL (23%) compared with PBK eyes in which a pre-operative ACIOL was retained post-operatively (59%) [28].

12.7.2.2 Descemet Stripping (Automated) Endothelial Keratoplasty

Descemet's stripping endothelial keratoplasty (DSEK) (if the donor is prepared manually) or Descemet's stripping automated endothelial keratoplasty (DSAEK) replaces host Descemet membrane and endothelium with a thin layer of donor posterior stroma, Descemet membrane, and endothelium. This technique is an improved and easier version of an earlier surgery known as deep lamellar endothelial keratoplasty (DLEK) that required posterior host lamellar dissection. DSAEK ushered in an era of more rapid visual recovery after keratoplasty. It can result in best-corrected visual acuities of 20/25 or better. Thin DSAEK grafts (<80 μm) may outperform in terms of visual acuity compared to thicker DSAEK. DSAEK grafts have significantly lower immunological rejection rates than PKP [29].

12.7.2.3 Descemet's Membrane Endothelial Keratoplasty (DMEK)

DMEK is an exact anatomical replacement of diseased corneal Descemet membrane and endothelium. DMEK is a technically more challenging surgery and may result in more complications such as graft detachments and failures, but since 2014, the number of DMEK procedures has been rapidly catching up with DSAEK due to standardization of technique and eye bank preparation of grafts in western countries [9]. By eliminating donor stromal tissue, DMEK probably results in more rapid recovery and better vision than DSAEK [30] and lower initial immunologic rejection rates than DSAEK and PK for similar indications [29].

12.7.3 Alternatives to Corneal Transplantation

In eyes with limited or poor visual outcome or awaiting corneal transplantation, these alternative options can be utilized to alleviate pain and some optimize cosmesis.

12.7.3.1 Phototherapeutic and Superficial Keratectomy (PTK and STK)

PTK excimer laser energy provides symptomatic relief from painful bullae. The mechanism is multifactorial and likely related to a reduction in corneal thickness which lowers the osmotic load of the corneal stroma and enhances the efficacy of remaining endothelial cells [31]. Ablation of the subepithelial nerve plexus reduces corneal sensation and subsequent corneal scarring and stabilizes epithelial adhesion to the underlying Bowman layer decreasing recurrent bullae formation [32]. Superficial epithelial keratectomy (STK) combined with corneal cautery, and amniotic membrane transplantation may be effective [33]. In one case, resolution of pain was noted at a 42-month follow-up.

12.7.3.2 Corneal Crosslinking (CXL)

CXL with riboflavin and ultraviolet radiation was originally introduced as a photochemical treatment for corneal ectatic disorders such as Keratoconus and Post-LASIK ectasia [34] but is a theoretical management option for bullous keratopathy. Improvements in ocular pain may be observed from a reduction in CCT and corneal stromal strengthening reducing the potential space for fluid accumulation and bullae formation. However, at least one randomized controlled trial has shown no effectiveness in improvement of pain, corneal clarity, or vision [35].

12.7.3.3 Anterior Stromal Puncture (ASP)

ASP provides symptomatic relief for patients with pain from early localized edema. It is performed at the slit lamp by using a needle to create multiple stromal punctures. This may promote epithelial adhesion to the underlying stroma by stimulating the production of extracellular matrix proteins and can be used in conjunction with amniotic membrane or bandage contact lens to promote epithelial healing [31].

12.7.3.4 Conjunctival Flap

A thin conjunctival flap, also known as a Gundersen Flap, can be transposed over the cornea after removing the corneal epithelium. This technique relieves pain from exposed corneal nerves, while providing metabolic and mechanical support for corneal healing [36]. While not as cosmetically appealing, it is a historically effective way to reduce pain in an eye with poor vision.

12.8 Future Directions and Conclusions

Bullous keratopathy remains a challenging condition for cornea specialists. While advancements in cataract surgical technique and IOL design have reduced the incidence of PBK, a common indication for a corneal transplant in many parts of the world remains corneal edema following cataract surgery [3]. The introduction of novel intraocular devices may be an emerging etiology for endothelial decompensation. The rapid evolution of endothelial keratoplasty over the past few decades has improved surgical management of bullous keratopathy. Current therapies are being investigated to treat endothelial dysfunction using cell-based therapy. Cultured endothelial cells treated with Rho-associated kinase (ROCK) inhibitors and injected into the anterior chamber show promise for resolution of PBK [37] but data collection from phase 1/2 multicenter randomized controlled trials are underway (clinicaltrials.gov). While topical treatment of (ROCK) inhibitors may promote endothelial migration [38], it is unclear whether they will provide any stimulus for endothelial proliferation which would be an essential step in restoring clarity to a cornea with PBK. Other biological factors such as engineered fibroblast growth factor may have the potential to activate both endothelial cell proliferation and migration to restore endothelial pump function in cases of PBK [39]. Artificial endothelial layers may also provide a means to bypass endothelial transplantation and central migration [40].

Progress in corneal transplantation, emerging pharmacological modalities, and innovations in surgical devices and instrumentation could collectively reduce the burden of blindness from bullous keratopathy.

Acknowledgments Supported by grant P30 EY010572 from the National Institute of Health (Bethesda, MD), and by unrestricted departmental funding from Research to Prevent Blindness (New York, NY).

References

1. Narayanan R, Gaster RN, Kenney MC. Pseudophakic corneal edema: a review of mechanisms and treatments. Cornea. 2006;25(9):993–1004.
2. Chen X, Xu J, Chen X, Yao K. Cataract: advances in surgery and whether surgery remains the only treatment in future. Adv Ophthalmol Pract Res. 2021;1(1):100008.
3. Matthaei M, et al. Changing indications in penetrating keratoplasty: a systematic review of 34 years of global reporting. Transplantation. 2017;101(6):1387–99.
4. Geroski DH, et al. Pump function of the human corneal endothelium. Effects of age and cornea guttata. Ophthalmology. 1985;92(6):759–63.
5. Ali M, et al. Biomechanical relationships between the corneal endothelium and Descemet's membrane. Exp Eye Res. 2016;152:57–70.
6. DelMonte DW, Kim T. Anatomy and physiology of the cornea. J Cataract Refract Surg. 2011;37(3):588–98.
7. Szentmary N, Szende B, Suveges I. Epithelial cell, keratocyte, and endothelial cell apoptosis in Fuchs' dystrophy and in pseudophakic bullous keratopathy. Eur J Ophthalmol. 2005;15(1):17–22.
8. Cohen EJ, et al. Pseudophakic bullous keratopathy. Am J Ophthalmol. 1988;106(3):264–9.
9. Eye Bank Association of America. 2021 Eye banking statistical report. Eye Bank Association of America, W., D.C, p. 10. https://restoresight.org; 2021. Accessed 5 Sept 2022.
10. Mathews PM, et al. Etiology of global corneal blindness and current practices of corneal transplantation: a focused review. Cornea. 2018;37(9):1198–203.
11. Vasavada AR, et al. Impact of high and low aspiration parameters on postoperative outcomes of phacoemulsification: randomized clinical trial. J Cataract Refract Surg. 2010;36(4):588–93.
12. Foulks GN, et al. Histopathology of silicone oil keratopathy in humans. Cornea. 1991;10(1):29–37.
13. Pastor SA, et al. Corneal endothelial cell loss following trabeculectomy with mitomycin C. J Glaucoma. 1993;2(2):112–3.
14. Koo EB, et al. Effects of glaucoma tube surgery on corneal endothelial cells: a review. Eye Contact Lens. 2016;42(4):221–4.

15. Sirinek PE, Lin MM. Intracameral sustained release bimatoprost implants (Durysta). Semin Ophthalmol. 2022;37(3):385–90.
16. Seah I, Sng CCA, Ang M. Endothelial cell loss associated with minimally invasive glaucoma surgery. Curr Opin Ophthalmol. 2022;33(2):119–29.
17. Price MO, et al. Corneal endothelial dysfunction: evolving understanding and treatment options. Prog Retin Eye Res. 2021;82:100904.
18. Jeng BH, et al. Amantadine-associated corneal edema potentially irreversible even after cessation of the medication. Ophthalmology. 2008;115(9):1540–4.
19. Madreperla SA, Johnson M, O'Brien TP. Corneal endothelial dysfunction in digoxin toxicity. Am J Ophthalmol. 1992;113(2):211–2.
20. Arslan OS, et al. Histologic findings of corneal buttons in decompensated corneas with toxic anterior segment syndrome after cataract surgery. Cornea. 2013;32(10):1387–90.
21. Arthur SN, et al. Uveitis-glaucoma-hyphema syndrome and corneal decompensation in association with cosmetic iris implants. Am J Ophthalmol. 2009;148(5):790–3.
22. Alio JL, et al. Corneal graft failure: an update. Br J Ophthalmol. 2021;105(8):1049–58.
23. Doughty MJ, Zaman ML. Human corneal thickness and its impact on intraocular pressure measures: a review and meta-analysis approach. Surv Ophthalmol. 2000;44(5):367–408.
24. American Academy of Ophthalmology et al. 2019–2020 BCSC: Basic and Clinical Science Course. External Disease and Cornea 2019: American Academy of Ophthalmology.
25. Zander D, et al. Predicting edema resolution after Descemet membrane endothelial keratoplasty for Fuchs dystrophy using Scheimpflug tomography. JAMA Ophthalmol. 2021;139(4):423–30.
26. Gasset AR, Kaufman HE. Bandage lenses in the treatment of bullous keratopathy. Am J Ophthalmol. 1971;72(2):376–80.
27. Thompson RW Jr, et al. Long-term graft survival after penetrating keratoplasty. Ophthalmology. 2003;110(7):1396–402.
28. Writing Committee for the Cornea Donor Study Research, G, et al. Factors associated with corneal graft survival in the cornea donor study. JAMA Ophthalmol. 2015;133(3):246–54.
29. Mannis MJ, Holland E. The evolution of contemporary keratoplasty, Cornea, vol. 5. New York: Elsevier; 2021.
30. Chamberlain W, et al. Descemet endothelial thickness comparison trial: a randomized trial comparing ultrathin Descemet stripping automated endothelial keratoplasty with Descemet membrane endothelial keratoplasty. Ophthalmology. 2019;126(1):19–26.
31. Siu GD, Young AL, Jhanji V. Alternatives to corneal transplantation for the management of bullous keratopathy. Curr Opin Ophthalmol. 2014;25(4):347–52.
32. Hart CT, Cleary G, Chan E. Long-term outcomes of phototherapeutic keratectomy for bullous keratopathy. Cornea. 2022;41(2):155–8.
33. Shalabi N, et al. Superficial epithelial keratectomy, cautery, and amniotic membrane transplant for the treatment of painful bullous keratopathy in eyes with poor visual potential. Cornea. 2014;33(7):755–9.
34. D'Oria F, Palazon A, Alio JL. Corneal collagen cross-linking epithelium-on vs. epithelium-off: a systematic review and meta-analysis. Eye Vis (Lond). 2021;8(1):34.
35. Choy BNK, et al. Randomized control trial on the effectiveness of collagen cross-linking on bullous keratopathy. Cornea. 2020;39(11):1341–7.
36. Guell JL, et al. Treatment of symptomatic bullous keratopathy with poor visual prognosis using a modified Gundersen conjunctival flap and amniotic membrane. Ophthalmic Surg Lasers Imaging. 2012;43(6):508–12.
37. Kinoshita S, Koizumi N, Ueno M. Cultured cells and ROCK inhibitor for bullous keratopathy. N Engl J Med. 2018;379(12):1185.
38. Syed ZA, Rapuano CJ. Rho kinase (ROCK) inhibitors in the management of corneal endothelial disease. Curr Opin Ophthalmol. 2021;32(3):268–74.
39. Pizzuto S, et al. A human corneal organ culture model of Descemet's stripping only with accelerated healing stimulated by engineered fibroblast growth factor 1. J Vis Exp. 2022;185
40. Auffarth GU, et al. Implantation of an artificial endothelial layer for treatment of chronic corneal edema. Cornea. 2021;40(12):1633–8.

Congenital Hereditary Endothelial Dystrophy

13

Neet Mehta and Muralidhar Ramappa

Congenital hereditary endothelial dystrophy (CHED) [1, 2] is a rare autosomal recessive corneal endothelial dystrophy that presents as early onset childhood corneal clouding, typically manifesting at birth or immediately thereafter. It has a high predilection in areas with high rates of parental consanguinity and is commonly seen in Asian and Middle Eastern countries. CHED is characterized by bilateral, diffuse, noninflammatory, and ground glass cloudy cornea, and a mutation of SLC4A11 [3], an abundant corneal solute transporter, has been attributed to its causation. SLC4A11 is a large multi-domain integral membrane protein encoded by the SLC4A11 gene, which was earlier thought to be a bicarbonate transporter-related protein 1 (BTR1) [4] but was later found to be a sodium-borate cotransporter [5]. CHED cases have also been associated with progressive, postlingual sensorineural hearing loss (SNHL), a condition known as the Harboyan Syndrome [6]. The ocular manifestation is indistinguishable from the normal forms of CHED, and the overlap is due to the presence of SLC4A11 gene products in the spiral ligament fibrocytes of the inner ear.

The embryonic development of the anterior segment per se comprises the separation of the lens vesicle from the surface ectoderm, followed by three waves of neural crest cell migration. After 12 weeks of gestation, the corneal endothelium produces Descemet's membrane composed of an anterior banded zone produced before the

N. Mehta
Academy of Eye Care Education, L V Prasad Eye Institute, Hyderabad, Telangana, India

M. Ramappa (✉)
Institute for Rare Eye Diseases and Ocular Genetics, L V Prasad Eye Institute, Hyderabad, Telangana, India

The Cornea Institute, L V Prasad Eye Institute, Hyderabad, Telangana, India

Jasti V Ramanamma Children's Eye Care Center, L V Prasad Eye Institute, Hyderabad, Telangana, India
e-mail: muralidhar@lvpei.org

F. A. Woreta, R. B. Singh (eds.), *Cornea Casebook*, Current Practices in Ophthalmology, https://doi.org/10.1007/978-981-96-0495-1_13

fifth month of gestation and a posterior non-banded zone produced later. CHED, which characteristically has a normal anterior banded zone and an abnormal posterior non-banded zone, is postulated to arise from an abnormality in "neural crest cell terminal differentiation," manifested by degeneration of corneal endothelial cells after synthesizing a normal anterior banded zone in the fifth month of gestation [7].

Prompt management of cases with corneal cloudiness in this particular young age group is vital to minimizing the risk of amblyopia and secondary corneal changes that can lead to poor postsurgical functional outcomes in this subset of cases.

This chapter focuses on the varied presentation of CHED that can commonly be seen in our clinics, with a special focus on optimizing treatment strategies.

13.1 Case 1

13.1.1 Summary

- Mild to moderate CHED have better visibility of anterior segment details and minimum secondary corneal scarring due to chronic corneal edema.
- Mild to moderate cases can benefit from undergoing DSAEK.
- DSAEK at a younger age group will have better patient compliance as compared to penetrating keratoplasty.

An 8-year-old girl was brought to the clinic, her mother complaining of bluish discoloration of both eyes since birth. The girl had difficulty seeing and managing her routine activities. She had a normal birth history and normal developmental milestones. There was a positive history of parental consanguinity. Her visual acuity was limited to counting fingers at 1 m in both eyes. On examination, she had ground glass corneal cloudiness in both her eyes, with anterior segment details very hazily seen (Fig. 13.1).

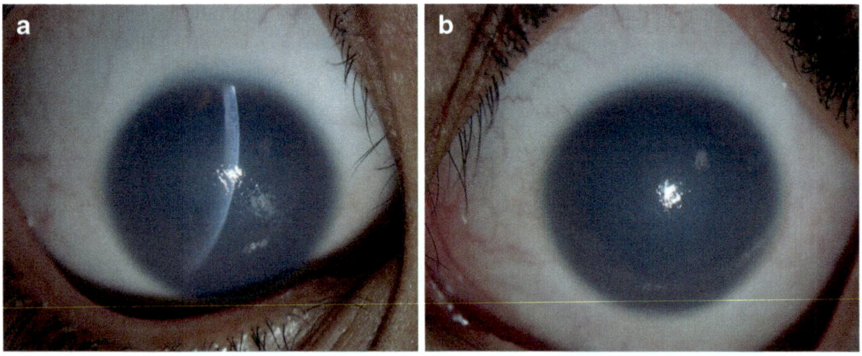

Fig. 13.1 Slitlamp photographs of both the eyes showing a diffuse ground glass corneal haze with poor visualization of the anterior chamber details

Proceeding with such a case, it is important to rule out other conditions that can present as Congenital Corneal clouding. These may result from hereditary, developmental, infectious, or metabolic causes. They can be bilateral and can be seen in isolation or in association with other ocular or systemic abnormalities. It is very important for an ophthalmologist to accurately diagnose the condition, predict the natural history of the disorder, look for associated ocular and systemic abnormalities, provide genetic counseling, and begin appropriate medical or surgical therapy promptly.

The prevalence of congenital corneal opacity (CCO) is approximately 3:100,000 newborns, and this figure increases to 6:100,000 if congenital glaucoma is included [8]. Although CHED is rare, it needs to be differentiated from other causes that might mimic a similar presentation. Out of these, those that very closely mimic CHED include Primary Congenital Glaucoma (PCG), X-linked Endothelial Corneal Dystrophy (XECD), posterior polymorphous dystrophy (PPMD), Congenital Hereditary stromal Dystrophy (CHSD), and Mucopolysaccharidosis (MPS).

A thorough clinical history of the onset of the corneal clouding, other associated systemic factors, family history, birth history, history of trauma, and medication use all help point out the diagnosis. Apart from these, numerous investigations aid us in coming to a diagnosis.

Coming back to the case, Anterior-segment Optical coherence tomography (AS-OCT) shows the following characteristic features (Fig. 13.2):

1. A generalized increase in corneal thickness.
2. Thickened epithelial layer with a few epithelial bullae with underlying irregular Bowman's membrane.
3. Increased stromal thickness.
4. Abnormally thickened and hyporeflective Descemet's membrane.

A diagnosis of CHED was made, and the patient was offered the option of surgical intervention in the form of Descemet's stripping automated endothelial keratoplasty (DSAEK). She underwent sequential DSAEK with superficial keratectomy—first in the right eye and then in the left—due to persistent corneal edema that led to an overlying secondary epithelial degenerative pannus.

Apart from AS-OCT, there are other diagnostic aids that can help in reaching the diagnosis and selecting the appropriate management:

1. *Pachymetry*: CHED cases will show 2–3 times more central corneal thickness than the age-matched normal.
2. *Slit-lamp Subjective grading system* for corneal haze: A study by Ramappa et al. [9] graded corneal clouding in CHED based on the visibility of iris structures and the presence or absence of anterior stromal scarring into; mild-minimal corneal cloudiness not obscuring the iris details (Fig. 13.3a), moderate-obscured iris details, but visible pupillary silhouette (Fig. 13.3b) and severe iris and pupillary details obscured (Fig. 13.3c).

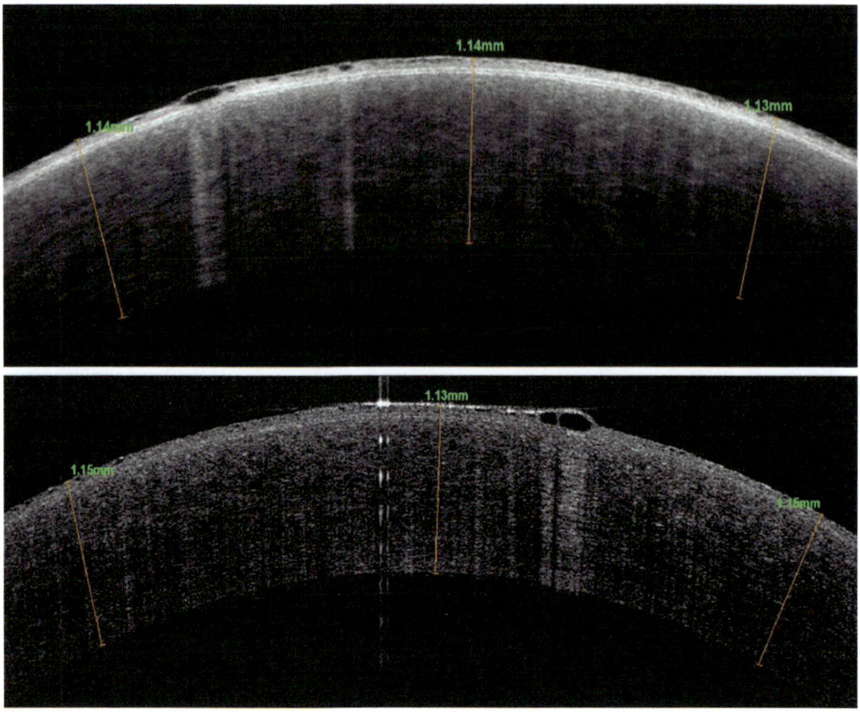

Fig. 13.2 Anterior Segment-Optical Coherence Tomography (ASOCT) of the patient

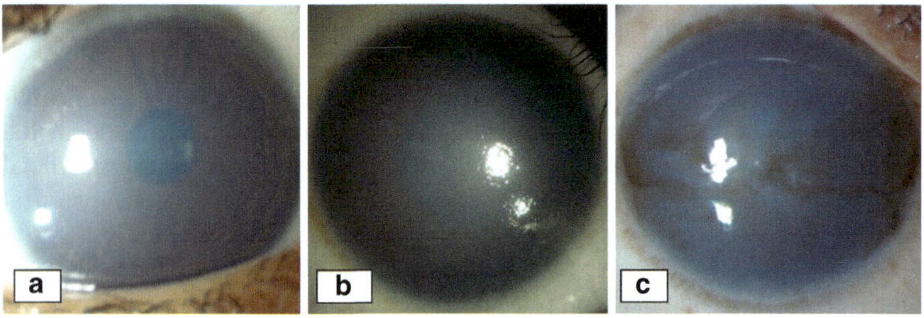

Fig. 13.3 Showing the various grades of corneal haze. (**a**) Mild disease with minimal corneal cloudiness not obscuring the iris details. (**b**) Moderate corneal haze obscures the iris details, but the pupillary silhouette could be seen. (**c**) Severe disease wherein the iris, and pupillary details both are obscured. (Ramappa et al. [9])

3. *Densitometry Using Scheimpflug Imaging*: Measures the reflectance pattern using a Scheimpflug imaging device, giving an objective measurement of the amount of corneal haze. The densitometry readings are standardized from a scale of 0 to 100 grayscale units (GSU). Based on this, one can get a quantitative estimation of the corneal cloudiness the patient has at individual layers (Fig. 13.4) [13, 14].

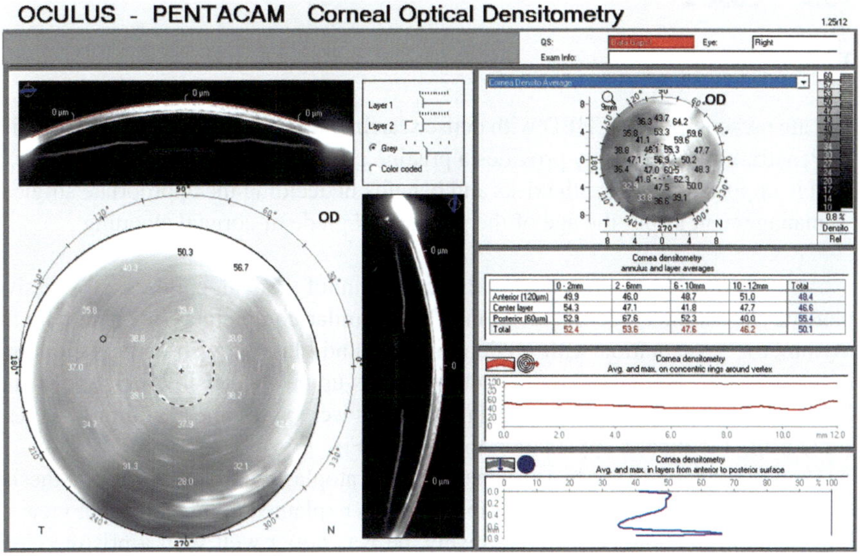

Fig. 13.4 Corneal densitometry [10] quantifies the corneal clouding based on reflectivity pattern. Here, densitometry values are calculated after dividing the cornea into Anterior (120 µm), central and Posterior (60 µm) divisions, using the Pentacam

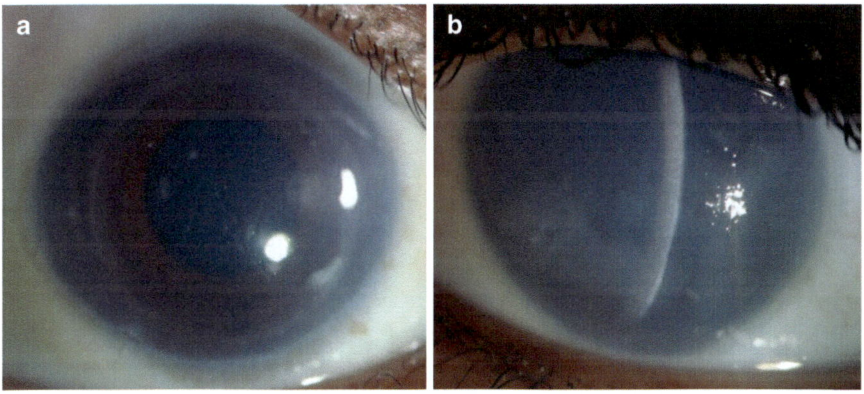

Fig. 13.5 (**a**) Right eye post DSAEK showing a well central clear corneal lenticule; (**b**) Left eye of the same patient

The patient underwent DSAEK in the right eye initially and post-operatively the lenticule was well attached and centered and she was started on postoperative regimen of antibiotics and tapering doses of topical steroids. At 1 month visit, she achieved an unaided visual acuity of 20/50 in the operated eye (Fig. 13.5).

13.2 Case 2

13.2.1 Summary

- Late presentation of CHED with dense scarring may have underlying amblyopia.
- Penetrating keratoplasty provides a pristine clear graft and better visual acuity.
- It is important to titrate the risks and benefits in deciding the appropriate surgical management as per the age of the patient and grade of corneal clouding.

An 18-year-old boy presented with a complaint of gradual, painless, progressive blurring of vision. Three of his siblings have similar complaints. He came with an asymmetric presentation with predominant ground glass greyish corneal clouding in his right eye. His vision was counting fingers up to 1 meter in his right eye and 20/60p in his left eye. His intra-ocular pressures were within normal limits as measured using Goldmann applanation tonometer (Fig. 13.6).

He was planned for right eye penetrating keratoplasty under general anesthesia, and the possibility of underlying amblyopia was explained to the parents in view of long-standing pathology. Postoperatively, he was doing well with a pristine clear graft, a visual acuity of 20/40p, and normal intraocular pressures. He was asked to follow a strict regimen of regular monthly follow-ups, and compliance with medication was explained (Fig. 13.7).

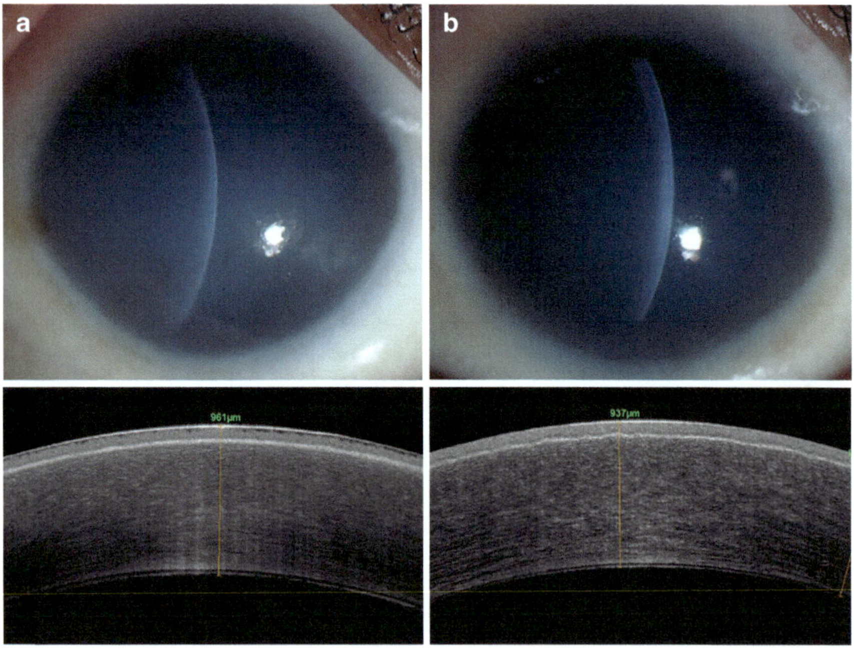

Fig. 13.6. Asymmetrical presentation of CHED with right eye (**a**) showing more corneal cloudiness than the left eye (**b**)

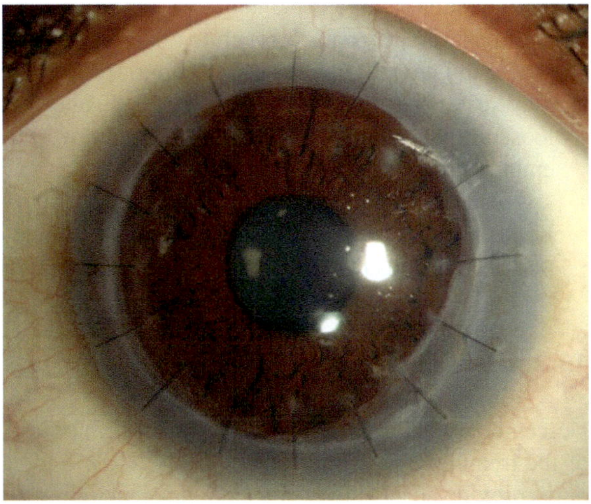

Fig. 13.7 Right eye post penetrating keratoplasty in a case of CHED

13.2.2 Decision Makers in the Management of CHED

Managing corneal opacification in CHED has been a challenge due to the lack of a conservative approach and surgical management being the only definitive treatment modality available. The various surgical modalities include conventional full-thickness penetrating keratoplasty (PK) [12], Descemet's stripping automated endothelial keratoplasty (DSAEK) [14–16], and Descemet membrane endothelial keratoplasty (DMEK) [17–19].

13.2.3 PK in CHED

Penetrating keratoplasty (PK) was the standard treatment for children with CHED. Still, the decision to proceed with PK is complex due to the challenges of pediatric PK. Pediatric PK presents unique preoperative, intraoperative, and postoperative issues that must be addressed.

1. Preoperatively, the timing and risk-benefit ratio of surgery must be considered. Also, assessing the degree of visual impairment is difficult in the pre-verbal age group.
2. Intraoperative challenges [20] in PK for CHED in younger age groups include:
   (a) Low scleral rigidity.
   (b) Tendency for anterior rotation of the lens iris diaphragm leading to shallowing of the anterior chamber, peripheral anterior synechiae (PAS) formation, iris incarceration in the wound, endothelial trauma, and glaucoma.
   (c) Expulsion of intraocular contents due to an "open to sky" procedure.

3. Postoperatively, high demand of care is needed with regular, frequent follow-ups and a more stringent postoperative steroid regimen to counter the rapid and severe inflammatory response or allograft rejection. The robust wound healing may result in corneal neovascularization, uneven contraction of tissue, early loosening of sutures, irregular astigmatism, overriding of graft tissue with poor epithelialization, and ulceration.

   However, having said the drawbacks, the full-thickness Penetrating Keratoplasty does provide a pristine clear cornea that can amount to superior postoperative visual acuity compared to selective endothelial keratoplasty.

13.2.4 DSAEK in CHED

Descemet-stripping automated endothelial keratoplasty (DSAEK) is currently one of the treatments of choice in cases of CHED. Endothelial transplantation procedures provide an edge over conventional penetrating keratoplasty in providing:

1. Faster visual rehabilitation.
2. Fewer sutures-and-suture-related complications.
3. "Closed-system" technique, thus reducing the risk of sight-threatening intraoperative complications, particularly suprachoroidal hemorrhage.
4. Preserves the structural integrity of the globe, so, postoperative wound dehiscence is infrequent.

Long-term outcomes of DSAEK in corneal endothelial disorders in children less than 14 years of age, in a study by Ramappa et al. [9], showed a pediatric DSAEK survival probability at 1, 3, 5, and 7 years to be 92%, 87%, 78%, and 78%, respectively which was superior to the results reported for pediatric Penetrating Keratoplasty (PK). In this series, CHED was the most common indication for pediatric DSAEK (116 eyes, that is 69.5%), which had a long-term graft survival probability of 97%, 95%, 90%, and 90% at 1, 3, 5, and 7 years, respectively.

This study also suggested that CHED, with no previous interventions, influenced long-term graft survival in a positive way. In previously failed graft cases, also DSAEK gave excellent visual outcomes and could be a superior alternative to performing a repeat PK in a pediatric population. Besides, recent evidence has shown that DSAEK produces lower rates of intraocular pressure elevation when compared to PK. Some authors also believe that DSAEK is associated with lower rates of acute graft rejection. This would translate into reduced postoperative visits with fewer examinations under anesthesia and a less frequent steroid dosage with an early tapering of steroids, thus avoiding the side effects of steroid use.

However, the drawbacks of DSAEK include technical difficulty, poor visibility during peeling off the Descemet membrane, thickened Descemet endothelial complex, and more robust stromal adhesions.

13.2.5 DMEK in CHED

Descemet's membrane endothelial keratoplasty (DMEK) [21] further refines the posterior Lamellar approaches; however, the procedure is much more demanding and challenging to manage among infants and leads to more endothelial cell loss and dislocation than other EK techniques.

13.3 Summary of Management

Analyzing the outcomes from various studies with different surgical modalities in CHED, the cases of CHED with significant secondary corneal changes like stromal and Descemet's level scarring, band-shaped keratopathy, etc., appear to benefit more from undergoing a full-thickness keratoplasty than undergoing a DSAEK. DSAEK can be the treatment of choice in cases of CHED with a relatively clearer cornea with minimal to nil secondary corneal changes.

Nevertheless, some cases of CHED with a very mild haze and near-normal visual acuity do not warrant any surgical management. These cases may benefit from non-invasive management with the use of topical NSAIDs and anti-glaucoma agents. One review of CHED proposed algorithm [11] to help decide the appropriate management based on the subjective corneal grading and AS-OCT parameters (Fig. 13.8). Apart from these, amblyopia management and appropriate genetic counseling are crucial to the success of surgical interventions. Newer management modalities like the use of NSAIDs, and gene editing could have a potential in the future of managing cases of CHED.

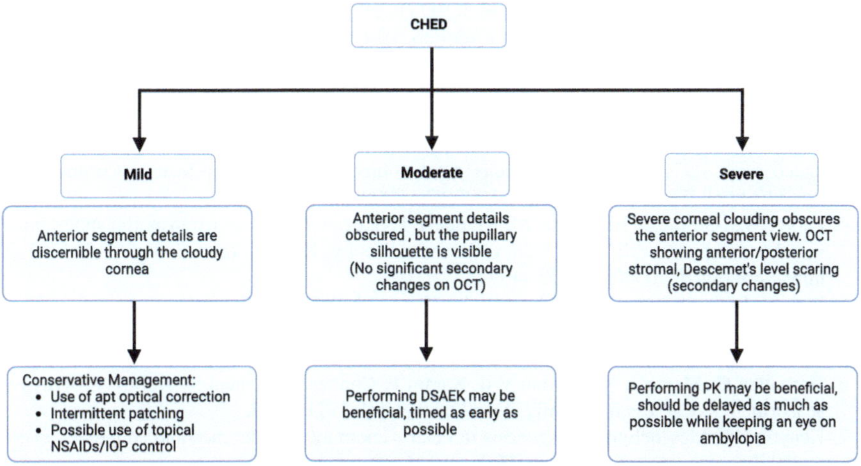

Fig. 13.8 Flowchart of proposed algorithm for congenital hereditary endothelial dystrophy

13.4 Summary

1. CHED Type 2 is an Autosomal recessive corneal endothelial dystrophy that presents as early onset corneal cloudiness.
2. Differentiating from other masquerades of congenital corneal cloudiness is of vital importance.
3. One can take the help of AS-OCT, pachymetry, and Densitometry in quantitative grading of corneal clouding.
4. Definite management includes PK, DSAEK, and DMEK, which can be decided after a thorough benefit-risk-to-benefit assessment.
5. DSAEK outscores PK taking into consideration the not so stringent post-operative steroid regimen and follow-up schedule and less suture-related complication.
6. PK however does provide a superior visual outcome but has its own set of complications.
7. Conservative approaches are generally limited to cases of CHED with early corneal edema and no secondary changes and are still under experiment.

Financial support Hyderabad Eye Research Foundation and Hyderabad Eye Institute, Hyderabad, India.

Financial Disclosure(s) The authors have no proprietary or commercial interest in any materials discussed in this article.

References

1. Weiss JS, Møller HU, Aldave AJ, et al. IC3D classification of corneal dystrophies–edition 2. Cornea. 2015 Feb;34(2):117–59. https://doi.org/10.1097/ICO.0000000000000307.
2. Mehta N, Verma A, Achanta DS, Kannabiran C, Roy S, Mishra DK, Chaurasia S, Edward DP, Ramappa M. Updates on congenital hereditary endothelial dystrophy. Taiwan J Ophthalmol. 2023;13(4):405–16. https://doi.org/10.4103/tjo.TJO-D-23-00135.
3. Roy S, Praneetha DC, Vendra VP. Mutations in the corneal endothelial dystrophy-associated gene SLC4A11 render the cells more vulnerable to oxidative insults. Cornea. 2015 Jun;34(6):668–74. https://doi.org/10.1097/ICO.0000000000000421.
4. Parker MD, Ourmozdi EP, Tanner MJ. Human BTR1, a new bicarbonate transporter superfamily member and human AE4 from kidney. Biochem Biophys Res Commun. 2001;282(5):1103–9. https://doi.org/10.1006/bbrc.2001.4692.
5. Park M, Li Q, Shcheynikov N, Zeng W, Muallem S. NaBC1 is a ubiquitous electrogenic Na+-coupled borate transporter essential for cellular boron homeostasis and cell growth and proliferation. Mol Cell. 2004;16(3):331–41.
6. Harboyan G, Mamo J, Kaloustian V d, Karam F. Congenital corneal dystrophy. Progressive sensorineural deafness in a family. Arch Ophthalmol. 1971;85:27.
7. Kenyon KR. Mesenchymal dysgenesis in Peter's anomaly, sclerocornea and congenital endothelial dystrophy. Exp Eye Res. 1975;21(2):125–42.
8. Nichal KK, Naor J, Jay V, et al. Clinicopathological correlation of congenital corneal opacification using ultrasound biomicroscopy. Br J Ophthalmol. 2002;86:62–9.

9. Ramappa M, Mohamed A, Achanta DSR, Tumati CSK, Chaurasia S, Edward DP. Descemet stripping automated endothelial keratoplasty in pediatric age group: a decade of our experience. Cornea. 2021;40(12):1571–80. https://doi.org/10.1097/ICO.0000000000002811.
10. Lopes B, Ramos I, Ambrósio R Jr. Corneal densitometry in keratoconus. Cornea. 2014;33(12):1282–6. https://doi.org/10.1097/ICO.0000000000000266.
11. Neet Mehta & Muralidhar Ramappa. Novel proposed algorithm in congenital hereditary endothelial dystrophy. Semin Ophthalmol. 2022;38:108. https://doi.org/10.1080/08820538.2022.2094713.
12. Aasuri MK, Garg P, Gokhle N, et al. Penetrating keratoplasty in children. Cornea. 2000;19(2):140–4. https://doi.org/10.1097/00003226-200003000-00004.
13. Ashar JN, Pahuja S, Ramappa M, et al. Deep anterior lamellar keratoplasty in children. Am J Ophthalmol. 2013;155(3):570–574 e1. https://doi.org/10.1016/j.ajo.2012.09.029.
14. Ramappa M, Ashar J, Vaddavalli PK, et al. Endothelial keratoplasty in children: surgical challenges and early outcomes. Br J Ophthalmol. 2012;96(8):1149–51. https://doi.org/10.1136/bjophthalmol2011-300941.
15. Ashar JN, Ramappa M, Chaurasia S. Endothelial keratoplasty without Descemet's stripping in congenital hereditary endothelial dystrophy. J AAPOS. 2013;17(1):22–4. https://doi.org/10.1016/j.jaapos.2012.09.013.
16. Ashar JN, Ramappa M, Vaddavalli PK. Paired-eye comparison of Descemet's stripping endothelial keratoplasty and penetrating keratoplasty in children with congenital hereditary endothelial dystrophy. Br J Ophthalmol. 2013;97(10):1247–9. https://doi.org/10.1136/bjophthalmol-2012-302602.
17. Saad A, Ghazzal W, Keaik M, Indumathy TR, Fogla R. Outcomes of Descemet's membrane endothelial keratoplasty for congenital hereditary endothelial dystrophy. J AAPOS. 2020;24(6):358.e1–6. https://doi.org/10.1016/j.jaapos.2020.07.018. Epub 2020 Nov 27
18. Sharma N, Agarwal R, Jhanji V, Bhaskar S, Kamalakkannan P, Nischal KK. Lamellar keratoplasty in children. Surv Ophthalmol. 2020;65(6):675–90. https://doi.org/10.1016/j.survophthal.2020.04.002.
19. Mittal V, Sehdev N, Mittal R. Descemet membrane endothelial keratoplasty in congenital hereditary endothelial dystrophy: initial experiences. Cornea. 2021;40(8):972–6. https://doi.org/10.1097/ICO.0000000000002701.
20. AlArrayedh H, Collum L, Murphy CC. Outcomes of penetrating keratoplasty in congenital hereditary endothelial dystrophy. Br J Ophthalmol. 2018;102(1):19–25. https://doi.org/10.1136/bjophthalmol2016-309565.
21. Stuart AJ, Romano V, Virgili G, Shortt AJ. Descemet's membrane endothelial keratoplasty (DMEK) versus Descemet's stripping automated endothelial keratoplasty (DSAEK) for corneal endothelial failure. Cochrane Database Syst Rev. 2018;6(6):CD012097. https://doi.org/10.1002/14651858.CD012097.pub2.

Part IV

Ectatic Disorders

Keratoconus & Corneal Ectasia

14

Lorena Barros, Alexandre Batista da Costa Neto, Guilherme Portas-Almeida, and Renato Ambrósio Jr

14.1 Introduction

Keratoconus (KC) is a bilateral disease that is usually asymmetric. It is characterized by progressive thinning and bulging of the cornea, caused by a continuous cycle of biomechanical decompensation of the stroma, leading to progressive myopia and irregular astigmatism [1, 2]. The prevalence varies among studies, ranging from 0.05% to 5.4%. These differences may be related to ethnic and environmental factors—for example, a higher prevalence among people from the Middle East and Eastern Asia, and in regions with hot, dry climates. There is consensus that there are essential triggers, mainly eye rubbing [3–5]. Also, secondary ectasia may occur due to a purely mechanical insult, whereas primary ectasia is related to intrinsic biomechanical and genetic factors (reflecting stress susceptibility), in line with McGhee's two-hit hypothesis [1, 5, 6].

L. Barros (✉)
Department of Ophthalmology, Federal University of the State of Rio de Janeiro (UNIRIO), Rio de Janeiro, Brazil

A. B. da Costa Neto
Department of General Surgery, Federal University of the State of Rio de Janeiro (UNIRIO), Rio de Janeiro, Brazil

G. Portas-Almeida
Department of Ophthalmology, São José Local Health Unit, Lisbon, Portugal

R. Ambrósio Jr
Department of Ophthalmology, Federal University of the State of Rio de Janeiro (UNIRIO), Rio de Janeiro, Brazil

Instituto de Olhos Renato Ambrósio, Rio de Janeiro, Brazil

F. A. Woreta, R. B. Singh (eds.), *Cornea Casebook*, Current Practices in Ophthalmology, https://doi.org/10.1007/978-981-96-0495-1_14

A recent mixed-methods study on parental knowledge about KC found that not only was literacy regarding their children's disease generally unsatisfactory, but also that increased KC severity was statistically associated with lower parental education levels [7]. With that being said, lack of information about the disease should be fought with the help of global campaigns, to raise awareness about the disease and give effective strategies to address KC, relieving the suffering of the patients and reducing disease burden [8]. The diagnosis of KC and corneal ectasia is nowadays based on Scheimpflug-based tomography and biomechanical assessments, using cutting-edge algorithms that offer additional diagnostic power, especially on forme fruste or cases with high susceptibility of developing clinical ectasia [9–13]. The higher diagnostic capacity helped clinicians bring better care to KC patients, changing the paradigmatic therapeutic modalities of the previous era—spectacle correction, contact lens (CL) prescription, and Penetrating Keratoplasty (PK)—and better chances to rehabilitate vision on such complex cases. The big challenge nowadays relies on deciding when to or not to indicate surgery [14, 15]. A prospective study by experienced physicians showed us that classical CXL procedures could achieve complication rates of up to 3%. Thus, the cost-benefits of every invasive procedure must always be measured to provide the best healthcare possible [14, 16].

14.2 Clinical Case 1

Two 19-year-old monozygotic females presented for a second opinion about KC diagnosis. They had no systemic disease, no allergies, and no previous history of eye surgery. The family history was negative for any ophthalmic disease. On examination, the best spectacle-corrected Visual Acuity (BSCVA) of twin n° 1 was 20/25 in the right eye (OD) (sph −2.50 cyl −2.00@15°) and 20/25 in the left eye (OS) (sph −1.75 cyl −1.25@155°), and 20/20 in OD (sph +0.25 cyl −0.70@8°) and 20/20 in OS (sph −0.25 cyl −1.50@137°) of twin n° 2. The intraocular pressure (IOP) was 8 mm Hg in both eyes (OU) of twin n°1 and 15.0 mmHg in OD, and 14.5 mmHg in OS of twin n°2. Slit-lamp examination (SLE), Fundoscopic examination (FE), and specular microscopy were routine on both eyes.

Diagnose of KC was confirmed on OU of twin n° 1 and VAE-NT (very asymmetric Ectasia with normal tomography) on OD of twin n° 2 using the Placido disk-based topography (Oculus Keratograph 5®), Pentacam HR® corneal tomography (Oculus Optikgeräte GmbH, Wetzlar, Germany; Figs. 14.1 and 14.2) and Corvis-ST® (Oculus Optikgeräte GmbH, Wetzlar, Germany; Figs. 14.3 and 14.4). Transepithelial corneal crosslinking (TE-CXL) was done on both eyes in 10/2019 of twin n° 1. Medical management, disease education, and control of risk factors were adopted to halt ectasias progression in both eyes. The patient was followed for 2.5 years. Pentacam HR of OD and OS showed discreet flattening of anterior curvatures in twin n°1 and long-term stability in twin n°2.

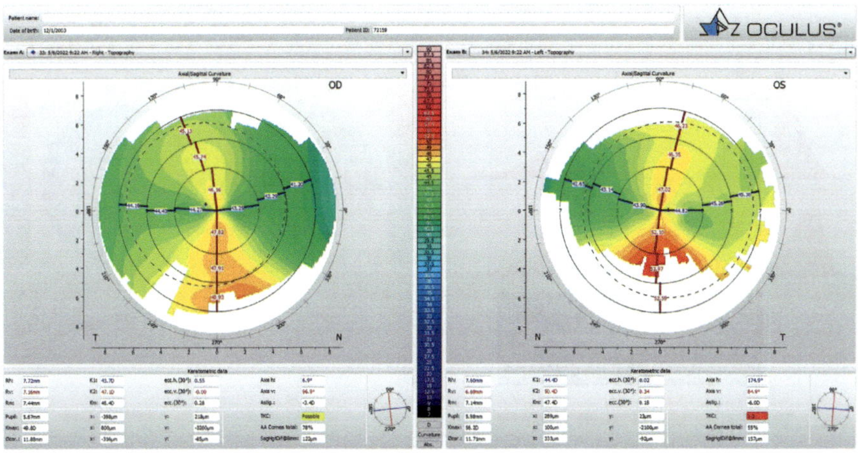

Fig. 14.1 Placido's topography: (OCULUS Keratograph®5 M) bilateral irregular and asymmetric astigmatism in the twin n°1

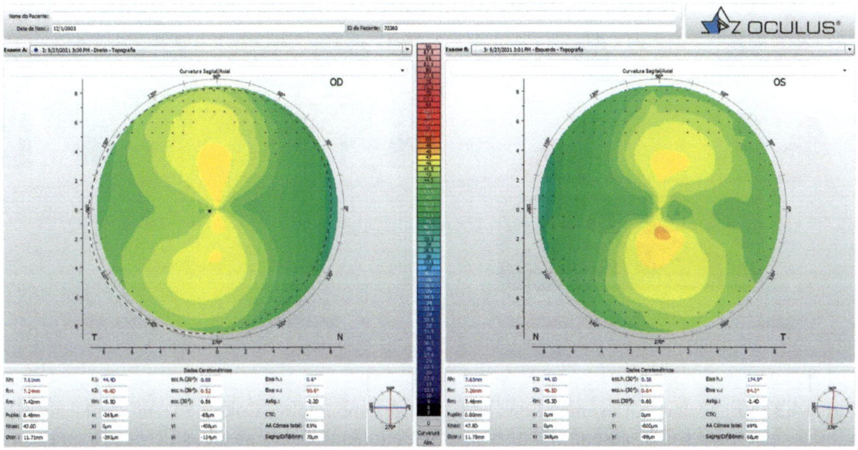

Fig. 14.2 Placido's topography: (OCULUS Keratograph®5 M) bilateral regular and symmetric astigmatism in the twin n°2

14.2.1 Discussion

As mentioned in the chapter introduction, the multimodal examination is critical to evaluate and characterize ectasia and ectasia susceptibility. If possible, patients with KC and their first-degree relatives must undergo genetic screening because there are strong indicators of genetic etiology in the pathogenesis of KC [17]. In the future genetic study will enable us to understand the underlying mechanisms that cause these associations. Integration of parameters from different exams showed a more accurate and precise capacity for detecting forme fruste ectasia than topographic,

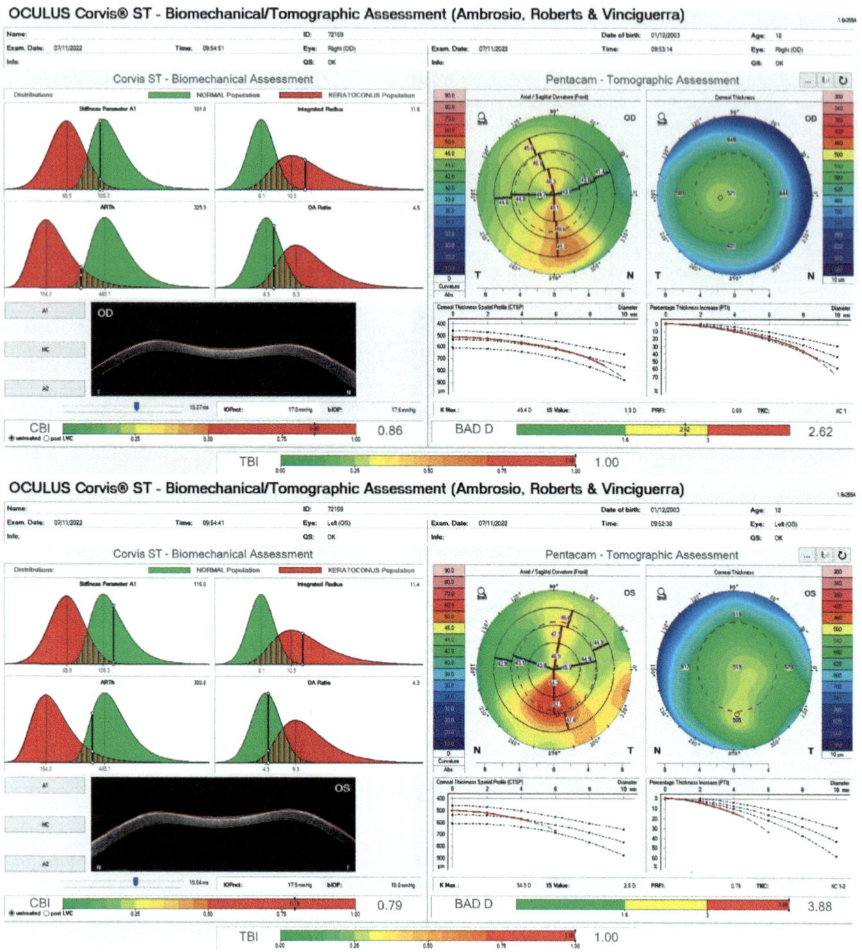

Fig. 14.3 Biomechanical examinations and corneal tomography (Corvis ST and Pentacam HR, Oculus) identified KC disease in OU of twin n°1: Belin/Ambrósio Enhanced Ectasia Display total deviation (BAD-D) OD 2.62 and OS 3.88; Tomographic and Biomechanical Index (TBI_V2) (Ambrosio, 2022) OD 1.00 and OS 1.00; Pentacam Random-Forest Index (PRFI) of OD 0.69 and OS 0.79; Corvis Biomechanical Index (CBI) OD 0.86 and OS 0.79; Kmax OD 49.4D and OS 54.5D; thinnest point thickness of OD 521 μm and OS 505 μm

tomographic, or biomechanical parameters alone [13]. What we would like to highlight with the study of these cases is to suspect ectasia in first-degree parents of patients diagnosed with clinical KC. This also highlights the importance of multimodal imaging for both the diagnosis and treatment of ectasia. The second twin had the diagnosis of VAE-NTB (Normal topography/biomechanic) on OS. Just BAD-D index from tomography and TBI from the integration of tomography with biomechanics were to characterize the Ectasia susceptibility of OS. All topography indexes like I-S, TKC, and the CBI from Corvis-ST were average. This ectasia

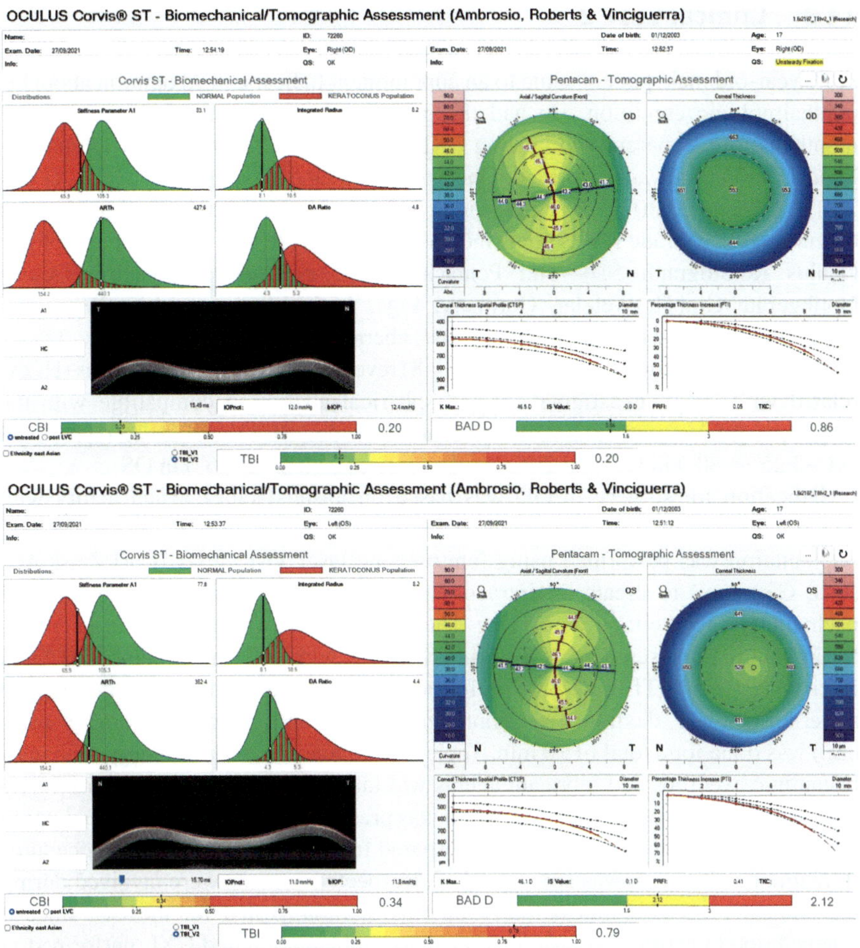

Fig. 14.4 Biomechanical examinations and corneal tomography (Corvis ST and Pentacam HR, Oculus), respectively, of twin n°2: BAD-D OD 0.86 and OS 2.12; TBI_V2 (Ambrosio, 2022) of OD 1.00 and OS 0.20; PRFI of OD 0.41 and OS 0.05; CBI of OD 0.20 and OS 0.34; Kmax of OD 46.5 D and OS 46.1 D; thinnest point thickness of OD 553 μm and of OS 529 μm

susceptibility characterization is essential once the twin n°2 should be highly discouraged from performing LVC and eye rubbing.

Overview

KC is associated with genetics as an ectatic dystrophy of the cornea and is aggravated by extrinsic biomechanical weakening factors on the cornea.

Ectasia Susceptibility is a novel concept related to the increase in sensitivity or enhanced ectasia diagnostics.

14.3 Clinical Case 2

A 14-year-old male patient came to an appointment to hear a third opinion about his ophthalmologic condition. He had the presumptive diagnosis of bilateral KC 3 months before, apparently indicating CXL in both eyes. The thorough ophthalmological evaluation was performed. Uncorrected distance visual acuity (UDVA) was 20/150 OD and 20/30 OS. With the aid of complementary multimodal imaging, the diagnosis of KC grade II was confirmed using the Placido disk-based topography—Oculus Keratograph 5®)—and Pentacam HR® corneal tomography (Oculus Optikgeräte GmbH, Wetzlar, Germany; Figs. 14.5, 14.6, and 14.7). Wavefront Analysis (WFA) with Raytracing-based aberrometer iTrace® (HOYA, Tracey Technologies, Houston, TX, USA; Fig. 14.8) revealed high-order aberrations (HOA) related with irregular astigmatism and spherical aberration compatible with the diagnosis. WFA-assisted manifest refraction provided BCSVA of 20/25 (sph −0.50 cyl −3.25 @ 80°) in OD and 20/20 (sph −0.25 cyl −1.25 @ 95°) in OS.

Indication for surgery in OD was based on unsatisfactory visual acuity with glasses and contact lens intolerance. The intrastromal corneal ring segment (ICRS) implantation was performed using femtosecond laser VisuMax® (Carl Zeiss AG, Jena, Germany) to create an intracorneal tunnel at 75% depth of the minimal pachymetry on Scheimpflug imaging. The main incision was made at the steep axis for implanting one segment of Keraring SI6 150° with 200 μm (Mediphacos, Belo Horizonte, Brazil). TE-CXL was performed, using the tunnel traject to impregnate a sterile, isotonic, dextran-free Riboflavin solution and UVA irradiation (9 mW/ cm^2) was done for a total of 10 min. Topical treatment for chronic allergy with antihistaminic eyedrops and lubricant agents was taken on and omega-3 essential fatty acid and riboflavin oral supplementation was prescribed. The patient was told not to rub the eyes, advising that OS could be spared from additional invasive procedures if treatment adherence was accomplished. Respective parents were involved during the clinical process. Clinical follow-up was then suggested for the OS, since it retained good uncorrected vision. After ICRS implantation and CXL performed in OD, UDVA improved to 20/40 and remained stable from the sixth month, as the BSCVA improved to 20/25 (+0.50 sph −2.0 cyl at 85°). Flattening of anterior corneal shape was demonstrated by Scheimpflug-based tomography (Fig. 14.7). OCT-AS (RTVue-100®, Optovue Inc., Fremont, CA) showed growth of central epithelial thickness on surrounding areas of the ICRS (Fig. 14.9). The patient has been followed for over 8 years and 3 months (99 months), with yearly follow-up with complementary imaging (tomography and biomechanical evaluation with Pentacam HR® and Corvis ST®; Fig. 14.10). Anatomical and biomechanics parameters remained stable OU, with Belin ABCD Progression display showing unchanged anterior and posterior curvature values (Fig. 14.11), retaining BSCVA of 20/20.

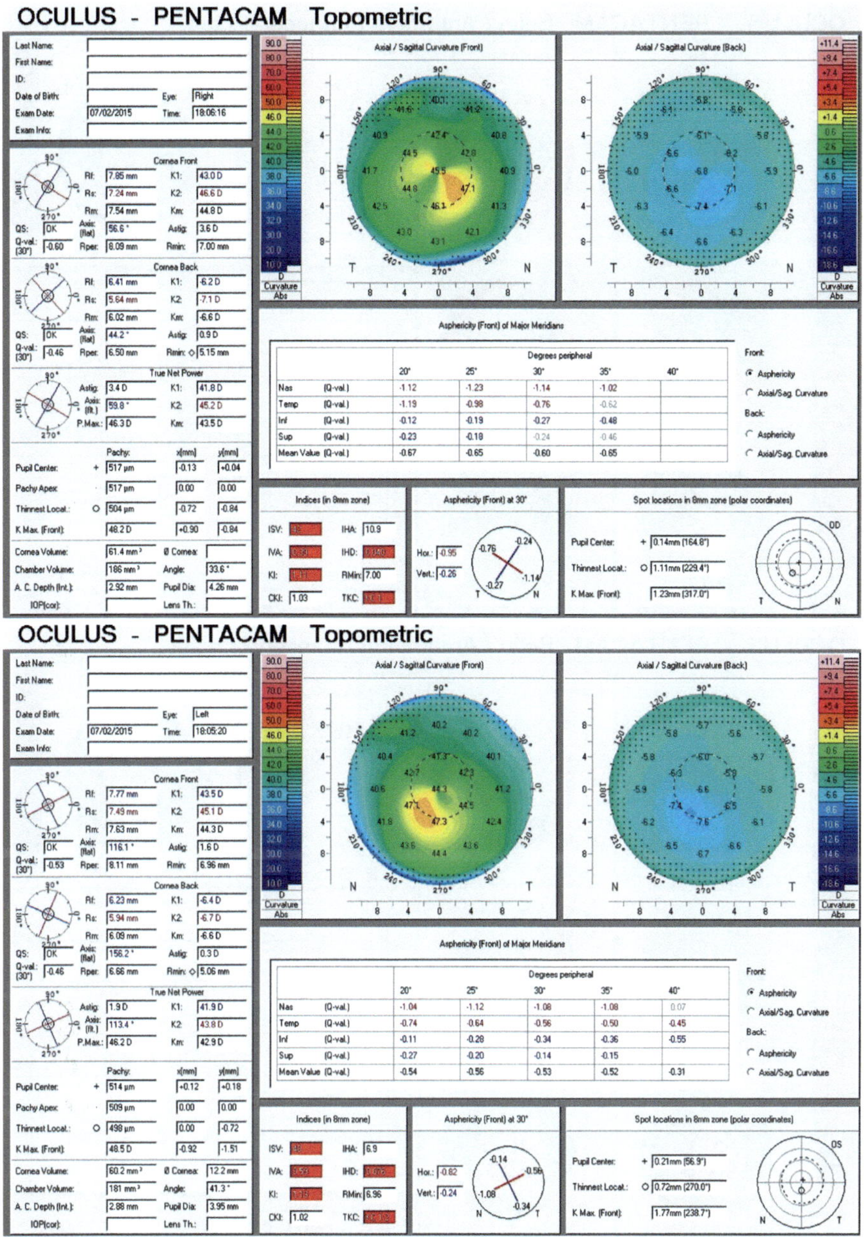

Fig. 14.5 Pentacam topometric display of OU showing relatively symmetric KC (slightly worse OD > OS), with asymmetric bow-tie appearance

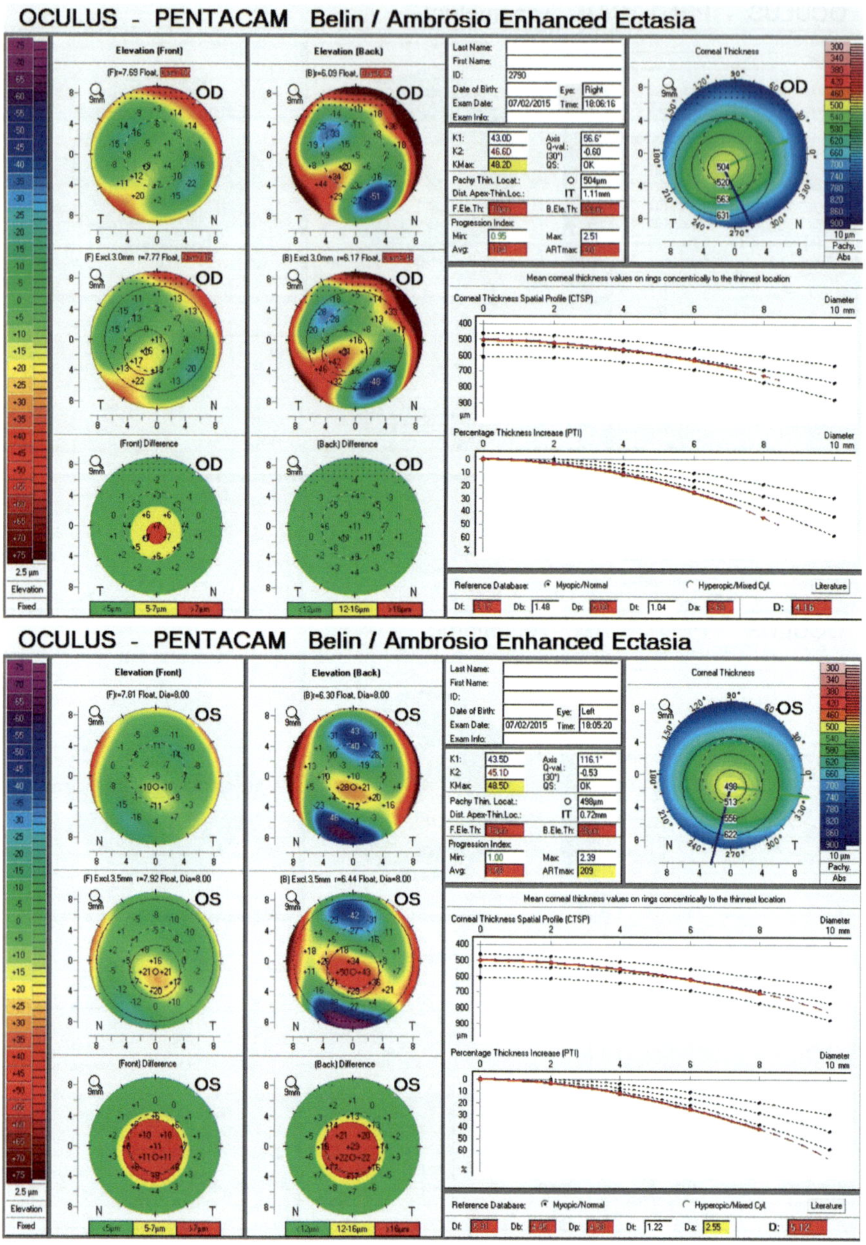

Fig. 14.6 Belin-Ambrósio Enhanced Ectasia display of OU showing alteration of both. Front and back elevation and pathologic pachymetry map progression with BAD-D > 1.45

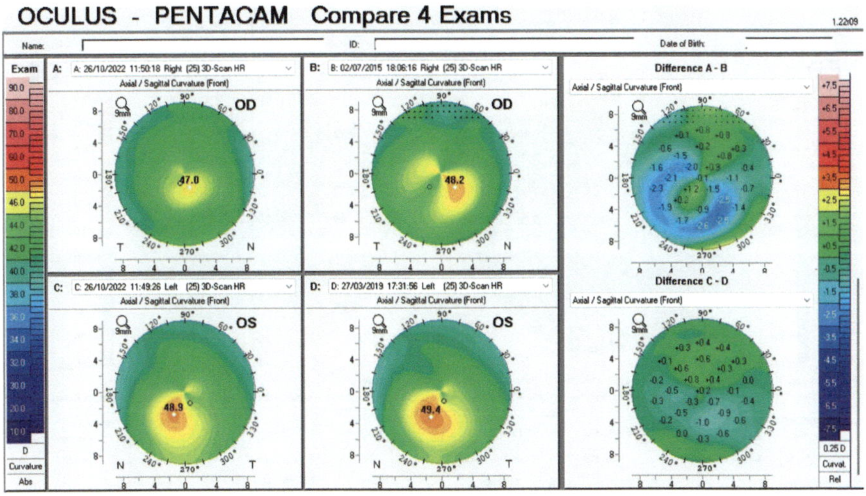

Fig. 14.7 Topometric evolution of both eyes. (**a**) OD after implantation of ICRS and TE-CXL; (**b**) same eye, baseline exam; (**a-b**) Difference of corneal surface topography after the procedure, showing flattening effect of anterior curvature; (**c**): OS on the last visit exam; (**d**): OS, 3 years and half ago; (**c-d**): Difference of topographic aspect of the cornea, showing irrelevant alterations

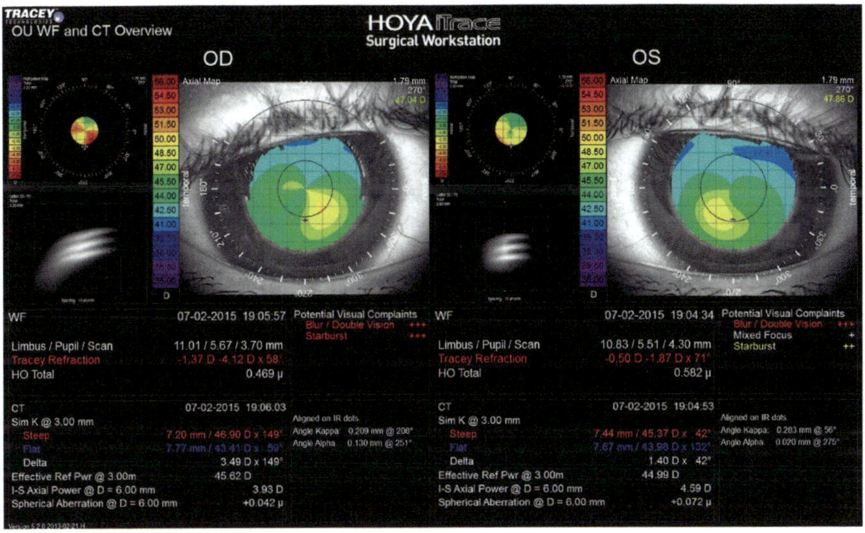

Fig. 14.8 Raytracing aberrometry of both eyes (OU) shows considerable high-order aberrations (HOA) related to irregular astigmatism and spherical aberration

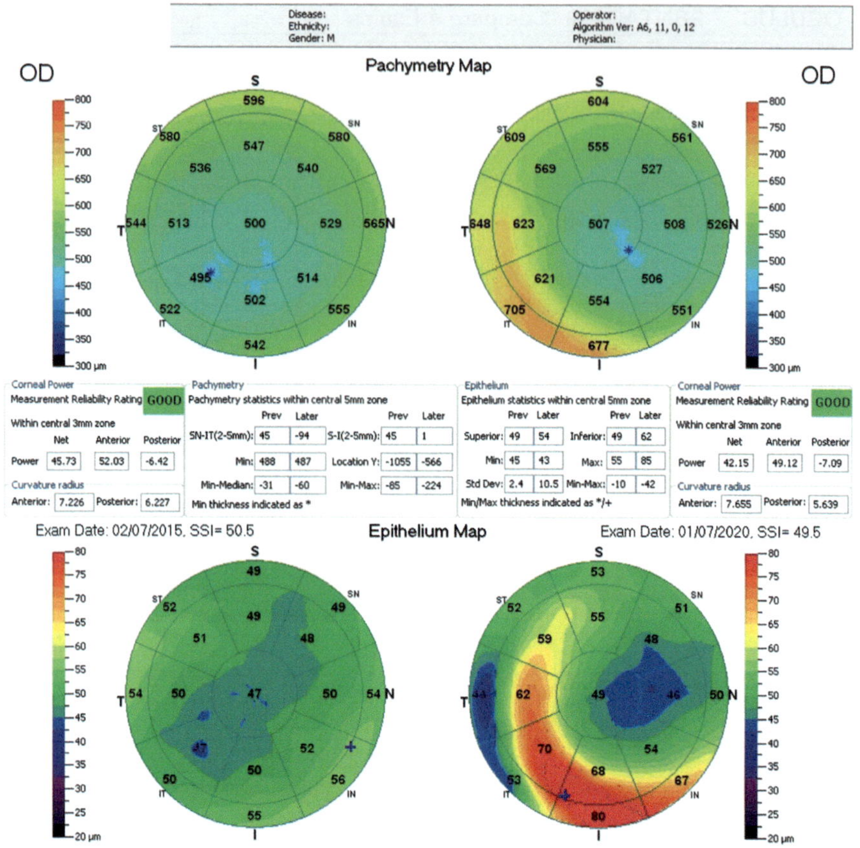

Fig. 14.9 Pachymetry map (total and sectorial), showing the reactive thickening effect after ICRS implantation on the central epithelium. Of note, the relative thinning of corneal epithelium of area overlying the ICRS

14.3.1 Discussion

This case illustrates an early stage clinical KC on OU. Topographic indexes on the Pentacam display showed values compatible with a clinical diagnosis of KC. According to Fernando Faria-Correia et al., cut-offs of ISV > 38, IHD > 0.021, and IVA > 0.32 demonstrated high reliability as diagnostic tools for KC, with Areas Under Curvature (AUC) of 0.977, 0.974, and 0.958, respectively [18]. Tomographic assessment also showed altered parameters, namely, Best-Fit Sphere (BFS) anterior and posterior elevation maps and BAD-D higher than 1.62. The area under receiver operating curvatures (AUROC) of the BAD-D and its logistic regression-based index (BAD-DI) was significantly lower than that for the Tomographic and Biomechanical Index (TBI), as was published in 2017 [13]. TBI is a random-forest, Artificial Intelligence (AI) parameter based on the sum of Scheimpflug-based corneal tomography and biomechanical assessment. Previous studies had first raised

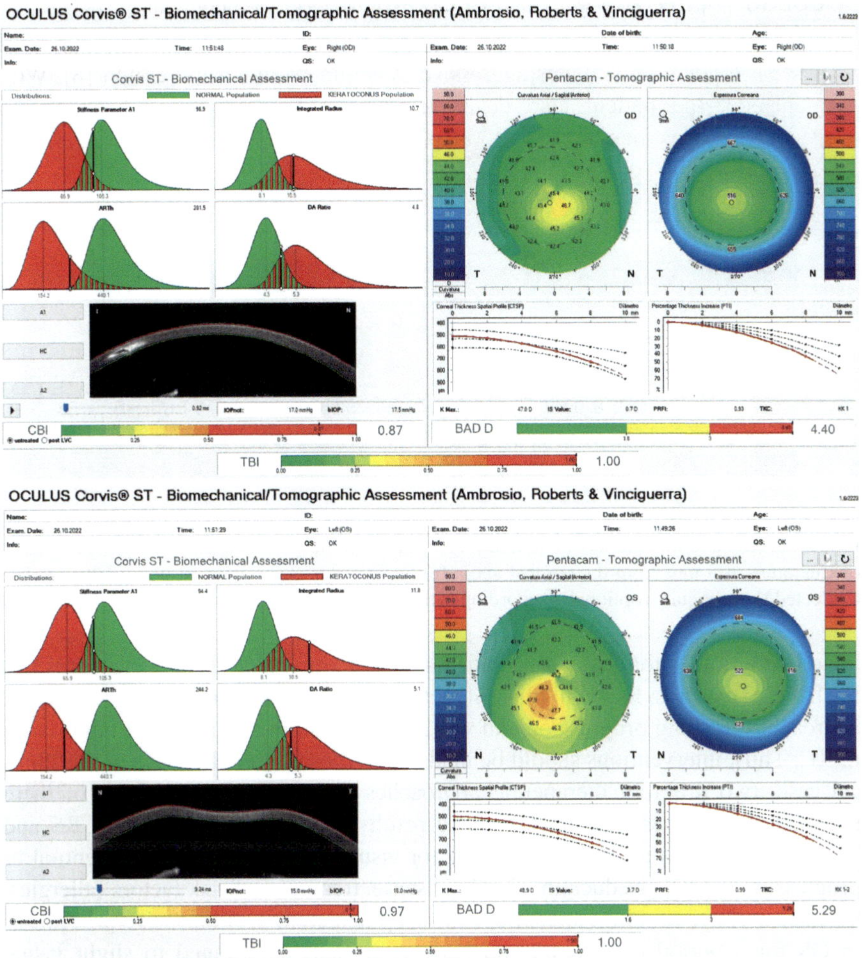

Fig. 14.10 Biomechanical and tomographic assessment of both eyes, showing altered biomechanical and tomographic indexes. TBI had the maximum value possible (1.00), showing absolute certainty on the diagnosis of KC

the possibility and showed its more accurate and precise capacity for detecting forme fruste ectasia than topographic, tomographic, or biomechanical parameters alone [10, 13]. Invasive procedures such as ICRS and CXL should be cautiously offered to KC patients, as these can rarely cause complications. High-risk factors associated with CXL-associated complications include age over 35 and DCVA >20/25 [16]. Managing KC and corneal ectasia cases demands high diagnostic power, requires good clinical decisions, and, last but not least, exhaustive comprehension of the condition [8, 15]. The clinician's role is vital in bringing parents and patients to the decision-making process, raising awareness of risk factors for disease progression, and showing strategies to help them manage their disease. He must

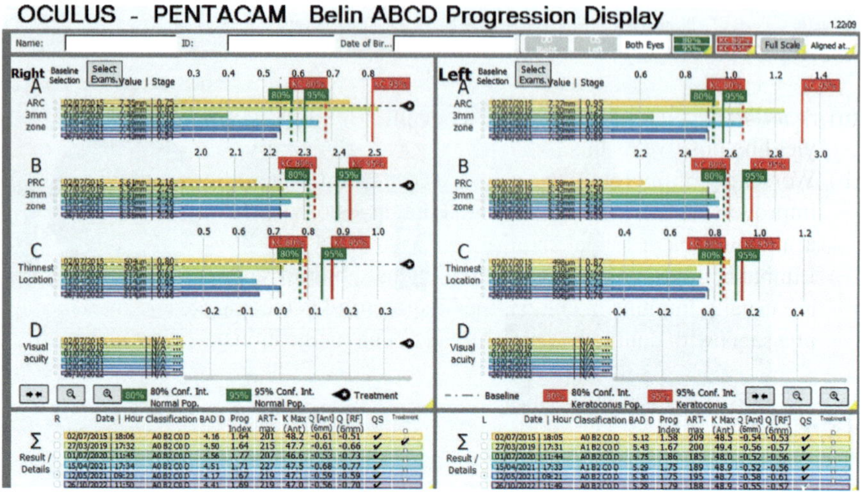

Fig. 14.11 Belin ABCD progression scale, showing structural stability of KC OU over 7 years of follow-up. (**a**) Anterior Radius of Curvature at 3 mm from the corneal apex; (**b**) Posterior Radius of Curvature at 3 mm from the corneal apex; (**c**) Pachymetry at the thinnest point; (**d**) Distance Corrected Visual Acuity (optional). According to the scale, KC of OU are both classified as A0B2C0

underline attitudes that can spare patients from additional surgical procedures [8]. Each case requires its own plan of action, as each eye might need different approaches. Halting progression and visual rehabilitation are of utmost importance in KC. Thus, interventions should be made upon those principles [14]. In this clinical case, two different therapeutic approaches were adopted, and both of them revealed effectiveness and very positive results: the associated use of ICRS and TE-CXL acted as a therapeutic strategy for visual rehabilitation and prevention of progression in OD, as education for the disease, treatment of risk factors (allergies, avoidance of eye rubbing) and strict follow-up helped to avoid invasive procedures in OS for a period of 7 years and half, as well as contributed to slight visual improvement.

Overview

Surgery in KC is indicated if there is unsatisfactory corrected visual acuity (with CL or glasses) and/or if there is documented or high risk of progression of the disease.

Clinical treatment and close monitoring are the ideal approach if good vision is present in a stable ectatic cornea.

Risks and benefits of surgery must always be considered and explained to KC patients.

14.4 Clinical Case 3

A 40-year-old woman was diagnosed with KC by her previous ophthalmologist 2 years ago. She came searching for a second opinion. She had no systemic disease and no allergies. The patient had no previous history of eye surgery or treatment for her KC. The family history was negative for any ophthalmic disease. On examination, the BSCVA was 20/20 in OD (sph +0.25 cyl −0.25@8°) and 20/20 in OS (sph −0.25 cyl −1.50@137°). The IOP was 14 mm Hg in OU. The slit-lamp examination demonstrated bilateral central guttata, confirmed by specular microscopy showing corneal guttae bilaterally. (Fig. 14.12). The Placido's topography, corneal anterior segment tomography, and biomechanics are shown in Figs. 14.13, 14.14, and 14.15.

14.4.1 Discussion

KC is an ectatic corneal disorder that typically manifests in young adulthood with decreasing visual acuity associated with progressive corneal ectasia, myopia, and irregular astigmatism. Most previous studies analyzing the pedigrees of familial KC have reported an AD (autosomal dominant) mode of inheritance [19, 20].

Fuchs' endothelial corneal dystrophy (FECD) is characterized by a decrease in endothelial cell density and regularity and in advanced cases, leads to progressive corneal edema. Decreased visual acuity (VA) is mainly due to corneal guttae and edema formation. In some cases, FECD may be hereditary and has a female preponderance of 3:1, with onset typically in the fourth decade of life and a prevalence of 4–10% in adults over 40 [21].

KC can occur in association with other dystrophies. In general, corneal dystrophies are a group of genetically determined corneal diseases. More than 12 chromosomes have been associated with corneal dystrophies [19]. The evidence of familial inheritance, dizygotic twins' discordance, and variable association of the pathology with other known genetic disorders are strong indicators of genetic etiology, at least in a subset of patients [22].

KC has been described as associated with posterior polymorphous dystrophy, ICE (irido corneal endothelial) syndrome, Fuchs, and anterior basement membrane dystrophy [20]. There are also a few sporadic instances of triple corneal dystrophy association—KC, FD, and epithelial basement membrane corneal dystrophy, three cases reported by Cremona et al. [20] and another case reported by Mazzotta et al. [23] In a recent review, association with FECD + KC was found in 15 papers presenting 69 cases [24].

Some authors hypothesize that the two clinical entities (KC and FECD) may have a common genetic descent [22]. Although the two pathologies are commonly seen in day-to-day clinical practice, and their coexistence has been reported rarely.

Corneal central thickness measurements do not represent the extent of stromal lamellae loss and endothelial function. KC is linked with corneal thinning, and FECD increases corneal thickness. Jurkunas and Azar [25] analyzed this important

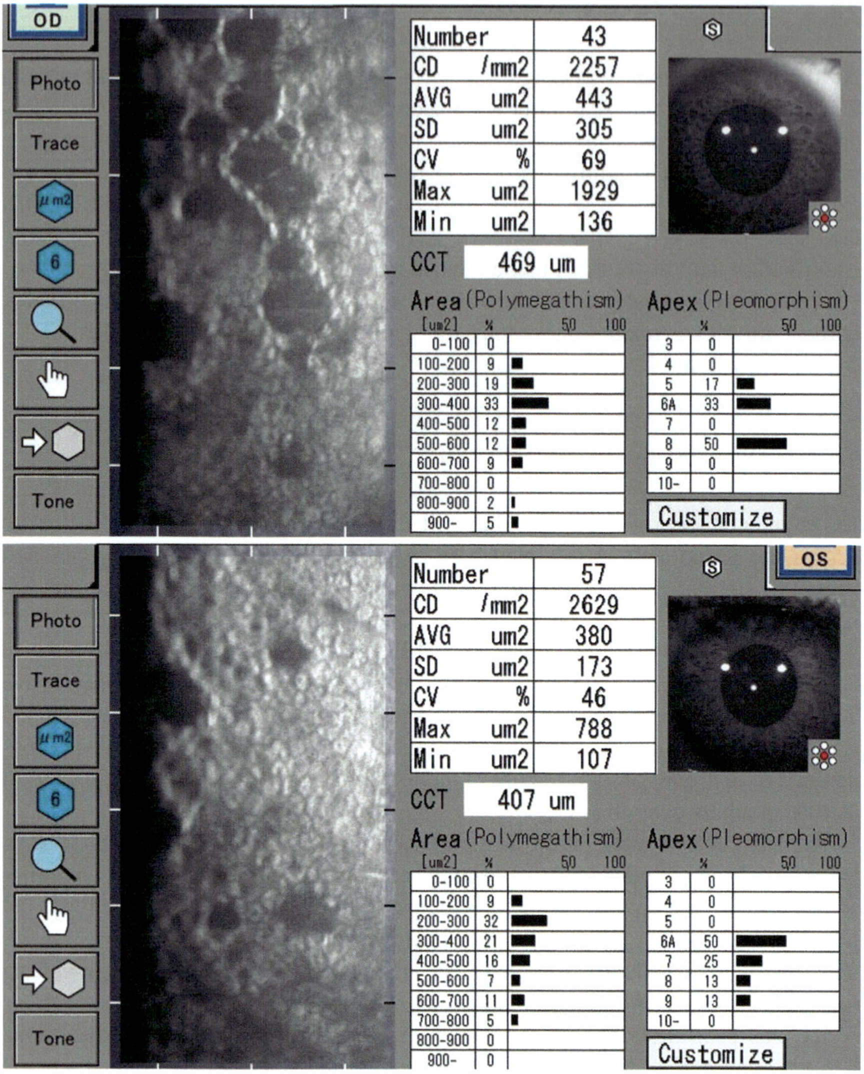

Fig. 14.12 Specular microscopy showing corneal guttata, polymegathism, pleomorphism and areas of excrescence in both eyes

critical issue and highlighted that corneal thinning due to KC and thickening due to FECD may give false pachymetry readings [20]. Also, there was a negative correlation between the amount of guttata and keratometry (K) readings: the more advanced the guttata, the lower the K readings [26]. When these two dystrophies coexist, the disease severity or progression of each one can be underestimated.

Careful slit lamp examination, corneal specular microscopy, topography, and tomography combined with biomechanical characterization are critical to evaluate and characterize the coexistence of both diseases. If possible, patients with

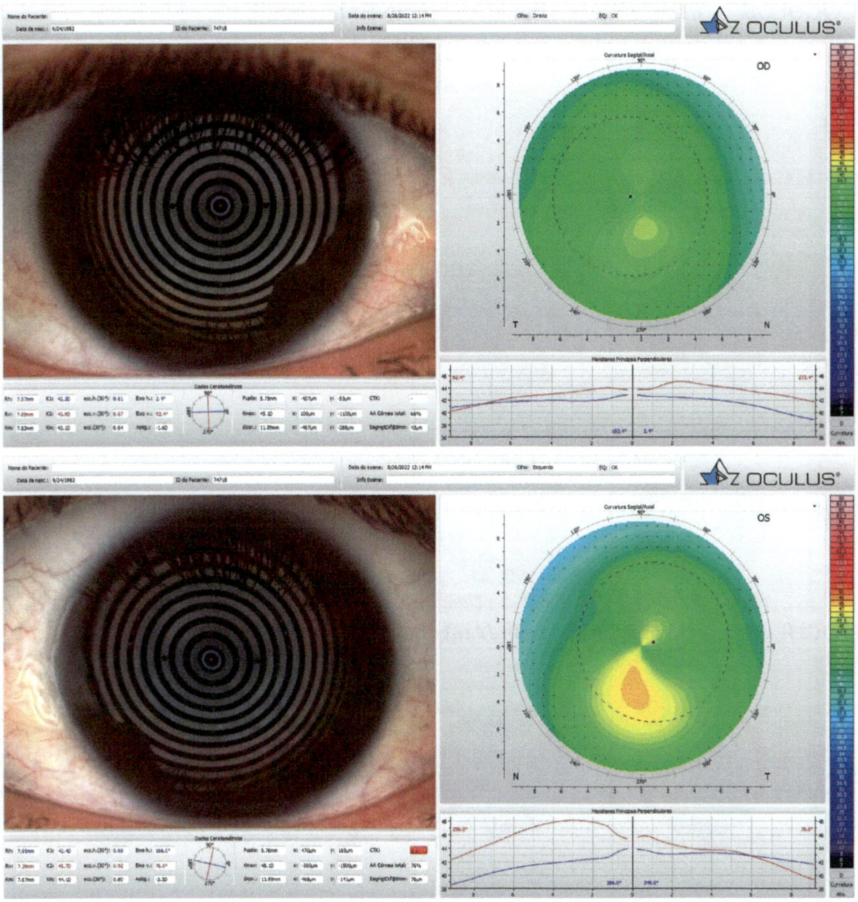

Fig. 14.13 Placido's topography: (OCULUS Kerato-graph®5M) bilateral irregular and asymmetric astigmatism

combined KC and FECD and their first-degree relatives must undergo genetic screening. The gene study will help us to identify the mechanisms involved with these associations.

> **Overview**
> KC can appear in association with other corneal dystrophies.
>
> Further investigation of the co-appearance of corneal dystrophies is essential and might lead to the discovery of gene mutations responsible for it.
>
> In cases of coexistence of KC and FECD, pachymetric measurements can be falsely high and so don't represent the true thinning of stromal lamellae.

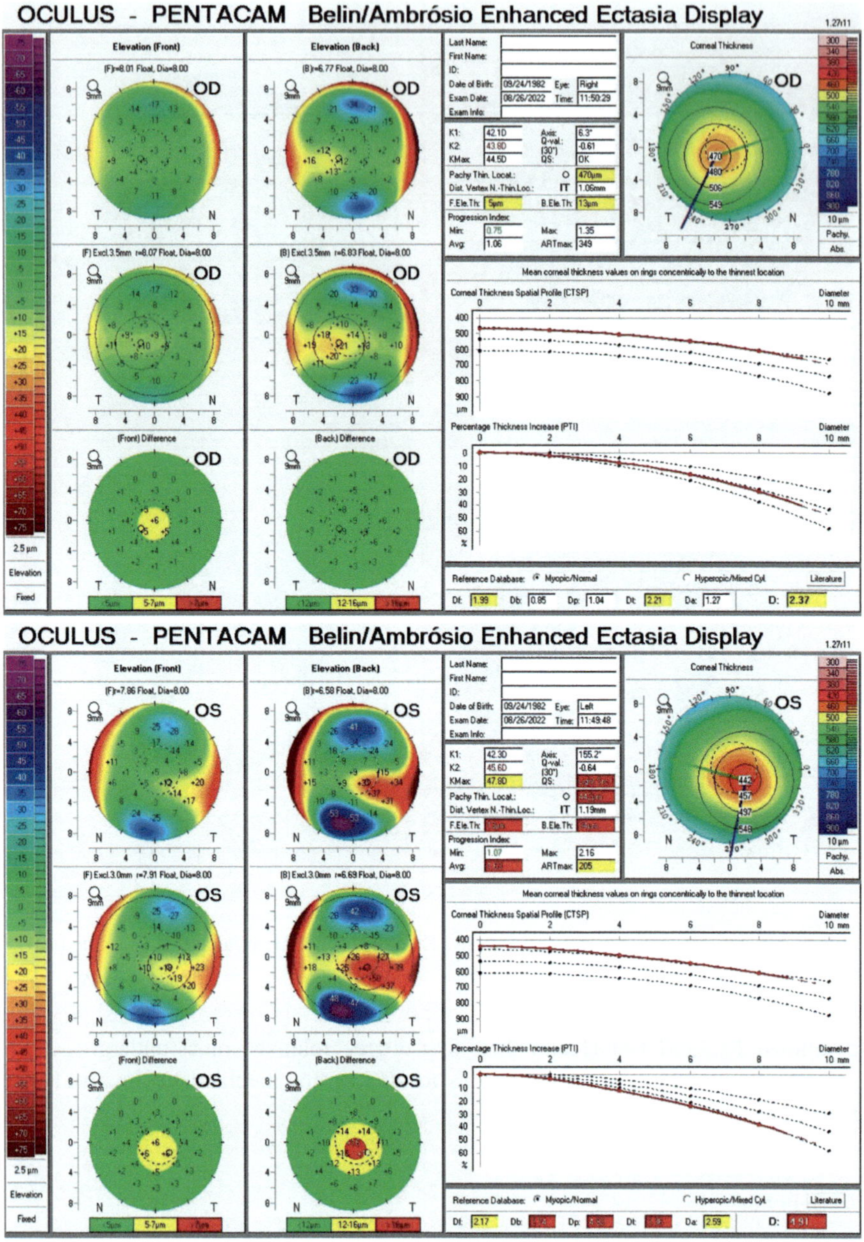

Fig. 14.14 Belin-Ambrósio Enhanced Ectasia display of OU showing alteration of both front and back elevation, as well as pathologic pachymetry map progression, compatible with the diagnosis of KC

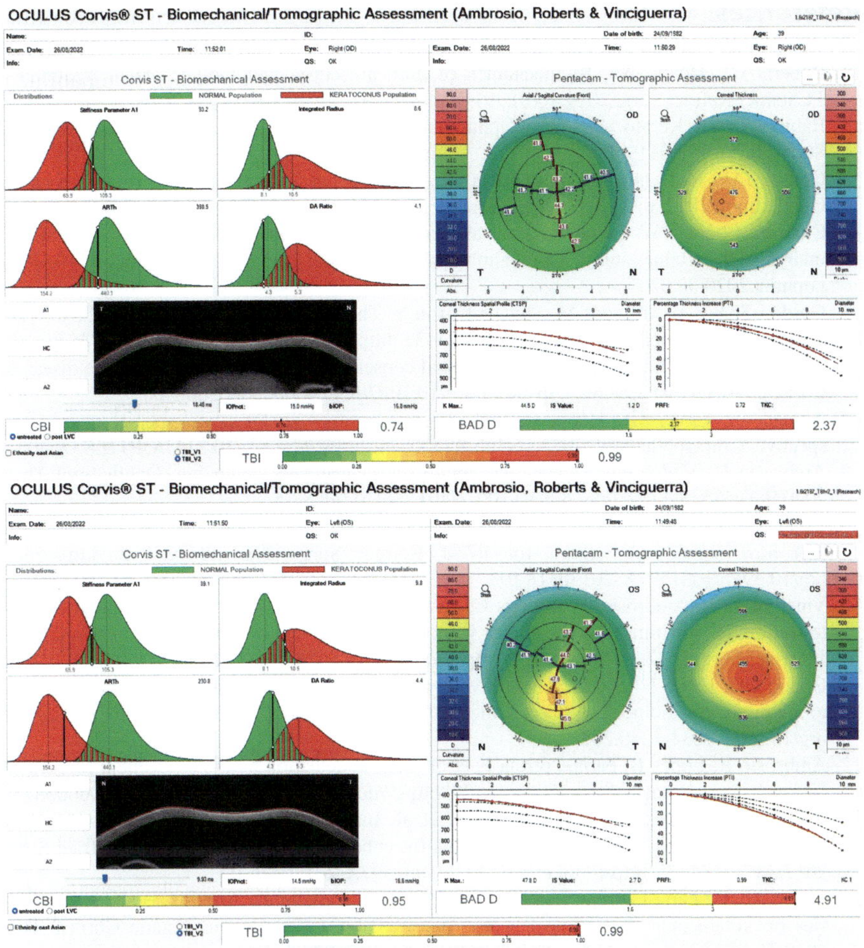

Fig. 14.15 Biomechanical examination with corneal tomography (Corvis ST and Pentacam HR, Oculus) identified KC disease in both eyes: BAD-D OD 2.37 and OS 4.91; Tomographic and Biomechanical Index (TBI_V2) (Ambrosio, 2022) OD 0.99 and OD 0.99; CBI OD 0.74 and OE 0.95

References

1. Roberts CJ, Dupps WJ. Biomechanics of corneal ectasia and biomechanical treatments. J Cataract Refract Surg. 2014;40(6):991–8. https://doi.org/10.1016/j.jcrs.2014.04.013.
2. Rabinowitz YS. Keratoconus. Surv Ophthalmol. 1998;42(4):297–319. https://doi.org/10.1016/S0039-6257(97)00119-7.
3. Gomes JAP, Rodrigues PF, Lamazales LL. Keratoconus epidemiology: a review. Saudi J Ophthalmol. 2022;36(1):3–6. https://doi.org/10.4103/sjopt.sjopt_204_21.
4. Chan E, Chong EW, Lingham G, et al. Prevalence of keratoconus based on Scheimpflug imaging: the Raine study. Ophthalmology. 2021;128(4):515–21. https://doi.org/10.1016/j.ophtha.2020.08.020.
5. Gordon-Shaag A, Millodot M, Shneor E, Liu Y. The genetic and environmental factors for keratoconus. Biomed Res Int. 2015;2015:24–32. https://doi.org/10.1155/2015/795738.
6. Gomes JAP, Tan D, Rapuano CJ, et al. Global consensus on keratoconus and ectatic diseases. Cornea. 2015;34(4):359–69. https://doi.org/10.1097/ICO.0000000000000408.
7. Ahmad TR, Turner ML, Hoppe C, et al. Parental keratoconus literacy: a socioeconomic perspective. Clin Ophthalmol. 2022;16(July):2505–11. https://doi.org/10.2147/OPTH.S375405.
8. Ambrósio R. Violet June: the global keratoconus awareness campaign. Ophthalmol Ther. 2020;9(3):685–8. https://doi.org/10.1007/s40123-020-00283-5.
9. Ambrósio R, Randleman JB. Screening for ectasia risk: what are we screening for and how should we screen for it? J Refract Surg. 2013;29(4):230–2. https://doi.org/10.3928/1081597X-20130318-01.
10. Vinciguerra R, Ambrósio R, Roberts CJ, Azzolini C, Vinciguerra P. Biomechanical characterization of subclinical keratoconus without topographic or tomographic abnormalities. J Refract Surg. 2017;33(6):399–407. https://doi.org/10.3928/1081597X-20170213-01.
11. Criado GG, Júnior NBS, Mazzeo TJMM, et al. Of subclinical ectasia with integrated corneal tomography and biomechanics assessments. Rev Bras Oftalmol. 2021;80(1):71–6. https://doi.org/10.5935/0034-7280.20210014.
12. Ambrósio R, Lopes B, Faria-Correia F, et al. Ectasia detection by the assessment of corneal biomechanics. Cornea. 2016;35(7):e18–20. https://doi.org/10.1097/ICO.0000000000000875.
13. Ambrósio R, Lopes BT, Faria-Correia F, et al. Integration of Scheimpflug-based corneal tomography and biomechanical assessments for enhancing ectasia detection. J Refract Surg. 2017;33(7):434–43. https://doi.org/10.3928/1081597X-20170426-02.
14. Ambrósio R, Faria-Correia F, Silva-Lopes Í, et al. Paradigms, paradoxes, and controversies on keratoconus and corneal ectatic diseases. Int J Keratoconus Ectatic Corneal Dis. 2018;7(1):35–49. https://doi.org/10.5005/jp-journals-10025-1158.
15. Ambrósio R, Lopes B, Amaral J, et al. Keratoconus: breaking paradigms and contradictions of a new subspecialty. Rev Bras Oftalmol. 2019;78(2):81–5. https://doi.org/10.5935/0034-7280.20180101.
16. Koller T, Mrochen M, Seiler T. Complication and failure rates after corneal crosslinking. J Cataract Refract Surg. 2009;35(8):1358–62. https://doi.org/10.1016/j.jcrs.2009.03.035.
17. Guerra G, de Oliveira VB, Ferreira I, Ramos I, Belin MW, Ambrósio R Jr. Subclinical keratoconus detection in identical twins. Int J Keratoconus Ectatic Corneal Dis. 2016;5(1):35–9. https://doi.org/10.5005/jp-journals-10025-1119.
18. Correia FF, Ramos I, Lopes B, Salomão MQ, Correa RO. Topometric and tomographic indices for the diagnosis of keratoconus. Int J Keratoconus Ectatic Corneal Dis. 2012;1(2):92–9. https://doi.org/10.5005/jp-journals-10025-1018.
19. Edwards M, McGhee CN, Dean S. The genetics of keratoconus. Clin Experiment Ophthalmol. 2001;29(6):345–51. https://doi.org/10.1046/j.1442-9071.2001.d01-16.x.
20. Cremona FA, Ghosheh FR, Rapuano CJ, et al. Keratoconus associated with other corneal dystrophies. Cornea. 2009;28(2):127–35. https://doi.org/10.1097/ICO.0b013e3181859935.

21. Wang N, McKelvie J. Coincident keratoconus and Fuchs' endothelial dystrophy: dual dystrophies mask progression. Indian J Ophthalmol. 2020;68(12):3074. https://doi.org/10.4103/ijo.IJO_1783_20.
22. Gurnani B, Kaur K, Tripathy K. Is there a genetic link between keratoconus and Fuch's endothelial corneal dystrophy? Med Hypotheses. 2021;157:157. https://doi.org/10.1016/j.mehy.2021.110699.
23. Mazzotta C, Traversi C, Raiskup F, Lo Rizzo C, Renieri A. First identification of a triple corneal dystrophy association: keratoconus, epithelial basement membrane corneal dystrophy and Fuchs' endothelial corneal dystrophy. Case Rep Ophthalmol. 2014;5(3):281–8. https://doi.org/10.1159/000367937.
24. Mylona I, Tsinopoulos I, Ziakas N. Comorbidity of keratoconus and Fuchs' corneal endothelial dystrophy: a review of the literature. Ophthalmic Res. 2020;63(4):369–74. https://doi.org/10.1159/000505579.
25. Jurkunas U, Azar DT. Potential complications of ocular surgery in patients with coexistent keratoconus and Fuchs' endothelial dystrophy. Ophthalmology. 2006;113(12):2187–97. https://doi.org/10.1016/j.ophtha.2006.06.036.
26. Ramos IC, Valbon BF, Pimentel LN, Caldas DL. Keratoconus associated with corneal guttata. Int J Keratoconus Ectatic Corneal Dis. 2012;1(3):173–8. https://doi.org/10.5005/jp-journals-10025-1033.

Pellucid Marginal Degeneration

15

Jennifer A. Tran, Kathryn M. Hatch, and Nandini Venkateswaran

15.1 Introduction

Pellucid marginal degeneration (PMD) is a rare type of corneal ectasia of unclear etiology. Typically characterized by inferior corneal thinning with a superior protrusion that spares the central cornea, it is the second most common corneal ectasia after keratoconus [1, 2]. Epidemiologically, PMD tends to affect men more than women [3], can occur in the second to fifth decade of life [1, 3], and is commonly bilateral [1, 3]. Vision decreases proportionally with worsening astigmatism. Pathology studies on PMD demonstrate a disruption of Bowman's layer associated with stromal thinning, with otherwise normal corneal structures [4]. On a molecular level, collagen abnormalities may also play a role in the pathophysiology [5]. The overall diagnosis of PMD is primarily clinical based on the slit lamp exam with supporting topographic or tomographic evidence (Fig. 15.1). Once advanced, PMD can lead to acute hydrops or spontaneous corneal perforation. Corneal scarring often follows hydrops in patients with PMD.

J. A. Tran · K. M. Hatch · N. Venkateswaran (✉)
Massachusetts Eye and Ear, Boston, MA, USA
e-mail: Jennifer_Tran@meei.harvard.edu; Kathryn_Hatch@MEEI.HARVARD.EDU; Nandini_Venkateswaran@MEEI.HARVARD.EDU

F. A. Woreta, R. B. Singh (eds.), *Cornea Casebook*, Current Practices in Ophthalmology, https://doi.org/10.1007/978-981-96-0495-1_15

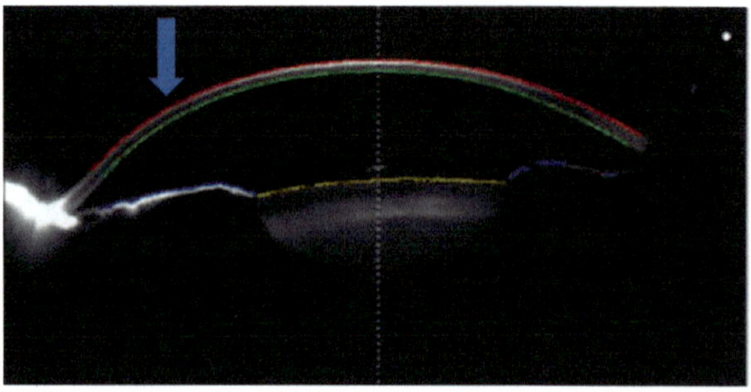

Fig. 15.1 Scheimpflug cross-sectional image showing corneal ectasia (blue arrow) consistent with PMD

15.2 Case 1

Case Summary

- The typical finding in PMD is a cornea that exhibits a protrusion—both central and inferior—spanning several clock hours, accompanied by a peripheral band of thinning.
- PMD and keratoconus may be confused with one another, especially if the latter is more inferior-involving.
- Corneal topographies of patients with PMD often demonstrate a "crab-claw" appearance.
- PMD can be monitored annually with topography for worsening that may require intervention.

A 72-year-old male presented to the cornea clinic for evaluation of glare and haloes. His ocular history was significant for PMD in both eyes, previously misdiagnosed as keratoconus in his 40s. He had previously used rigid gas-permeable lenses which he ultimately was not able to tolerate and switched to Novakone (Bausch and Lomb, New Jersey) custom soft contact lenses. He enjoyed monovision with his contact lenses, with his right eye set for distance and his left eye set for reading (off set of −1.00 diopter in the left eye). His visual acuity at his first presentation was 20/40–1 in the right eye and 20/60 in the left eye with mixed astigmatic correction. The initial examination revealed bilateral inferior corneal thinning and a visually significant cataract in both eyes.

The initial tomography demonstrated inferior steepening in a "crab-claw" pattern bilaterally (Fig. 15.2a and b), overall consistent with PMD. The maximum keratometry value was 51.1 diopters in the right eye and 53.9 diopters in the left eye. There was a high degree of astigmatism in both eyes, with 6.3 diopters of astigmatism at 176 degrees in the right eye and 7.1 diopters of astigmatism at 172 degrees in the left eye; the pattern of astigmatism was regular in the central 3 mm of the cornea but grew irregular in the inferior cornea in both eyes.

The patient opted to undergo cataract surgery in his right eye. Although the patient had a high degree of regular astigmatism in the central cornea. A toric intraocular lens was not chosen because the patient, a long-term contact lens wearer, planned to continue using contact lenses postoperatively. A toric intraocular lens

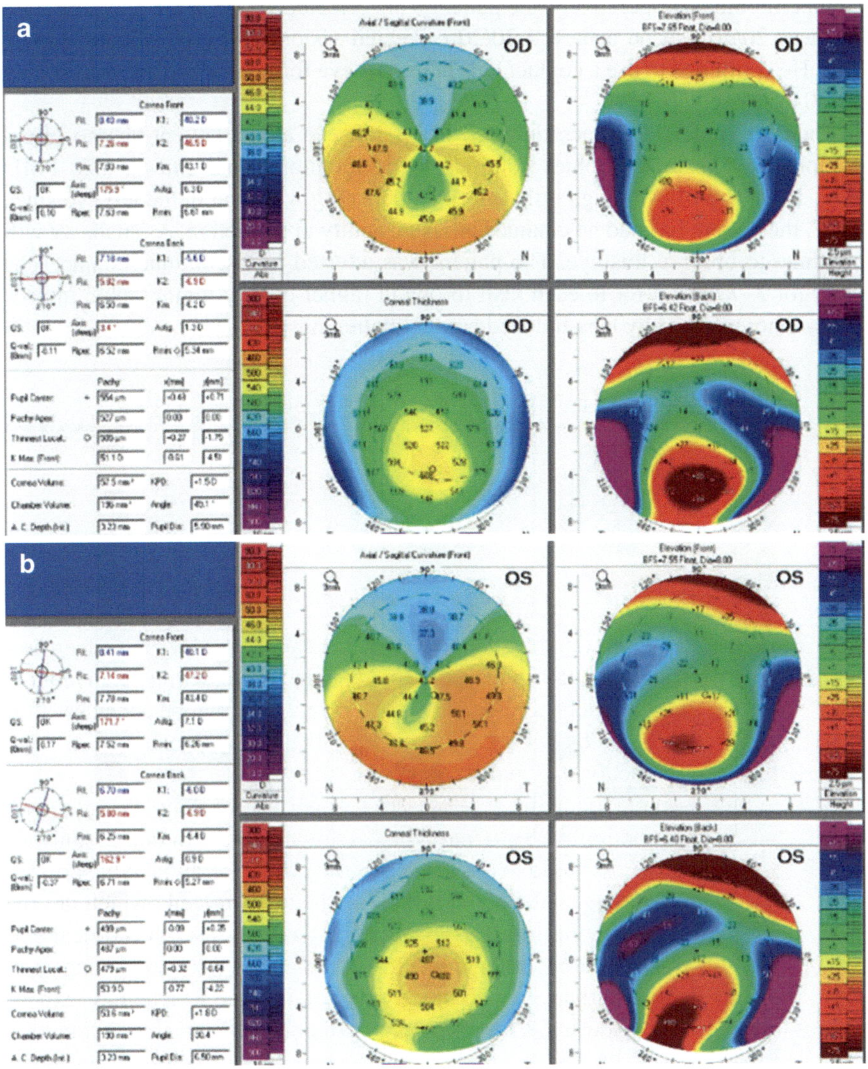

Fig. 15.2 (a and **b**) Tomographic images showing the crab-claw appearance of PMD with anterior and posterior corneal elevations

would induce lenticular astigmatism rendering a contact lens fitting far more complex. As such, a monofocal intraocular lens aimed for plano was implanted in the right eye. The patient was also advised that if his PMD progressed, his vision could potentially worsen, even with contact lenses; however, his PMD had been stable for many years and did not require pre-operative crosslinking to arrest the progression of underlying ectasia. Intraoperatively, a scleral tunnel wound was used to avoid further manipulation of the ectatic cornea as well as to minimize induction of additional corneal astigmatism.

One-month postoperatively, the patient's uncorrected vision in the operated right eye was 20/40 and he achieved 20/20 corrected vision with a Novakone contact lens. He continued to use a contact lens in his left eye for near vision and was seeing 20/20 up-close.

Cataract surgery has been deferred in his left eye as the patient has no visual complaints. His tomographies continue to be monitored and show stable PMD (Fig. 15.3a and b). Although mild inferior steepening was seen in the left eye since 2017, the patient has had no changes in visual acuity or refraction. As such, we will continue to observe this eye. The patient was advised to discontinue contact lens wear for 3–7 days prior to each visit to obtain higher-quality tomographic images that are not affected by lens-induced corneal flattening.

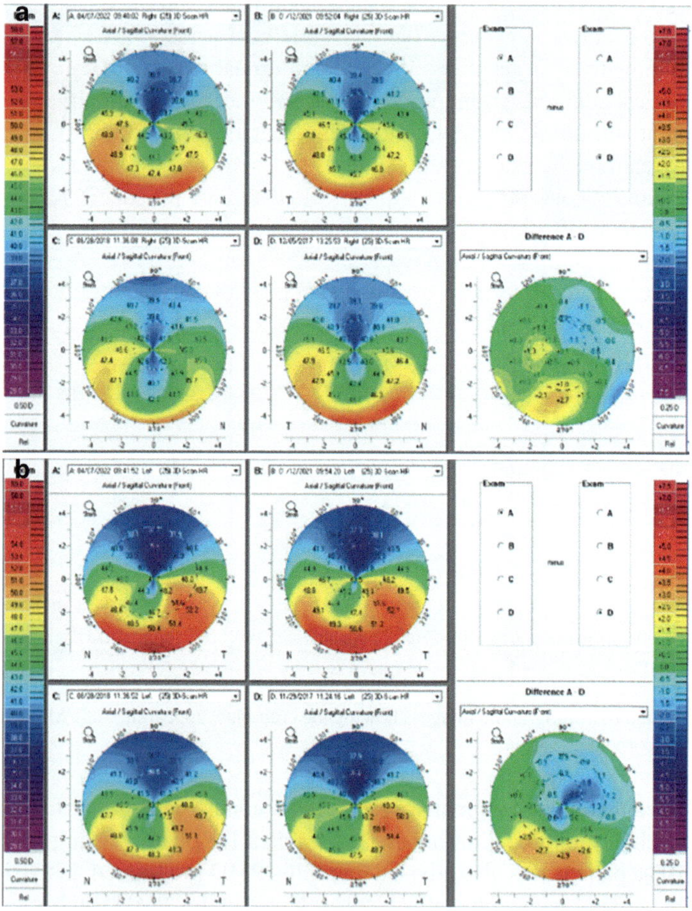

Fig. 15.3 (**a** and **b**) Tomographic images showing stable comparison corneal maps from 2017 to 2022 of the patient's right and left eyes. There is some overall corneal flattening but this is likely a result of intermittent contact lens wear before image acquisition. This patient did not undergo corneal collagen cross-linking

15.3 Case 2

Case Summary

- Corneal collagen cross-linking may play a role in arresting the progression of PMD.
- Epithelium-on vs epithelium-off crosslinking techniques can be used in PMD.

A 57-year-old male presented to cornea clinic for evaluation of unstable PMD in both eyes, diagnosed in the 1990s. He reported fluctuations in his vision for several months with bilateral worsening of his corneal keratometry values. Visual acuity was 20/25 with mixed astigmatic correction in both eyes. Slit lamp exam was notable for inferior corneal thinning bilaterally without scarring. Tomographically, there was inferior crab-claw steepening of both corneas, with a maximum keratometry value of 52.6 diopters in the right eye and 53.3 diopters in the left eye (Fig. 15.4a and b). The decision was made to proceed with epithelium-off collagen crosslinking (CXL) of both corneas beginning with the left eye as it was considered more significantly affected.

The patient underwent uncomplicated sequential CXL one week apart. Bandage contact lenses were placed for one week and he was started on antibiotic and steroid eyedrops with close follow-up.

Three months later, the patient presented with subjectively stable vision. Visual acuities were 20/25 in the right eye and 20/20 in the left eye with correction. Subsequent tomographies demonstrated stabilization of the corneal architecture of each eye 4 months after CXL along with mild corneal flattening effect (Fig. 15.5a and b).

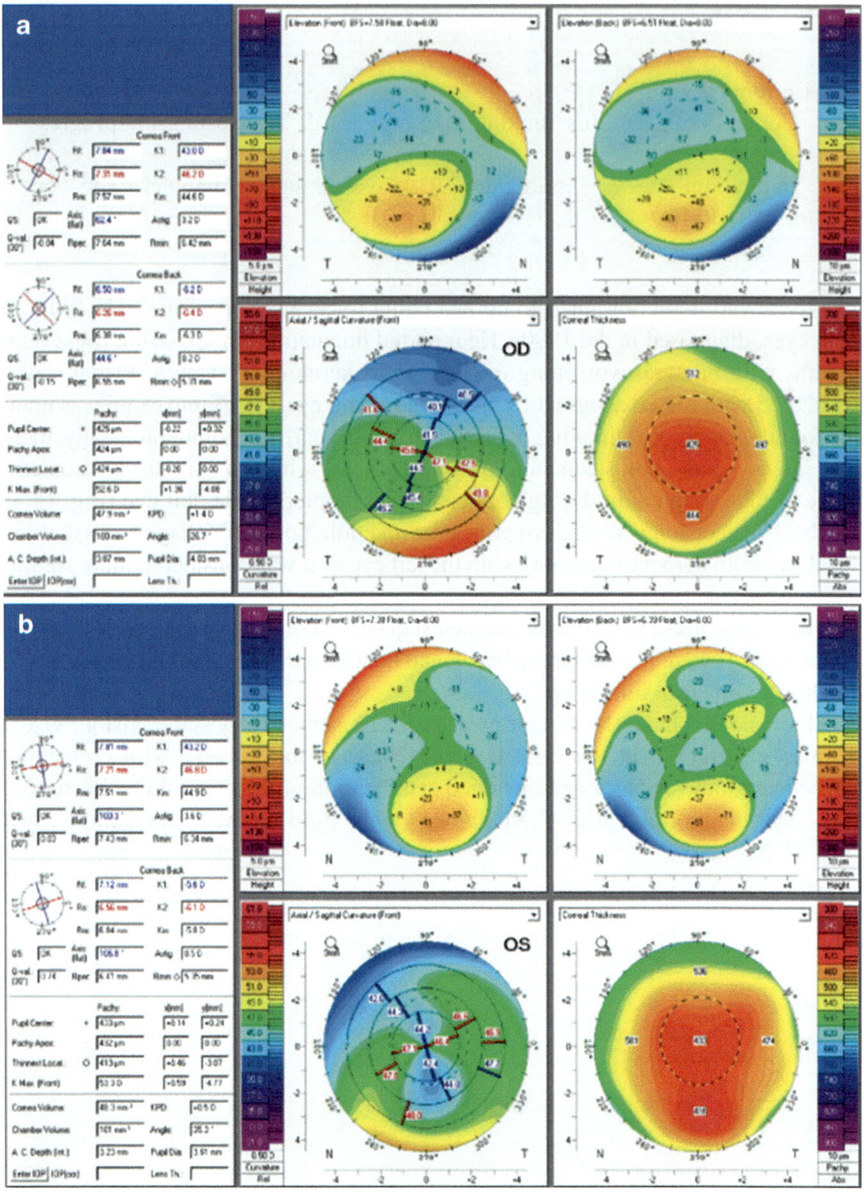

Fig. 15.4 (**a** and **b**) Tomographic images showing the crab-claw appearance of PMD with anterior and posterior corneal elevations in both eyes

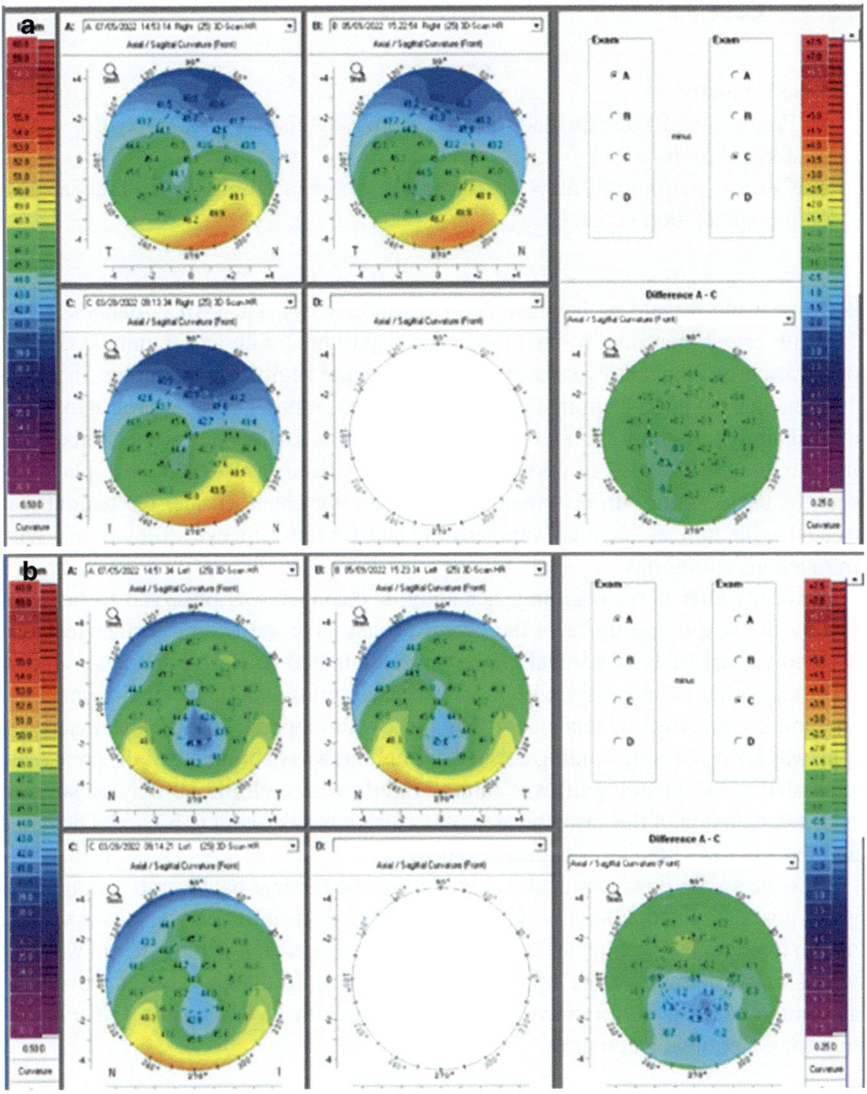

Fig. 15.5 (**a** and **b**) Tomographic images showing stable comparison corneal maps from pre and 4 months post CXL in both eyes. Corneal keratometry values show stability with mild corneal flattening as well

15.4 Case #3

Case Summary

- Progressive PMD can lead to corneal thinning and subsequent hydrops or corneal perforation.
- Corneal perforation may be treated with corneal gluing or with corneal transplantation surgery.

A 43-year-old female with a history of severe dry eye and PMD (diagnosed just 1 month prior) presented to the emergency department with an atraumatic corneal perforation of the right eye. At presentation, visual acuity was counting fingers at 10 feet. Her slit lamp examination revealed inferotemporal corneal protrusion with a focal area of thinning found to be Seidel positive, a shallow anterior chamber, and iris plugging to the area of corneal perforation. Cyanoacrylate glue was placed to seal the perforation with reformation of the anterior chamber, and the patient was treated with topical fortified vancomycin and tobramycin eye drops along with intravenous antibiotics.

Six days after corneal gluing, her anterior chamber was observed to be completely flat despite presence of the cyanoacrylate glue, indicating further leakage. Two additional trials of corneal gluing were attempted but failed. She then underwent a lamellar keratoplasty with a corneal patch graft using irradiated corneal tissue and conjunctival advancement (Fig. 15.6). Intraoperatively, all cyanoacrylate glue was removed, surrounding corneal epithelium was debrided, and the crescentic irradiated corneal patch graft was sutured tightly with multiple 10-0 nylon sutures. At the conclusion of the case, the area of perforation was found to be seidel negative and the anterior chamber remained formed.

Despite some retraction of the conjunctiva, the corneal patch graft remained in good position postoperatively. Her best corrected visual acuity at postoperative month two was 20/70. She has since been fit for a scleral contact lens to aid with her visual rehabilitation by her optometrist. She has unfortunately suffered from an atraumatic corneal perforation in her fellow eye with PMD as well 3 years later, requiring a corneal patch graft.

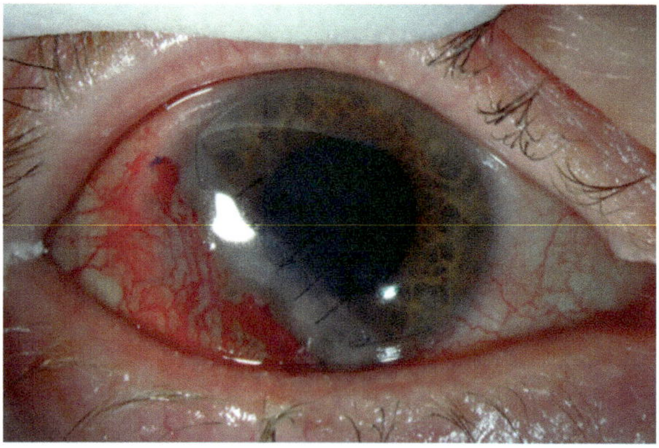

Fig. 15.6 Slit-lamp photograph of the patient's eye at postoperative week #2 status post right eye lamellar corneal patch graft and conjunctival advancement due to corneal perforation from progressive PMD

15.5 Discussion

15.5.1 PMD as Compared with Other Ectasias

Corneal ectasias are bilateral, noninflammatory, progressive structural abnormalities featuring corneal thinning that include conditions such as keratoconus, PMD, and keratoglobus. As shown by the cases above, there exists a wide range of presentations and outcomes of PMD.

PMD may be confused or co-exist with other ectatic disorders such as keratoconus. The classic slit lamp findings for keratoconus include a conical corneal appearance, Fleischer ring (iron line surrounding the cone), and Vogt's striae (linear vertical striae involving the stroma). In corneas with PMD, there is a "beer belly"-like protrusion superior to the circumferential thinning at the corneal periphery from 4 o'clock to 8 o'clock, separated from the corneal limbus by 1–3 mm of uninvolved corneal tissue [2, 5, 6].

Unlike keratoconus which tends to stop progressing in the third and fourth decades of life, PMD can be progressive throughout a patient's lifetime. Keratoconus also is typically diagnosed at younger ages (adolescence or early 20 s) while PMD tends to be diagnosed more commonly during the third decade of life [1, 3, 7]. Studies have also shown that patients with keratoconus are more likely to have mixed hyperopic astigmatism while patients with PMD tend to be more myopic [8].

Corneas with the so-called "crab-claw" appearance on topography, where there is marked flattening in the vertical meridian with accompanying steepening in the inferior periphery and midperipheral oblique meridians, can have either condition. However, one study demonstrated that corneas with "crab-claw" topography have a three-fold higher probability of having keratoconus compared to the probability of having PMD [9]. It is important to remember that the area of corneal pathology in PMD extends beyond that affected in keratoconus [10].

15.5.2 Progression

There are no accepted approaches for grading or scoring the severity of PMD. However, many publications categorizing mild, moderate, and advanced cases of PMD exist [3, 11–16].

The progression of PMD can occur with corneal steepening and thinning over years, although the exact timeframe is unclear [17]. When left unchecked, severe PMD can rarely result in acute hydrops or spontaneous corneal perforation as shown in Case 3. Regular topographic examinations allow clinicians to detect worsening keratometry values, progressive pachymetric thinning, and the development of irregular astigmatism.

Intervention should be considered if the patient endorses significant subjective changes in vision, demonstrates increasing astigmatism or worsening spherical equivalents on manifest refraction, steepening of topographic keratometric measurements on serial follow-ups, or progressive corneal thinning with associated corneal edema or scarring [17].

15.5.3 Management

The majority of PMD cases are treated medically. A recent study reported that out of 559 patients formally diagnosed with PMD over an 8-year period, approximately 88% were managed with glasses or contact lenses, 5% underwent corneal crosslinking, and 4% underwent cataract surgery [17].

Specially fitted contact lenses are often utilized as a first-line management option in cases of PMD to correct irregular astigmatism. Rigid gas-permeable lenses or scleral lenses have been shown to significantly improve visual acuity and are overall well-tolerated [7, 18]. There also exist hybrid contact lenses featuring a rigid gas-permeable optic with a soft lens skirt. Alternatively, there are soft contact lens options for patients unable to tolerate hard lenses, such as the Novakone lenses worn by the patient in Case 1. For the subset of patients unable to generally tolerate contact lenses, toric intraocular collamer lenses (ICLs) can be placed to reduce the patients' refractive error and are used in patients who have regular appearing central corneal astigmatism [19–21]. It should be emphasized that contact lenses and ICLs are principally used for vision correction and do not alter the progression of PMD overall.

For patients with documented progression of their ectasia, corneal collagen crosslinking may be indicated. Crosslinking is a procedure that strengthens collagen fibrils via the application of riboflavin and ultraviolet light. There are two main crosslinking techniques: epithelium-on and epithelium-off. In epithelium-off techniques, the corneal epithelium is first removed mechanically or chemically prior to instillation of riboflavin and application of ultraviolet light. In the transepithelial protocols, the epithelium is left intact during riboflavin instillation and ultraviolet light treatment. The epithelium-on protocols can include use of modified riboflavin solutions, increased riboflavin instillation time, partial epithelial disruption, as well as supplemental oxygen [22]. In the United States, CXL for PMD is considered an off-label procedure, and is only FDA approved for the treatment of progressive keratoconus and post-LASIK ectasia [23]. Its use in slowing or halting the progression of PMD has only recently started to gain traction. Patients with PMD evaluated 5 years after undergoing crosslinking demonstrated stable uncorrected visual acuity and keratometry values [24]. Other studies have similarly concluded that this procedure results in stable and/or improved visual acuity and keratometry [25–28]. Although CXL is a relatively understudied treatment option for PMD, there is evidence that it is a safe and effective treatment option [23, 24].

Intracorneal ring segments (ICRS) are synthetic polymer segments placed within the corneal stroma to counteract ectatic protrusion by steepening the periphery and subsequently flattening the central cornea. Multiple types of ICRS have been shown to be safe and effective in various ectasias [14, 29–31], although the procedure is limited to corneas with >450um thickness. There are various potential adverse sequelae such as epithelial ingrowth, segment extrusion [32], and corneal neovascularization, amongst others [33]. Few cases of ICRS implantation in corneas with PMD exist, likely because the area of greatest ectasia may fall outside of the zone of the intracorneal rings. One case report suggests inserting a thinner segment at the inferior cornea, especially where there is significant thinning in order to avoid corneal perforation [14].

Keratoplasty can be performed for PMD refractory to medical therapy or for more severe, vision-threatening cases.

- Full-thickness crescentic wedge resection is a technique in which the full-thickness, peripherally affected cornea is surgically excised and the adjacent tissue is closed, without the introduction of a donor graft.
- Crescentic lamellar wedge resection involves excision of the affected corneal stroma and subsequent re-approximation of the existing tissue.
- Crescentic lamellar keratoplasty is performed by dissecting the host lamella and placing lamellar donor tissue in the area of corneal thinning [34].
- Full-thickness intrastromal lamellar keratoplasty (FTILK) is a technique whereby a full-thickness donor stromal graft is inserted into a host intrastromal pocket [35]. This is a sutureless technique. However, the full-thickness graft confers additional bulk and astigmatism.
- Partial-thickness intrastromal lamellar keratoplasty (PTILK), which involves a partial-thickness stromal replacement with a donor graft in a similar manner to FTILK, has been demonstrated to improve visual acuity and reduce the bulk associated with FTILK, although against-the-rule astigmatism may remain [36].
- Tuck-in lamellar keratoplasty (TILK) features the insertion of a partial thickness, flanged stromal donor lenticule into a stromal pocket of the host cornea [37, 38]. This technique is thought to provide increased tectonic support to the graft.
- The full-thickness penetrating keratoplasty (PK) is considered a last-resort treatment due to the technical challenges of orienting the graft inferiorly, trephining large grafts due to the peripheral nature of PMD pathology, and the associated increased risks of graft rejection and corneal neovascularization when suturing large diameter grafts close to the corneal limbus.

Although several techniques have been described, there is no consensus on the definitive procedure type for PMD, owing to the rarity of this condition. One must weigh the potential risks and benefits of each procedure. The full-thickness keratoplasties generally confer the risks associated with an open-globe surgery and disrupt the host endothelium, thereby increasing the risk for graft rejection. The partial thickness keratoplasties tend to be better tolerated and have a decreased risk of rejection but may result in residual, uncorrected astigmatism. One recently developed technique, referred to as sclerocorneal intrastromal lamellar keratoplasty (SILK), addresses the insufficient astigmatic correction with a strategically placed scleral tunnel [39]. Overall, more studies need to be performed to assess the long-term outcomes of these surgical interventions.

Of note, recent trends in combining the above procedures have developed for cases of PMD. Kymionis et al. reported a successful combined corneal wedge resection and subsequent crosslinking procedure on one cornea, which had stabilized upon follow-up 8 months later [40]. The same group also reported simultaneously performing photorefractive keratectomy and crosslinking on eight corneas, demonstrating improved visual acuity without intraoperative or postoperative complications [41]. The long-term effectiveness of such combined procedures remains to be seen, although the results have been fairly positive in these reports.

Lastly, at the time of cataract surgery in cases with PMD, such as in Case 1, there are some important considerations. Obtaining accurate biometry and keratometry is crucial. Ensuring patients remain out of their contact lenses for weeks prior to obtaining measurement is recommended; we typically advise patients who have been in hard contact lenses to remain out of lenses for approximately one week per decade of lens wear time. To avoid a refractive surprise, targeting a slightly myopic refraction is beneficial, particularly in patients with highly irregular astigmatism, to minimize the risk of a hyperopic outcome. A myopic target refraction with a monofocal intraocular lens can be helpful for patients' near vision needs and also facilitates contact lens wear/fitting due to optics. Avoidance of toric intraocular lenses is recommended in patients who are dependent on contact lenses for the best quality of vision, as the lenticular astigmatism induced by a toric intraocular lens can be challenging to correct with a contact lens and lead to more aberrations. If patients have good spectacle-corrected vision and want to continue wearing spectacles after surgery, toric intraocular lenses can be implanted to debulk the magnitude of corneal astigmatism if the central corneal astigmatism is regular with a reproducible axis. Unlike keratoconus which can present with more central cones with irregular astigmatism, PMD can often have regular astigmatism in the central cornea due to the inferior corneal nature of the pathology and allow for better visual outcomes; however, the more ectatic the cornea, the less predictable intraocular lens calculations are.

Intraoperatively, trypan blue can aid with capsular visualization, especially if there is any significant corneal scarring. A temporal or superior limbal approach for cataract surgery will work well as the area of ectasia and thinning in PMD is typically in the inferior periphery of the cornea. A 10-0 nylon suture can be used to seal the wounds if there is concern about wound closure. However, a scleral tunnel can be utilized to reduce corneal tissue stress and minimize induction of additional corneal astigmatism.

15.5.4 Complications

Corneal hydrops occurs with the rupture of Descemet's membrane due to progressive corneal ectasia and thinning and is commonly associated with pain and vision loss. It is estimated that acute hydrops occurs between 1% and 6% of patients with PMD [3, 17]. Because many cases self-resolve within months, management is commonly conservative. Typical agents used in supportive care include hypertonic saline, intraocular pressure-lowering drops, topical steroids, and cycloplegic eyedrops.

Corneal perforation is a much rarer complication in PMD. At this time, there are only a few case reports describing this phenomenon [34, 42–46], and the overall incidence is unknown. The initial management of corneal perforation can also be conservative, e.g., corneal gluing with cyanoacrylate and/or the placement of a bandage contact lens [43, 46, 47]. However, care must be taken to identify and prevent infectious microbial keratitis thorough examinations, corneal culturing, and close monitoring.

The patient in Case 3 failed three trials of corneal gluing and the application of bandage contact lenses before undergoing a successful crescentic corneal patch graft. Symes et al. also described two similar cases in which crescentic lamellar keratoplasty was well-tolerated [34]. Other groups have reported repair via primary closure with corneal sutures [48], corneal patch graft [45], and penetrating keratoplasty [47], amongst other techniques. In rare cases, a patch graft can be employed in areas of significant corneal thinning to help prevent future corneal perforation.

15.6 Conclusion

PMD is a rare, typically bilateral, slowly progressive corneal ectasia that can result in visually significant complications. While much progress has been made in identifying the pathology, progression, and treatment options for PMD, there is more to learn. Studies are limited by the rarity of this condition. Nevertheless, further research needs to be done to address the underlying causes of PMD so that any deleterious vision loss may be prevented in the future.

Financial Disclosures Dr. Hatch is a consultant for Glaukos and CXLO. Dr. Venkateswaran is a consultant for Glaukos.

References

1. Krachmer JH, Feder RS, Belin MW. Keratoconus and related noninflammatory corneal thinning disorders. Surv Ophthalmol. 1984;28(4):293–322.
2. Robin JB, et al. Peripheral corneal disorders. Surv Ophthalmol. 1986;31(1):1–36.
3. Sridhar MS, et al. Pellucid marginal corneal degeneration. Ophthalmology. 2004;111(6):1102–7.
4. Zucchini G. Su di un caso di degerazione marginale della cornea-studio clinico ed istologico. Ann Ottalmol Clin Oculist. 1962;88:47–56.
5. Rodrigues MM, et al. Pellucid marginal corneal degeneration: a clinicopathologic study of two cases. Exp Eye Res. 1981;33(3):277–88.
6. Parker DL, et al. Pellucid marginal corneal degeneration. Cornea. 1986;5(2):115–24.
7. Kompella VB, Aasuri MK, Rao GN. Management of pellucid marginal corneal degeneration with rigid gas permeable contact lenses. CLAO J. 2002;28(3):140–5.
8. Lee BW, et al. Ectatic disorders associated with a claw-shaped pattern on corneal topography. Am J Ophthalmol. 2007;144(1):154–6.
9. Koc M, et al. Crab claw pattern on corneal topography: pellucid marginal degeneration or inferior keratoconus? Eye (Lond). 2018;32(1):11–8.

10. Belin MW, Boyd BM, Ambrosio R Jr. Pellucid marginal degeneration vs inferior keratoconus: why it matters. J Cataract Refract Surg. 2020;46(2):325–6.
11. Ambrosio R Jr, Wilson SE. Early pellucid marginal corneal degeneration: case reports of two refractive surgery candidates. Cornea. 2002;21(1):114–7.
12. Biswas S, et al. Management of pellucid marginal corneal degeneration. Eye (Lond). 2000;14(Pt 4):629–34.
13. Javadi MA, et al. Lamellar crescentic resection for pellucid marginal corneal degeneration. J Refract Surg. 2004;20(2):162–5.
14. Kymionis GD, et al. Intacs for early pellucid marginal degeneration. J Cataract Refract Surg. 2004;30(1):230–3.
15. Mularoni A, et al. Conservative treatment of early and moderate pellucid marginal degeneration: a new refractive approach with intracorneal rings. Ophthalmology. 2005;112(4):660–6.
16. Rasheed K, Rabinowitz YS. Surgical treatment of advanced pellucid marginal degeneration. Ophthalmology. 2000;107(10):1836–40.
17. Das AV, Pillutla LN, Chaurasia S. Clinical profile and demographic distribution of pellucid marginal corneal degeneration in India: a study of 559 patients. Indian J Ophthalmol. 2021;69(12):3488–93.
18. Ozek D, Kemer OE, Altiaylik P. Visual performance of scleral lenses and their impact on quality of life in patients with irregular corneas. Arq Bras Oftalmol. 2018;81(6):475–80.
19. Camoriano GD, et al. Toric collagen copolymer phakic intraocular lens to correct myopic astigmatism in eyes with pellucid marginal degeneration. J Cataract Refract Surg. 2012;38(2):256–61.
20. Kamiya K, et al. Posterior chamber toric phakic intraocular lens implantation for high myopic astigmatism in eyes with pellucid marginal degeneration. J Cataract Refract Surg. 2010;36(1):164–6.
21. Price MO, Price FW Jr. Evaluation of the toric implantable collamer lens for simultaneous treatment of myopia and astigmatism. Expert Rev Med Devices. 2015;12(1):25–39.
22. Caruso C, et al. Transepithelial corneal cross-linking with vitamin E-enhanced riboflavin solution and abbreviated, low-dose UV-A: 24-month clinical outcomes. Cornea. 2016;35(2):145–50.
23. Yong JJ, Hatch KM. Corneal cross-linking: an effective treatment option for pellucid marginal degeneration. Semin Ophthalmol. 2019;34(7–8):512–7.
24. Irajpour M, Noorshargh P, Peyman A. Corneal cross-linking in pellucid marginal degeneration: evaluation after five years. J Curr Ophthalmol. 2022;34(2):229–33.
25. Bikbov MM, et al. [Results of corneal crosslinking for pellucid marginal corneal degeneration]. Vestn oftalmol. 2017; 133(3): 58–66.
26. Hassan Z, et al. Collagen cross-linking in the treatment of pellucid marginal degeneration. Indian J Ophthalmol. 2014;62(3):367–70.
27. Mamoosa B, et al. Short-term result of collagen crosslinking in pellucid marginal degeneration. Adv Biomed Res. 2016;5:194.
28. Spadea L. Corneal collagen cross-linking with riboflavin and UVA irradiation in pellucid marginal degeneration. J Refract Surg. 2010;26(5):375–7.
29. Ertan A, Bahadir M. Intrastromal ring segment insertion using a femtosecond laser to correct pellucid marginal corneal degeneration. J Cataract Refract Surg. 2006;32(10):1710–6.
30. Jabbarvand M, et al. Outcome of complete intrastromal ring implantation using femtosecond laser in pellucid marginal degeneration. Eye (Lond). 2015;29(6):783–90.
31. Kubaloglu A, et al. A single 210-degree arc length intrastromal corneal ring implantation for the management of pellucid marginal corneal degeneration. Am J Ophthalmol. 2010;150(2):185–192 e1.
32. Moskwa R, et al. Spontaneous expulsion of intracorneal ring segment in pellucid marginal degeneration: a case report. J Fr Ophtalmol. 2021;44(1):e47–9.
33. Pinero DP, Alio JL. Intracorneal ring segments in ectatic corneal disease – a review. Clin Experiment Ophthalmol. 2010;38(2):154–67.
34. Symes RJ, et al. Corneal perforation associated with pellucid marginal degeneration and treatment with crescentic lamellar keratoplasty: two case reports. Cornea. 2007;26(5):625–8.

35. Jabbarvand M, et al. Intrastromal lamellar keratoplasty in patients with pellucid marginal degeneration. J Cataract Refract Surg. 2015;41(1):2–8.
36. Goncalves TB, et al. Partial-thickness intrastromal lamellar Keratoplasty for corneal pellucid marginal degeneration. Cornea. 2021;40(12):1620–3.
37. Kaushal S, et al. "Tuck In" Lamellar Keratoplasty (TILK) for corneal ectasias involving corneal periphery. Br J Ophthalmol. 2008;92(2):286–90.
38. Vajpayee RB, et al. Central penetrating keratoplasty with peripheral intrastromal tuck. Cornea. 2005;24(8):947–50.
39. Guindolet D, et al. Sclerocorneal intrastromal lamellar keratoplasty for pellucid marginal degeneration. Cornea. 2016;35(6):900–3.
40. Kymionis G, et al. Combined corneal wedge resection and corneal cross-linking for pellucid marginal degeneration: a first report. Ther Clin Risk Manag. 2019;15:1319–24.
41. Kymionis GD, et al. Simultaneous conventional photorefractive keratectomy and corneal collagen cross-linking for pellucid marginal corneal degeneration. J Refract Surg. 2014;30(4):272–6.
42. Akpek EK, et al. Spontaneous corneal perforation in a patient with unusual unilateral pellucid marginal degeneration. J Cataract Refract Surg. 2001;27(10):1698–700.
43. Forooghian F, Assaad D, Dixon WS. Successful conservative management of hydrops with perforation in pellucid marginal degeneration. Can J Ophthalmol. 2006;41(1):74–7.
44. Lucarelli MJ, Gendelman DS, Talamo JH. Hydrops and spontaneous perforation in pellucid marginal corneal degeneration. Cornea. 1997;16(2):232–4.
45. Orlin SE, Sulewski ME. Spontaneous corneal perforation in pellucid marginal degeneration. CLAO J. 1998;24(3):186–7.
46. Ueji N, et al. Case of unilateral pellucid marginal corneal degeneration progressing to corneal perforation with keratoconus in contralateral eye. Am J Ophthalmol Case Rep. 2022;25:101293.
47. Gharebaghi D, et al. Spontaneous corneal hydrops and perforation in pellucid marginal degeneration; a case report. J Ophthalmic Vis Res. 2009;4(3):174–6.
48. Chan E, Snibson GR, Poon A. Direct surgical repair of corneal perforation in pellucid marginal degeneration: a case series. Cornea. 2013;32(7):1058–62.

Post-keratorefractive Ectasia

16

Alejandro Arboleda and Edward E. Manche

Corneal keratoectasia is a serious complication after laser keratorefractive procedures including laser in situ keratomileusis (LASIK), photorefractive keratectomy (PRK), and small incision lenticule extraction (SMILE) [1–5]. Patients suffer from visual disability such as glare, halos, double images, ghosting, and reduced visual acuity due to the development of increased myopia and/or irregular astigmatism. Clinical examination and topographic analysis display asymmetric keratometric steepening and corneal thinning. Histopathologic studies suggest that ectasia is caused by a process termed interfiber fracture in which there is interlamellar and interfibrillar biomechanical slippage in the stress-bearing regions of the corneal stroma [6].

Known risk factors of keratoectasia include high myopia, abnormal corneal topography such as forme fruste keratoconus, and low residual stromal bed [1]. Management is aimed at preventing visual loss, reducing signs and symptoms of ectasia, and maintaining, restoring, and improving visual function [7]. Numerous treatments have been proposed including rigid gas permeable and/or scleral contact lens use, intracorneal ring segments (ICRS), and corneal cross-linking (CXL) with severe cases requiring corneal transplantation. These cases highlight key diagnostic features and management strategies for post-refractive ectasia, including the role of CXL.

A. Arboleda
Byers Eye Institute, Stanford University School of Medicine, Palo Alto, CA, USA

Department of Ophthalmology, Baylor College of Medicine, Houston, TX, USA
e-mail: alejandro.arboleda@bcm.edu

E. E. Manche (✉)
Byers Eye Institute, Stanford University School of Medicine, Palo Alto, CA, USA
e-mail: cornea@stanford.edu

F. A. Woreta, R. B. Singh (eds.), *Cornea Casebook*, Current Practices in Ophthalmology, https://doi.org/10.1007/978-981-96-0495-1_16

16.1 Case 1

- A diagnosis of corneal keratoectasia is made following prior keratorefractive procedure with slit lamp examination and the use of corneal topography and tomography imaging.
- Early intervention with CXL can maintain good spectacle-corrected visual acuity when progression of disease is halted at a mild stage.

A 42-year-old man was referred to the cornea clinic with decreased vision in the right eye for evaluation of corneal ectasia. The patient had a LASIK procedure in both eyes 12 years prior to presentation and had recent subjective changes in vision. Slit lamp examination of the right eye showed a LASIK flap with otherwise normal findings. The left eye showed a LASIK flap with vertical microstriae and fibrosis at the temporal edge without epithelial ingrowth. Corneal tomography showed irregular astigmatism of the right eye (Fig. 16.1). The patient was diagnosed with corneal ectasia, and corneal cross-linking was recommended for the right eye.

After discussion of risks and benefits, CXL was recommended in the right eye, and the patient agreed to proceed with treatment. One week later, the procedure was performed using the Dresden protocol without complication. In short, the corneal epithelium was debrided with a PRK spatula after topical anesthesia was instilled. Two drops of riboflavin were instilled every 2 min for 30 min, and UV-A light with a power of 3 mW/cm^2 was used to irradiate the cornea for 30 minutes for a final

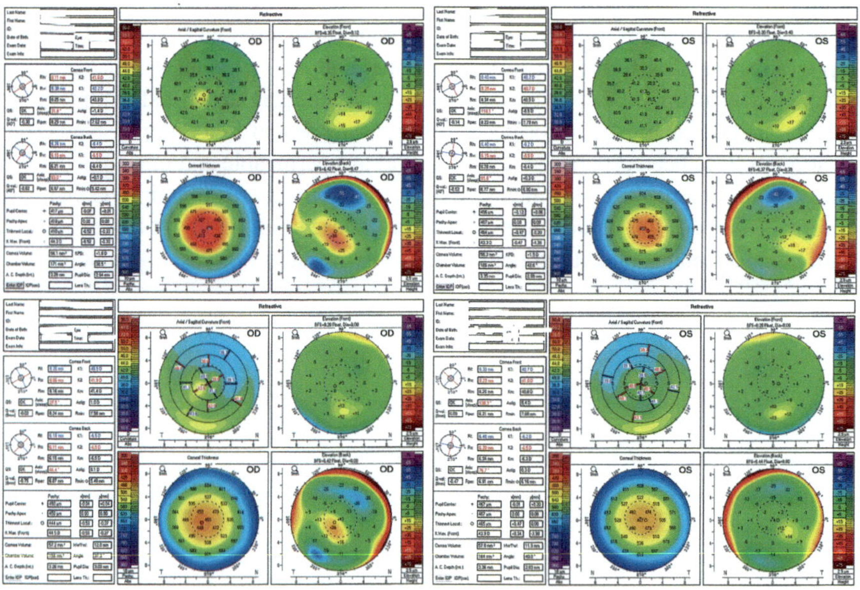

Fig. 16.1 Corneal tomography of patient 1 with mild post-LASIK ectasia. (Top) Initial corneal tomography images showing prior keratorefractive procedure and irregular astigmatism. (Bottom) Corneal tomography 3 years after CXL in the right eye. Scans display stable disease in both eyes

Table 16.1 Uncorrected visual acuity (UCVA), manifest refraction, and corrected distance visual acuity (CDVA) of patient 1 before and after CXL. Visual acuity is presented in Snellen form

	UCVA	Refraction	CDVA
Preoperative	20/32 20/25	−3.50 + 1.75 at 5 −2.00 + 1.00 at 7	20/20 20/20
Postoperative	20/20-1 20/32	−1.75 + 2.00 at 15 −2.25	20/16-1 20/12.5

energy density of 5.4 J/cm^2. After the procedure, a bandage contact lens was placed on the operated eye until the epithelium healed.

After CXL, the patient's right eye had a 1.75 D decrease in spherical error. Diagnostic testing also showed a 1 D decrease in keratometry in the steep axis and a 0.8 D decrease in maximum keratometry (Kmax). The patient has had serial examinations with stable refractive error and corneal tomography. At the most recent follow-up, 3 years after CXL and 15 years after initial LASIK procedure, visual acuity is excellent, and slit lamp examination shows mild anterior stromal haze in the right eye with no changes in the left eye. Early intervention was key in maintaining good CDVA that is correctable with spectacles and preventing further changes to the cornea (Table 16.1).

16.2 Case 2

- Patients undergoing PRK require screening evaluations before surgery as corneal keratoectasia can develop in these cases as well.
- Rigid contact lenses are a mainstay of therapy following surgical procedures to help correct irregular astigmatism.

A 45-year-old woman was referred to the cornea clinic due to concern for corneal ectasia in both eyes after undergoing PRK 5 years prior. Visual acuity was CF at 3′ in the right eye and 20/40 in the left eye. Slit lamp exam findings included Vogt's striae and iron lines which were more prominent in the right eye compared to the left eye. Corneal tomography displayed inferior steepening and irregular astigmatism.

The patient underwent CXL using the Dresden protocol in the right eye 3 months after the initial presentation and recovered without complication. The left eye was followed serially with frequent examinations and repeat diagnostic imaging. CXL was performed in the left eye using the Dresden protocol 2 years after initial presentation due to progression of astigmatism.

After CXL, corneal tomography has shown that the steep and flat keratometry readings have decreased and that Kmax has improved by 4.5 D in the right eye. Given that the surgery was performed with just a 3-month follow-up in the left eye, corneal remodeling is yet to be fully evaluated (see Fig. 16.2). This patient has benefitted from RGP lenses after surgery to help correct the irregular astigmatism and presently has a CDVA of 20/150 in the right eye and 20/30 in the left eye.

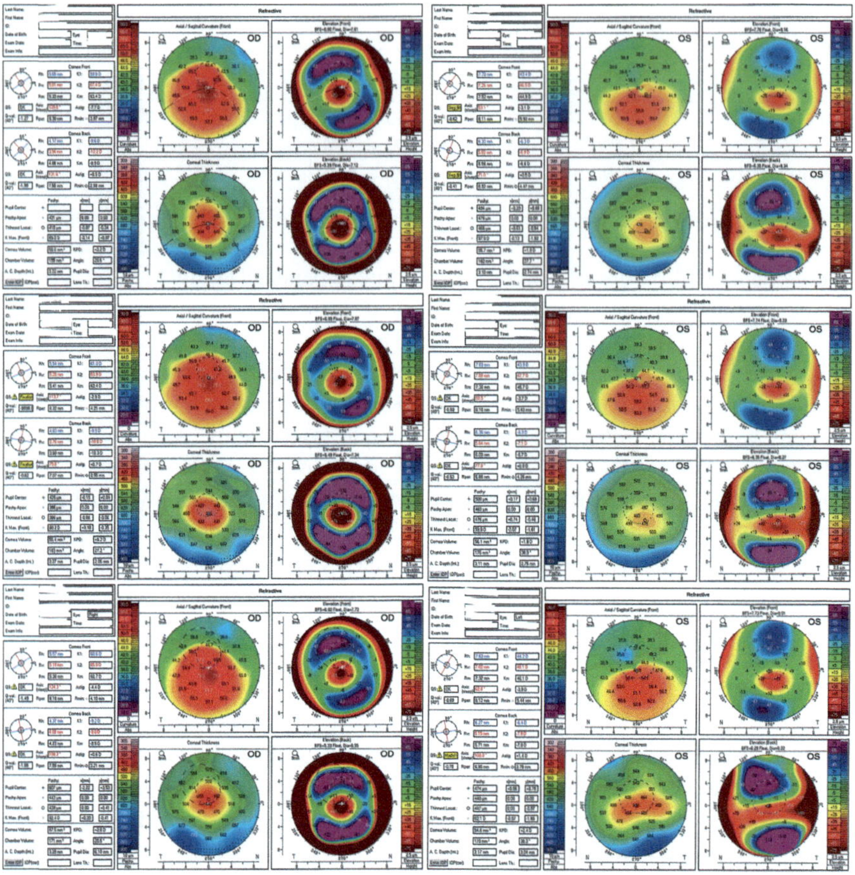

Fig. 16.2 Corneal tomography of patient 2 with post-PRK ectasia. (Top) Tomography at the initial visit. (Middle) Tomography 18 months after CXL in the right eye showing stable disease. There was mild progression in the left eye which subsequently underwent CXL. (Bottom) Tomography at the most recent visit. Keratometries in the right eye are stable with postoperative changes 2 years after CXL. The left eye is shown 3 months after CXL

16.3 Case 3

- Patients undergoing keratorefractive procedures require scheduled follow-ups, as corneal ectasia can develop many years after the procedure.
- Rigid contact lenses are useful in improving visual acuity but do not halt disease progression.

A 43-year-old man presented to the clinic with worsening vision in the left eye. The patient had undergone LASIK surgery 8 years prior. Slit lamp exam of both eyes showed well-centered LASIK flaps but an otherwise normal exam. Corneal tomography showed irregular astigmatism in the left eye (see Fig. 16.3) with manifest refraction showing astigmatism in the left eye (see Table 16.2). The patient was

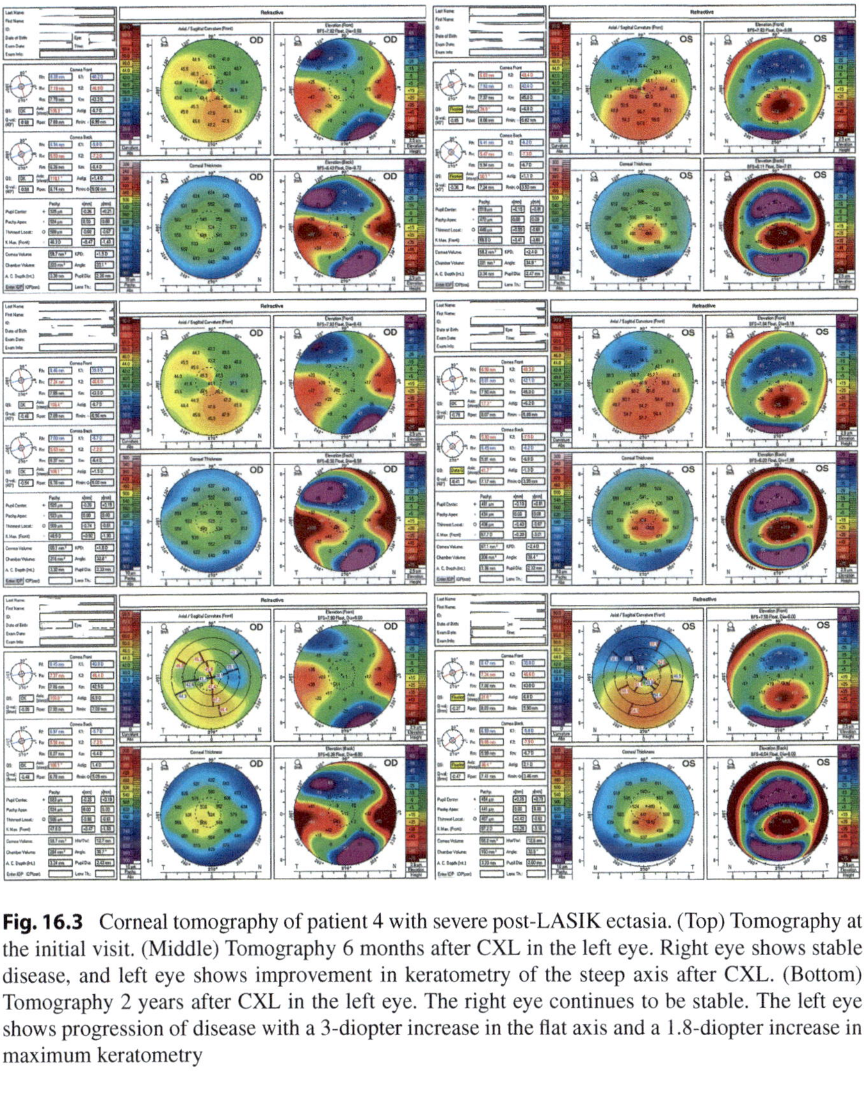

Fig. 16.3 Corneal tomography of patient 4 with severe post-LASIK ectasia. (Top) Tomography at the initial visit. (Middle) Tomography 6 months after CXL in the left eye. Right eye shows stable disease, and left eye shows improvement in keratometry of the steep axis after CXL. (Bottom) Tomography 2 years after CXL in the left eye. The right eye continues to be stable. The left eye shows progression of disease with a 3-diopter increase in the flat axis and a 1.8-diopter increase in maximum keratometry

using rigid gas permeable (RGP) lenses which improved vision. At this point, a diagnosis of corneal ectasia was discussed with the patient who opted for monitoring of disease.

At a follow-up visit 3 years later, the left eye was noted to have progression of astigmatism, and CXL was offered to the patient. The patient deferred the procedure, instead seeking correction with RGP lenses. The patient did not present to the cornea clinic for 5 years and followed up instead with optometry who referred him back for examination and possible intervention due to advanced progression of refractive error. At this next evaluation, 17 years after initial LASIK, the left eye had worsened visual acuity, increased refractive error, and notable changes to corneal

Table 16.2 Uncorrected visual acuity (UCVA), manifest refraction, and corrected distance visual acuity (CDVA) with rigid gas permeable contact lens correction for patient 3 at different time points. CXL was recommended in the left eye and deferred by the patient at the year 3 visit. CXL was performed in the left eye after the year 8 visit demonstrated severe progresion of myopic astigmatism. The patient has deferred CXL in the right eye. Visual acuity is presented in Snellen form

Time from diagnosis	UCVA	Refraction	CDVA (RGP lenses)
Initial diagnosis	20/15 20/20-1	−0.50 + 0.50 at 3 −0.50 + 2.00 at 33	20/15 20/15-2
Year 3	20/25-2 20/30-2	−1.00 + 1.25 at 170 −1.75 + 4.00 at 30	20/20+2 20/25-1
Year 8	20/30 + 1 20/125	−4.00 + 0.50 at 175 −7.75 + 6.00 at 20	20/30 20/50
CXL OS			
Year 10	20/40 20/80	−3.00 + 1.75 at 165 −2.50 + 6.75 at 30	20/12.5 20/20-1
Year 11	20/40 20/100	−3.00 + 1.75 at 165 −3.50 + 4.00 at 30	20/12.5 20/16

keratometry (Table 16.2). After discussion of options, the patient agreed for CXL of the left eye to halt progression.

Two years after CXL, there has been minimal change in corneal tomography in the operated left eye, and the patient has had a significant improvement in visual acuity. CDVA in the left eye with an RGP lens is 20/16, improved from 20/50 before CXL. Corneal tomography shows stabilization of disease without further keratometry changes. The right eye has gone through some astigmatic changes, but the patient has preferred to continue scheduled monitoring without intervention.

16.4 Case 4

- Intracorneal ring segments are a treatment option in keratoectasia but may be challenging to implant after previous LASIK surgery.
- CXL may be less effective in halting disease progression in eyes with post-LASIK ectasia compared to keratoconus.
- Contact lens intolerance can be a treatment challenge in patients with severe keratoectasia.

A 45-year-old woman presented to clinic with a chief complaint of decreased vision, worse in the left, for the previous 2 years. The patient had undergone LASIK in both eyes 17 years prior, followed by a PRK revision and anterior keratotomy in the right eye as well as radial keratectomy in the left eye at another institution. Slit lamp exam of the right eye showed a LASIK flap, paired AK incisions, an inferior iron line, and inferior steepening. Slit lamp exam of the left eye showed a LASIK flap, radial incision, iron ring, and inferior steepening with apical thinning. Corneal tomography showed irregular astigmatism in both eyes (see Fig. 16.1a).

The patient had previously been prescribed rigid gas permeable lenses but was not able to tolerate use due to irritation and dryness. At this point, options were discussed with the patient including CXL, and the patient decided to monitor with a serial evaluation in 3 months. At the follow-up visit, the corneal tomography showed progression of ectasia in the left eye (see Fig. 16.3). CXL was recommended in the left eye and the patient elected to proceed.

At the 1-year follow-up, the left eye had a 1.4 D decrease in steep keratometry and a 1 D decrease in Kmax. The patient continued to have issues with contact lenses: she reported ghost images with scleral lenses and was not able to tolerate RGP lenses. At the 2-year follow-up, there was progression of ectasia in the left eye with with a 3-diopter increase in the flat axis and a 1.8-diopter increase in maximum keratometry. At this point, she was recommended to follow up more frequently, and repeat CXL was suggested. She continued to follow up with optometry who attempted multiple contact lens changes. The patient then transferred her care to another cornea specialist. With the other specialist, intracorneal ring segment placement was attempted but had to be aborted mid-procedure due to incomplete formation of the channel with the femtosecond laser. She has continued to follow up at another academic institution where scleral lenses were prescribed. She continues to endorse difficulty wearing the lenses but has noted that the most recent lenses were more tolerable.

16.5 Discussion

Post-refractive keratoectasia was first reported by Seiler in 1998 and has been estimated to occur in 0.02% to 0.1% of patients undergoing refractive surgery [5, 8]. In a systematic review, Moshirfar et al. showed that incidence was highest after LASIK, followed by PRK and lastly by SMILE [5]. The four patients highlighted in this series review key aspects in the diagnosis, follow-up, and management of ectasia after keratorefractive procedures.

Diagnosis of ectasia consists of multiple criteria including a common historical pattern, slit lamp examination findings, and diagnostic imaging. Ectasia may occur at any point after keratorefractive procedure, so it is important to have a high index of suspicion regardless of time since surgery if patients have signs and symptoms of disease. Slit lamp examination findings include evidence of prior keratorefractive surgery, possible scarring and/or iron lines, inferior corneal thinning in the eyes, and advanced keratoectasia.

Diagnostic tools such as keratometry measurements, slit-scanning corneal topography, Scheimpflug imaging tomography, and optical coherence tomography (OCT) can help physicians with diagnosis and follow-up of these patients. Findings indicative of ectasia include inferior steepening, superior flattening, changes in anterior and posterior elevation, and changes in maximum keratometry [7, 9]. These findings were all highlighted in the patients presented. In recent years, these diagnostic tools have been used to pursue early disease detection on an individual basis and also in the setting of artificial intelligence with large data sets [10–12]. As these tools continue to develop, there may be the opportunity to develop more robust subclinical disease detection similar to keratoconus with a move toward early intervention prior to patient symptoms [13].

Conservative management with spectacles remains a first-line treatment but has limited success in cases of advanced astigmatism. Case 1 is an example of a mild case of ectasia that has been successfully managed with spectacle correction alone in the non-operated eye. Contact lenses remain a very important management tool with high success. Contact lens strategies include rigid gas permeable lenses, scleral lenses, custom wavefront-guided soft contact lenses, hybrid lenses, and tandem soft contact lens-RGP lenses [14]. RGP and scleral lenses provide a regular anterior refractive surface and improve CDVA [15]. Cases 2 and 3 show the visual improvement achieved with contact lenses despite severe myopic astigmatism with an irregular surface. However, contact lens intolerance remains a concern, with one study reporting that up to 20% of patients are unable to wear contact lenses on a regular basis [16]. Case 4 serves as an example of the difficulty patients can have with contact lens intolerance.

Corneal cross-linking is a procedure that has been FDA approved to diminish progression of ectasia. CXL has also been shown to improve Kmax, UCVA, CDVA, and corneal aberrations [17–19]. In four out of five eyes where CXL was performed in this series, the procedure successfully halted disease progression and allowed for functional vision with refractive correction. This is similar to the 78% success rate reported by Chanbour et al., who previously suggested that CXL may be less effective in post-LASIK ectasia compared to keratoconus [20]. Corneal haze is a known phenomenon after CXL that occurs and improves 3–12 months after onset. Studies have shown that this does not affect clinical outcomes [21]. All cases in this series displayed post-CXL haze on slit lamp exam, but patients did not report subjective complaints and maintained good visual acuity. It is also important to highlight the Athens protocol, in which patients undergo surface ablation immediately followed by CXL. This procedure improves topography and refractive error, and it has also been shown to have long-term stability [22, 23].

Contact lenses are also important after surgical intervention such as CXL or in cases of corneal transplantation. One interesting finding reported in the literature is reports of contact lens fitting changing after CXL in keratoconic eyes. Mandathar et al. reported a series of 34 eyes in which there were no changes in refraction and topography indices, but there were changes in contact lens fitting characteristics that suggest a change in shape or apex location after CXL [24]. Case 2 shows the impact that contact lenses can have in improving vision after CXL, with the patient's CDVA being greatly improved with contact lens use. This patient's diagnostic testing also demonstrated a decrease in keratometry readings and mild changes in post-CXL contact lens parameters that have been described in the literature.

Minimally invasive surgery with intrastromal corneal ring segments has been reported to improve keratoectasia [7, 25, 26]. However, patients whose corneas are too thin or who have rapidly progressive disease cannot undergo placement of the ring segments. Another issue with segment placement can be improper positioning due to the LASIK flap [27]. In case 4, there was difficulty placing the segments requiring aborting of the surgical procedure. Placement of intracorneal ring segments has also been combined with sequential cross-linking and shown to be successful in the management of ectasia patients [28]. One meta-analysis showed that patients undergoing simultaneous ring implantation with CXL had better spherical refractive error, flat keratometry reading, and steep keratometry reading compared to staging the procedure [29].

Successful corneal transplantation has also been reported to manage cases of post-keratorefractive ectasia [30, 31]. These procedures should be attempted after conservative management, and minimally invasive procedures have been attempted, as they carry lifelong risk of complications such as rejection and secondary glaucoma. The advent of treatments such as contact lenses, CXL, and intrastromal ring segments has significantly changed the management of corneal ectasias. Choi and Jeng report that corneal transplantation for ectasia has decreased by approximately 60% with the advent of modern treatment modalities [32].

Screening remains the only possible way to prevent disease. Reasons for exclusion from keratorefractive correction include abnormal corneal topography, low corneal thickness, high correction, and severe dry eye [33–35]. Using these criteria to reduce the risk of post-procedure keractoectasia has been successful, as the incidence has decreased [36, 37]. Ambrosio has highlighted the decreased incidence of 0.033% reported by Bohac et al. in 2018 compared to the incidence of 0.66% reported in an earlier series by Pallikaris in 2001 [37–39]. Despite these advances, cases of ectasia can still develop and will present a treatment challenge for corneal specialists.

Post-keratorefractive ectasia is a complex disease process that presents a treatment challenge for corneal specialists. Careful preoperative screening has reduced the incidence of disease, but patients continue to require serial examinations post-procedure and early intervention when there are signs of disease. Here we present four patients who underwent corneal cross-linking for the management of keratoectasia. As technologies continue to develop, the landscape of patient management may continue to change.

References

1. Randleman JB, Russell B, Ward MA, et al. Risk factors and prognosis for corneal ectasia after LASIK. Ophthalmology. 2003;110:267–75.
2. Randleman JB, Caster AI, Banning CS, et al. Corneal ectasia after photorefractive keratectomy. J Cataract Refract Surg. 2006;32:1395–8.
3. Randleman JB. Post-laser in-situ keratomileusis ectasia: current understanding and future directions. Curr Opin Ophthalmol. 2006;17:406–12.
4. Sachdev G, Sachdev MS, Sachdev R, et al. Unilateral corneal ectasia following small-incision lenticule extraction. J Cataract Refract Surg. 2015;41:2014–8.
5. Moshirfar M, Tukan AN, Bundogji N, et al. Ectasia after corneal refractive surgery: a systematic review. Ophthalmol Ther. 2021;10:753–76.
6. Dawson DG, Randleman JB, Grossniklaus HE, et al. Corneal ectasia after excimer laser keratorefractive surgery: histopathology, ultrastructure, and pathophysiology. Ophthalmology. 2008;115:2181–2191.e1.

7. Garcia-Ferrer FJ, Akpek EK, Amescua G, et al. Corneal ectasia preferred practice pattern®. Ophthalmology. 2019;126:P170–215.
8. Seiler T, Quurke AW. Iatrogenic keratectasia after LASIK in a case of forme fruste keratoconus. J Cataract Refract Surg. 1998;24:1007–9.
9. Imbornoni LM, McGhee CNJ, Belin MW. Evolution of keratoconus: from diagnosis to therapeutics. Klin Monatsbl Augenheilkd. 2018;235:680–8.
10. Koh S, Ambrósio R, Inoue R, et al. Detection of subclinical corneal ectasia using corneal tomographic and biomechanical assessments in a Japanese population. J Refract Surg. 2019;35:383–90.
11. Yilmaz FO, Yildiz BK, Demirok A. Detection of subclinical corneal ectasia after laser in situ Keratomileusis: Corvis ST. Beyoglu Eye Journal. 2021;6:145.
12. Lopes BT, Ramos IC, Salomão MQ, et al. Enhanced tomographic assessment to detect corneal ectasia based on artificial intelligence. Am J Ophthalmol. 2018;195:223–32.
13. Pérez-Rueda A, Jiménez-Rodríguez D, Castro-Luna G. Diagnosis of subclinical keratoconus with a combined model of biomechanical and topographic parameters. J Clin Med. 2021;10:2746.
14. Bromley JG, Randleman JB. Treatment strategies for corneal ectasia. Curr Opin Ophthalmol. 2010;21:255.
15. Maharana PK, Dubey A, Jhanji V, et al. Management of advanced corneal ectasias. Br J Ophthalmol. 2016;100(1):34–40.
16. Woodward MA, Randleman JB, Russell B, et al. Visual rehabilitation and outcomes for ectasia after corneal refractive surgery. J Cataract Refract Surg. 2008;34:383.
17. Hersh PS, Stulting RD, Muller D, et al. US multicenter clinical trial of corneal collagen crosslinking for treatment of corneal ectasia after refractive surgery. Ophthalmology. 2017;124:1475–84.
18. Vinciguerra P, Albè E, Trazza S, et al. Refractive, topographic, tomographic, and aberrometric analysis of keratoconic eyes undergoing corneal cross-linking. Ophthalmology. 2009;116:369–78.
19. Li G, Fan ZJ, Peng XJ. Corneal collagen crosslinking for corneal ectasia of post-LASIK: one-year results. Int J Ophthalmol. 2012;5:190.
20. Chanbour W, el Zein L, Younes MA, et al. Corneal cross-linking for keratoconus and post-LASIK ectasia and failure rate: a 3 years follow-up study. Cureus. 2021;13:e19552.
21. Greenstein SA, Fry KL, Bhatt J, et al. Natural history of corneal haze after collagen crosslinking for keratoconus and corneal ectasia: Scheimpflug and biomicroscopic analysis. J Cataract Refract Surg. 2010;36:2105–14.
22. Kanellopoulos AJ, Binder PS. Management of corneal ectasia after LASIK with combined, same-day, topography-guided partial transepithelial PRK and collagen cross-linking: the Athens protocol. J Refract Surg. 2011;27:323–31.
23. Kanellopoulos AJ. Ten-year outcomes of progressive keratoconus management with the Athens protocol (topography-guided partial-refraction PRK combined with CXL). J Refract Surg. 2019;35:478–83.
24. Mandathara PS, Kalaiselvan P, Rathi VM, et al. Contact lens fitting after corneal collagen cross-linking. Oman J Ophthalmol. 2019;12:177–80.
25. Rabinowitz YS. INTACS for KERATOCONUS and ectasia after LASIK. Int Ophthalmol Clin. 2013;53(1):27–39.
26. Piñero DP, Alio JL, Uceda-Montanes A, et al. Intracorneal ring segment implantation in corneas with post-laser in situ keratomileusis keratectasia. Ophthalmology. 2009;116:1665–74.
27. Abad JC. Management of slipped laser in situ keratomileusis flap following intrastromal corneal ring implantation in post-LASIK ectasia. J Cataract Refract Surg. 2008;34:2177–81.
28. Legare ME, Iovieno A, Yeung SN, et al. Intacs with or without same-day corneal collagen cross-linking to treat corneal ectasia. Can J Ophthalmol. 2013;48:173–8.
29. Hashemi H, Alvani A, Seyedian MA, et al. Appropriate sequence of combined Intracorneal ring implantation and corneal collagen cross-linking in keratoconus: a systematic review and meta-analysis. Cornea. 2018;37:1601–7.

30. McAllum PJ, Segev F, Herzig S, et al. Deep anterior lamellar keratoplasty for post-LASIK ectasia. Cornea. 2007;26:507–11.
31. Kucumen RB, Yenerel NM, Gorgun E, et al. Penetrating keratoplasty for corneal ectasia after laser in situ keratomileusis. Eur J Ophthalmol. 2008;18:695–702.
32. Choi JH, Jeng BH. Indications for keratoplasty in management of corneal ectasia. Curr Opin Ophthalmol. 2022;33:318–23.
33. Rubinfeld RS, Trattler WB, Talamo J, et al. Screening of refractive surgery candidates for LASIK and PRK. Cornea. 2015;34:e13–4.
34. Ambrósio R, Klyce SD, Wilson SE. Corneal topographic and pachymetric screening of keratorefractive patients. J Refract Surg. 2003;19:24–9.
35. Sharma N, Singhvi A, Sinha R, et al. Reasons for not performing LASIK in refractive surgery candidates. J Refract Surg. 2005;21:496–8.
36. Jin SX, Dackowski E, Chuck RS. Risk factors for postlaser refractive surgery corneal ectasia. Curr Opin Ophthalmol. 2020;31:288–92.
37. Ambrósio R. Post-LASIK ectasia: twenty years of a conundrum. Semin Ophthalmol. 2019;34:66–8.
38. Bohac M, Koncarevic M, Pasalic A, et al. Incidence and clinical characteristics of post LASIK ectasia: a review of over 30,000 LASIK cases. Semin Ophthalmol. 2018;33:869–77.
39. Pallikaris IG, Kymionis GD, Astyrakakis NI. Corneal ectasia induced by laser in situ keratomileusis. J Cataract Refract Surg. 2001;27:1796–802.

Keratoglobus

17

Varsha M. Rathi, Somasheila I. Murthy,
Pravin Krishna Vaddavalli, and Sunita Chaurasia

Keratoglobus is a rare, bilateral, noninflammatory globular protrusion of cornea, characterized by thinning of the whole cornea from limbus to limbus with a more marked thinning in the periphery [1]. The corneal diameter is of normal size. Congenital keratoglobus is associated with blue sclera, Leber's amaurosis, Ehlers-Danlos syndrome type VI, and brittle cornea syndrome [2–5]. Rathi et al. reported that the disease may be blinding in patients with blue sclera [6]. Sudden ruptures, perforations, or hydrops of the cornea—with or without trivial trauma—have been reported [7, 8]. Acquired keratoglobus has been reported in patients with vernal keratoconjunctivitis [9, 10] and dysthyroid ophthalmopathy [11].

A few cases of keratoglobus managed in different ways are described below.

17.1 Case 1

- Acute corneal hydrops
- Descemet's membrane detachment

V. M. Rathi (✉)
Allen Foster Community Eye Health Research Centre, Gullapalli Pratibha Rao International Centre for Advancement of Rural Eye care, LV Prasad Eye Institute, Hyderabad, Telangana, India

Indian Health Outcomes, Public Health and Economics (IHOPE) Research Centre, LVPEI, Hyderabad, Telangana, India

Shantilal Shanghvi Cornea Institute, LV Prasad Eye Institute, Hyderabad, Telangana, India
e-mail: varsharathi@lvpei.org

S. I. Murthy · P. K. Vaddavalli · S. Chaurasia
Shantilal Shanghvi Cornea Institute, LV Prasad Eye Institute, Hyderabad, Telangana, India
e-mail: somasheila@lvpei.org; pravin@lvpei.org; sunita@lvpei.org

F. A. Woreta, R. B. Singh (eds.), *Cornea Casebook*, Current Practices in Ophthalmology, https://doi.org/10.1007/978-981-96-0495-1_17

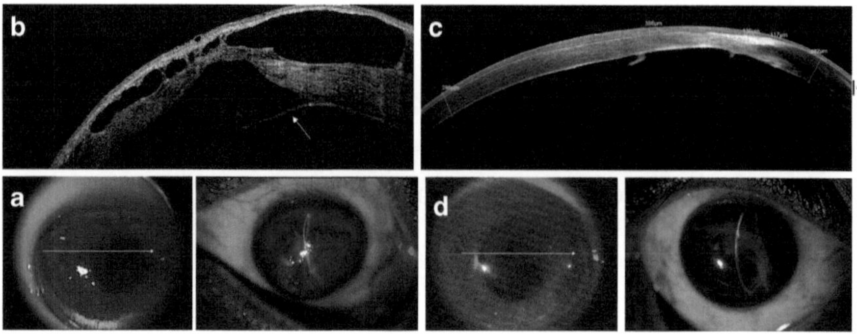

Fig. 17.1 (**a**) Shows the presence of stromal edema with bullae. (**b**) Shows the presence of increased corneal thickness, fluid pockets seen as empty spaces in the cornea and detached DM (arrow). (**c**) AS-OCT shows the compact cornea and the sutures are seen on the cornea. (**d**) Resolved corneal edema and thinning cornea with scarring

- Fluid pockets and thin cornea on AS-OCT
- Compression sutures just outside pupil in the area DM separation

A 47-year-old man presented with history of diminished vision in his right eye of a week's duration. His visual acuity in the right eye was hand movements, and in the left eye the vision improved to 20/50 with -5 D Sph -10.D Cyl@90 degrees. The right eye had corneal edema with Descemet's membrane detachment, and the left eye showed globular protrusion and thinning of the entire cornea. The clinical diagnosis was keratoglobus in both eyes with acute hydrops in the right eye. See Fig. 17.1a and b. Compression sutures were done in this patient. At 6-month follow-up, the cornea cleared (Fig. 17.1c and d). Patient's visual acuity improved to 20/200 with −11.50 DCyl@140 degrees.

17.2 Case 2

- Acute corneal hydrops
- Descemet's membrane detachment
- Air descemetopexy

A 23-year-old female presented with white opacity in her left eye of 20-day duration and had diminution of vision. She was diagnosed to have keratoglobus with acute hydrops in her left eye (Fig. 17.2a and b). She underwent descemetopexy in her left eye. A full-chamber air bubble was injected. After 10 minutes, saline was instilled, and a mobile air bubble was left at the end of the procedure. Over a year's follow-up, her visual acuity improved to 20/50 with −6 D Sph. Usually, descemetopexy with air is preferred to C3F8 gas as gas may cause

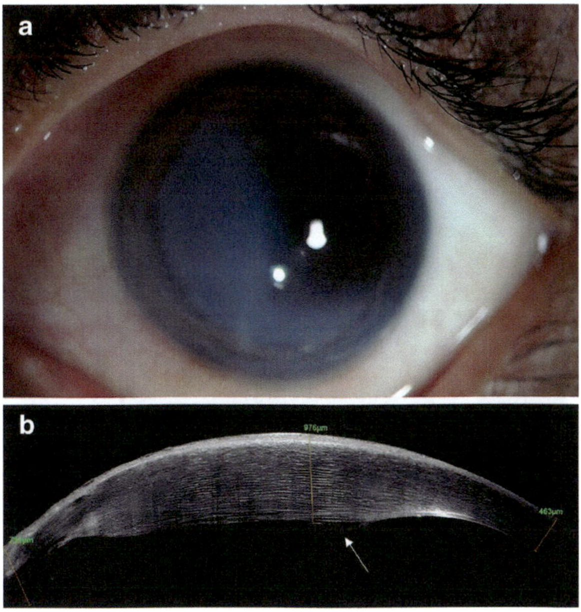

Fig. 17.2 (**a**) Cornea shows the presence of stromal edema. (**b**) Shows the increased thickness of the cornea with detached Descemet's membrane

increase in intraocular pressure and subsequent pupillary block glaucoma in patients of keratoglobus. The end outcome with air or C3F8 gas descemetopexy otherwise is similar [7].

17.3 Case 3

- Advanced keratoglobus.
- Epikeratoplasty.
- Especially in patients with healed hydrops.
- One may do endothelial keratoplasties if required in the future.

A 37-year-old gentleman had his right eye as atrophic bulbi due to repeated injuries in childhood and the left eye had advanced ectasia (Fig. 17.3a) showing the protruded cone. AS-OCT and corneal topography were done which showed advanced ectasia (Fig. 17.3b and c). His visual acuity in the right eye was 20/800. He underwent epikeratoplasty in his left eye. Conjunctival peritomy of 360 degrees was done at limbus along with extensive cauterization to control bleeding, and pannus resection was done. Following this, a 360-degree scleral tunnel was made at the limbus.

Donor button was trephined using 12-mm vacuum trephine, and dissection was done in the same to create a 360-degree scleral lip. This donor button was then placed over de-epithelialized host cornea and sutured to scleral tunnel with 24 9-0 nylon sutures (Fig. 17.3d)

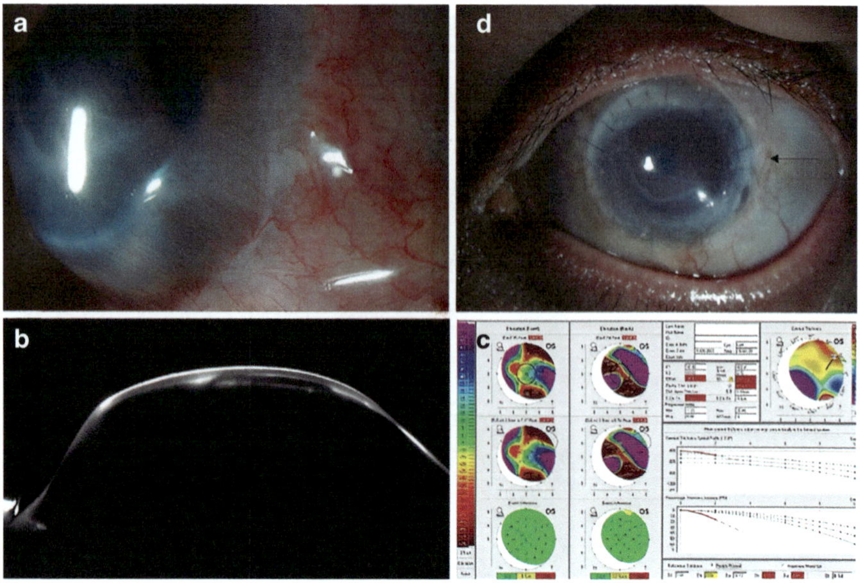

Fig. 17.3 (**a**) Advanced ectasia of the cornea. (**b**) AS-OCT showing the ectasia and thinning of the cornea. (**c**) Corneal topography shows thinning and steep cornea. (**d**) Cornea postoperatively shows the presence of sutures

17.4 Case 4 Delayed Diagnosis of Keratoglobus

- Corneal tear one eye.
- Adherent leukoma/corneal scars/healed hydrops in the other eye.
- Always check the other eye of the patients presenting with corneal tear or adherent leukoma.
- Joint hypermobility and facial examination.
- Delayed diagnosis.

An 8-year-old boy was brought by his parents with alleged history of trauma to his right eye with a pencil while studying in school. He had inferior full-thickness corneal tear of around 2 clock hours (5–7 o'clock) at the limbus with iris tissue prolapsing out of the tear. The child was diagnosed to have RE open globe injury, penetrating type, zone 1, and was subjected to corneal tear repair in the emergency clinic. In the postoperative period, he developed endophthalmitis and underwent pars plana lensectomy and vitrectomy and endolaser and silicone oil injection. Subsequently, his eye condition improved (Fig. 17.4a). The best corrected visual acuity in this eye was counting fingers close to the face, and the other eye was 20/50 with −5.00 D Sph. Over the follow-up, the child developed corneal edema in the

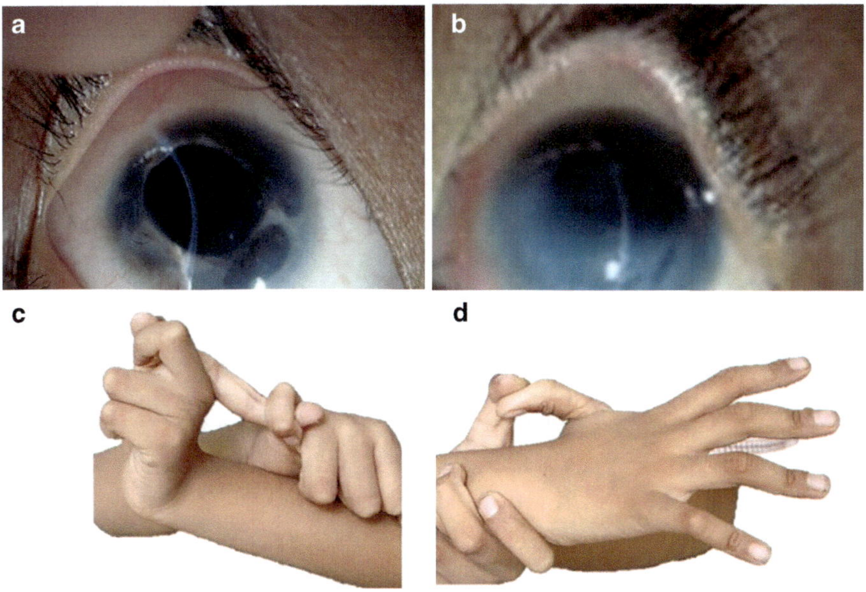

Fig. 17.4 (**a**) Presence of aphakia and thin cornea after the tear repair with adherent leukoma. (**b**) Presence of corneal edema. (**c** and **d**) Hypermobility of the joints

better left eye with reduced vision. He was referred to the cornea department for the presence of corneal edema (Fig. 17.4b) when the clinician diagnosed the case as keratoglobus and corneal hydrops. He had hypermobile joints (Fig. 17.4c and d). There is a possibility of missing the diagnosis, and looking up for the systemic features in such cases will give a clue for associated syndrome such as the Ehlers-Danlos syndrome.

17.5 Case 5 Primary Congenital Glaucoma

- Large eyeball
- Corneal edema—acute increase in intraocular pressure
- High intraocular pressure
- May mimic keratoglobus
- Trab with Trab

A mother brought her 3-month-old infant boy who had bluish white discoloration of his left eye of 1-day duration at one of our rural remote centers. There was no history of trauma to the eye and no history of parental consanguinity. Figure 17.5a shows the presence of corneal edema similar to keratoglobus with hydrops and with

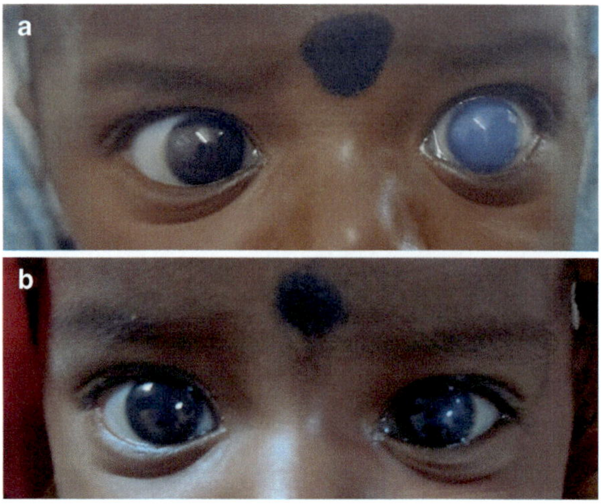

Fig. 17.5 (**a**) A diffuse photograph of both eyes showing large eyeballs with corneal edema in the left eye. (**b**) The cornea cleared after the glaucoma surgery in the left eye

large corneal diameter similar to megalocornea. The intraocular pressure was high digitally for both eyes. A diagnosis of hydrops in the left eye and primary congenital glaucoma in the right eye was made, and the infant was put on Dorzox eye drops thrice a day. He underwent examination under anesthesia, and the presence of Haab's striae was noted in both eyes. The IOP was 10 mmHg, and the cup/disc ratio was 0.7. The child was advised antiglaucoma medications for both eyes and subsequently underwent trabeculotomy + trabeculectomy for the left eye, and the cornea cleared (Fig. 17.5b). This case shows that one may get confused with acute hydrops of keratoglobus and timely intervention in a patient of primary congenital glaucoma will help prevent further deterioration of vision. See Table 17.1.

Table 17.1 Differentiating clinical features of keratoglobus

	Keratoglobus	Ectatic disorders		Nonectatic disorders		
	Keratoglobus	Keratoconus	Pellucid marginal degeneration	Megalocornea	Congenital glaucoma	Brittle cornea syndrome
Thinning	Generalized thinning	Thinning focal or globular	Thinning usually inferiorly, may be seen superiorly	No thinning	No, reported by some	Yes
Protrusion	Generalized	Protrusion of thinned out cornea	Ectasia above thinning	Protrusion present	Protrusion present	Generalized
Presentation time	At birth	Children	Adult	At birth	At birth	At birth
Progression	Yes	Yes	Yes	No	No	No
Fleischer's ring	Absent	Present	Absent	Absent	Absent	No
Corneal diameter	Normal	Normal	Normal	More	More	Normal
Disc					Glaucomatous disc changes	

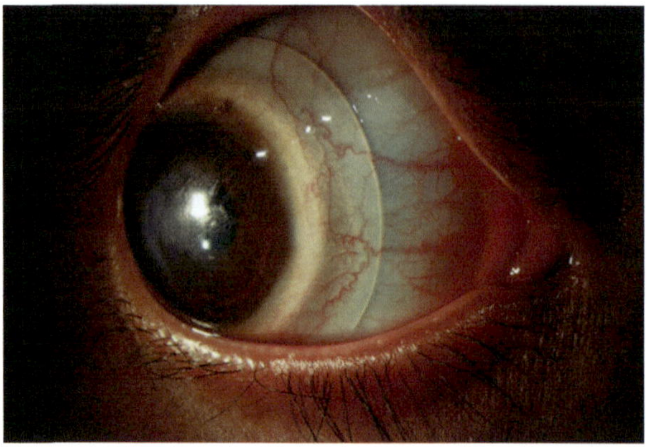

Fig. 17.6 Scleral contact lens (PROSE) resting on sclera post-epikeratoplasty

17.6 Discussion

The above cases highlight the importance of taking proper family history and examination of the other eye in case the patient presents with perforation, adherent leukoma, scars, and corneal edema—acute hydrops. This will help in the management of both eyes of the patients, with prevention of injuries in the future and proper management of the existing condition. Diagnosis is based on family history of consanguinity, family history of keratoglobus, thin protruded cornea, joint deformities, typical facial features such as flat face, blue sclera (not present in all patients), history of corneal perforations, and tears and white scars in the eyes during childhood. As trivial trauma to the eye may cause perforation of the cornea, the use of glasses would provide both functional vision and protection against trauma. Contact lenses are prescribed to the patients based on the risk of the trauma and visual improvement (Fig. 17.6). Although scleral lenses may be prescribed in some patients, it should be prescribed judiciously in the presence of blue sclera, or scleral lenses with fenestration may be used. Surgeries are indicated for the management of corneal hydrops, perforations, and tears [12, 13].

Funding Support (For all authors) Hyderabad Eye Research Foundation, Hyderabad.

References

1. Wallang BS, Das S. Keratoglobus. Eye (Lond). 2013;27(9):1004–12.
2. Cameron JA, Cotter JB, Risco JM, Alvarez H. Epikeratoplasty for keratoglobus associated with blue sclera. Ophthalmology. 1991;98(4):446–52.
3. Gillespie FD. Congenital amaurosis of Leber. Am J Ophthalmol. 1966;61(5 Pt 1):874–80.
4. Imamoglu S, Kaya V, Imamoglu EY, Gok K. Congenital keratoglobus with blue sclera in two siblings with overlapping Marshall/Stickler phenotype. Indian J Ophthalmol. 2016;64(11):856–9.
5. Gregoratos ND, Bartsocas CS, Papas K. Blue sclerae with keratoglobus and brittle cornea. Br J Ophthalmol. 1971;55(6):424–6.

6. Rathi VM, Murthy SI, Bagga B, Taneja M, Chaurasia S, Sangwan VS. Keratoglobus: an experience at a tertiary eye care center in India. Indian J Ophthalmol. 2015;63(3):233–8.
7. Basu S, Vaddavalli PK, Ramappa M, Shah S, Murthy SI, Sangwan VS. Intracameral perfluoropropane gas in the treatment of acute corneal hydrops. Ophthalmology. 2011;118(5):934–9.
8. Biglan AW, Brown SI, Johnson BL. Keratoglobus and blue sclera. Am J Ophthalmol. 1977;83(2):225–33.
9. Gupta VP, Jain RK, Angra SK. Acute hydrops in keratoglobus with vernal keratoconjunctivitis. Indian J Ophthalmol. 1985;33(2):121–3.
10. Cameron JA, Al-Rajhi AA, Badr IA. Corneal ectasia in vernal keratoconjunctivitis. Ophthalmology. 1989;96(11):1615–23.
11. Cameron JA. Keratoglobus. Cornea. 1993;12(2):124–30.
12. Vajpayee RB, Bhartiya P, Sharma N. Central lamellar keratoplasty with peripheral intralamellar tuck: a new surgical technique for keratoglobus. Cornea. 2002;21(7):657–60.
13. Vajpayee RB, Sharma N, Saxena R, Dada T. Epikeratoplasty for traumatic corneal ectasia. Cornea. 1999;18(2):237–9.

Part V

Autoimmune Disorders

Peripheral Ulcerative Keratitis

18

Virender Singh Sangwan, Manisha Acharya,
Kaustubh Wagh, and Abha Gour

18.1 Introduction

The cornea is a complex multicomponent structure that forms the clear outermost surface of the eye. Behind the tear film, the first layer of the cornea to see incoming light is the epithelium, which prevents foreign material from entering the eye. Unlike most cells, the corneal epithelium is nourished by the tear film rather than by the vasculature. Behind the corneal epithelium lie Bowman's layer and stroma, which consist of collagen fibrils embedded in a network of glycosaminoglycans. These layers provide mechanical strength and rigidity to the cornea. The innermost layers of the cornea are Descemet's membrane and the endothelium, which serve to remove water from the corneal stroma and maintain transparency [1] (Fig. 18.1).

Laterally, the cornea can be divided into the central cornea, the peripheral cornea, and the limbal region (Fig. 18.1b). The central cornea is ~0.5 mm thick and contains densely packed and regularly arranged collagen fibrils. On the other hand, the peripheral cornea is thicker (~ 1 mm) and contains more loosely packed and less regularly arranged collagen I fibers. The epithelial cells in the peripheral cornea more strongly adhere to the basement membrane than those in the central cornea. While the central cornea is largely devoid of vasculature, the peripheral cornea is

V. S. Sangwan · M. Acharya · A. Gour (✉)
Department of Cornea and Anterior Segment Services, Dr Shroffs Charity Eye Hospital, New Delhi, India

Department of Stem Cell Research, Dr Shroffs Charity Eye Hospital, New Delhi, India
e-mail: abha@sceh.net

K. Wagh
Department of Physics, University of Maryland, College Park, MD, USA

Laboratory of Receptor Biology and Gene Expression, National Cancer Institute, National Institute of Health, Bethesda, MD, USA

F. A. Woreta, R. B. Singh (eds.), *Cornea Casebook*, Current Practices in Ophthalmology, https://doi.org/10.1007/978-981-96-0495-1_18

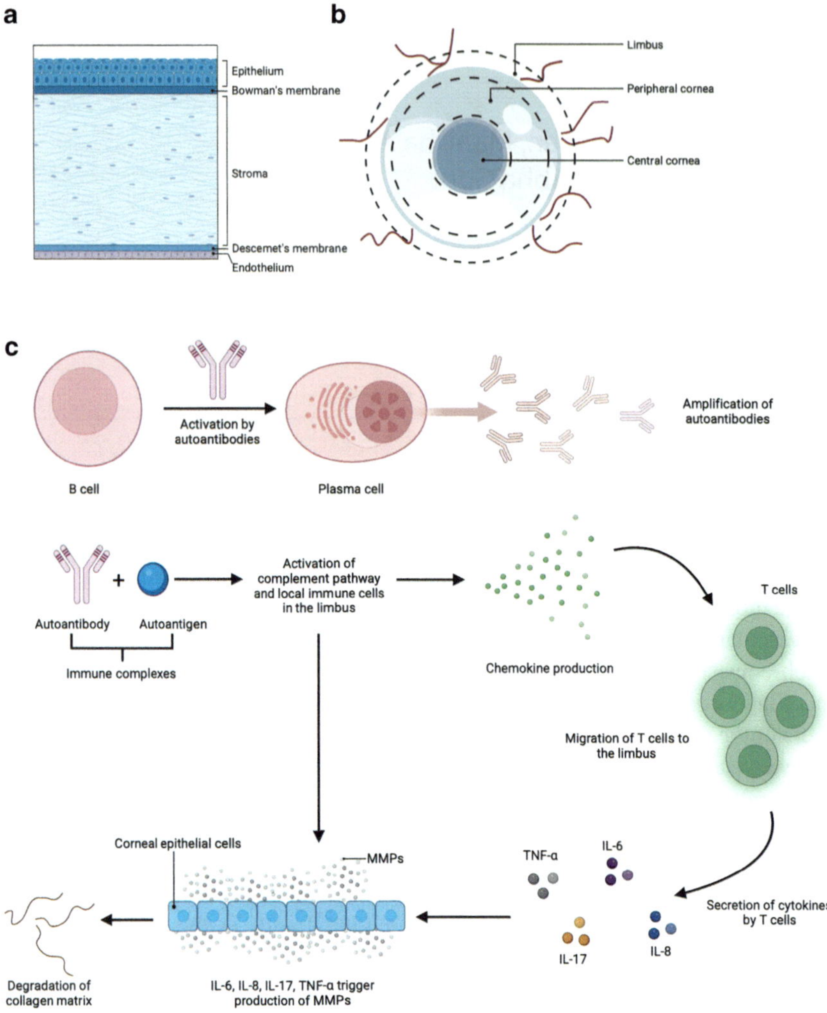

Fig. 18.1 Immunopathogenesis of peripheral ulcerative keratitis(**a**) Cross section of the cornea. (**b**) Lateral sectioning of the cornea. The limbal cornea contains vasculature, while the central and peripheral portions of cornea are avascular. (**c**) Autoantibodies activate B cells, causing their differentiation into plasma cells. These plasma cells amplify the number of autoantibodies, which, together with autoantigens, form immune complexes. These immune complexes are deposited in the limbal cornea through the vasculature, where they activate resident immune cells and the complement pathway. This triggers the production of chemokines, which attract helper T cells. Upon activation, these T cells secrete cytokines such as TNF-α, IL-6, IL-8, and IL-17, all of which promote the production of matrix metalloproteinases (MMPs) by cells in the corneal and conjunctival epithelium and cells in the lacrimal glands. Upregulation of MMPs triggers the degradation of the collagen matrix in the peripheral cornea and basement membrane (*Created using* Biorender.com)

surrounded by the limbus, which has a dense network of capillaries that provide a constant supply of blood, immune cells, and immune complexes [2].

Peripheral ulcerative keratitis (PUK) is a sight-threatening, acute-onset inflammatory condition of the peripheral cornea associated with progressive stromal thinning [3] and an overlying epithelial defect. This is due to the release of pro-inflammatory mediators from the associated corneal limbal vasculitis [4]. Studies estimate the incidence of PUK to be 0.2 to 3 cases per million people [5, 6] with a general predilection to the female sex. However, some have also reported an equal incidence in both. It is also essential to maintain a strong suspicion of infectious etiology in the management as a significant percentage of PUK cases are of an infectious origin [5].

In this chapter, we aim to discuss a series of cases to assist in better clinical understanding and management of this condition.

18.2 Case 1

- Acute onset
- Small perforation
- Managed with tissue adhesive and BCL
- Secondary to systemic disease [4]
- Managed with systemic antitubercular medication

This is a case of a 27-year-old female patient who presented with complaints of pain and redness in the left eye for 1 month, with no associated history of ocular trauma, fever, or joint pains. Her best corrected visual acuity was 20/30 in the left eye and 20/20 in the right eye.

Slit-lamp biomicroscopy examination of the left eye revealed congested conjunctiva, a 3 × 4 mm area of peripheral corneal perforation with iris prolapse, and a peaked pupil at the 9 o'clock position (Image 18.1). The anterior chamber was formed but shallow. The rest of the anterior and posterior segment examination was within normal limits. Right eye examination showed normal anterior and posterior segment. Diagnostic corneal scraping was performed, which showed no organism on staining. She was advised a detailed systemic workup, including complete blood count, erythrocyte sedimentation rate, C-reactive protein, RA factor, Mantoux test, and chest X-ray. She was scheduled for a procedure using tissue adhesive. A 14-mm Acuvue Oasys bandage contact lens was applied (Image 18.2).

On investigation, her erythrocyte sedimentation rate was raised. Chest X-ray showed increased markings in the right hilum, and the Mantoux test was strongly positive for tuberculosis. Further contrast-enhanced computed tomography (CECT) chest showed nodular calcific lesion, and fine needle aspiration cytology (FNAC) of the right cervical lymph node revealed necrotizing granulomatous lymphadenitis suggestive of tubercular etiology.

She was diagnosed as having PUK with corneal perforation secondary to tuberculosis [7], and a course of antitubercular treatment was given. After 3 months, the cornea was epithelized with no recurrence in the further course of follow-up (Images 18.3 and 18.4).

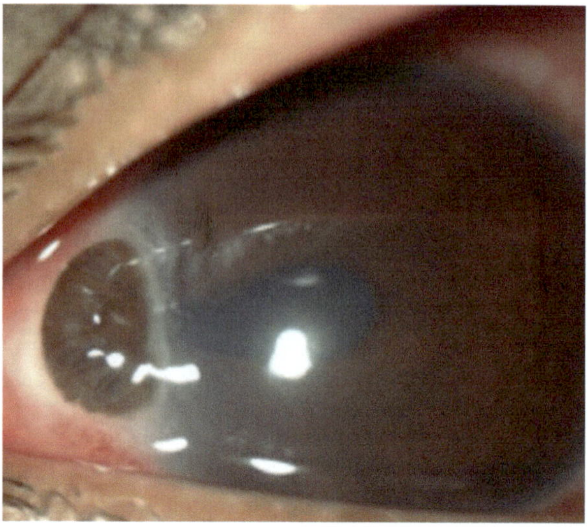

Image 18.1 At presentation, PUK-like picture with 3 × 2 mm defect with iris prolapse and surrounding corneal edema extending over one clock hour. Iris prolapse was present at 9 o'clock with a stretched pupil margin

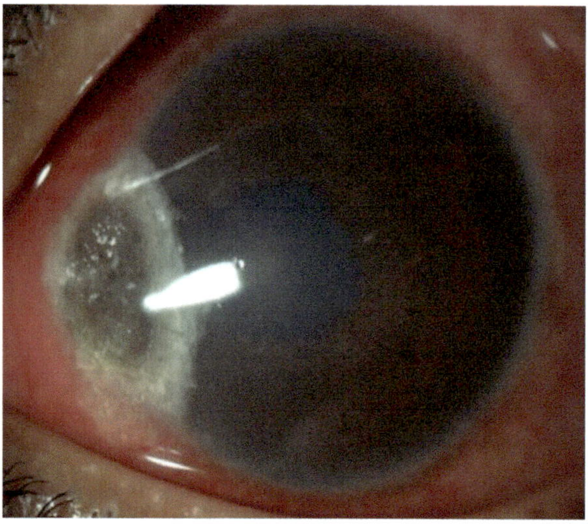

Image 18.2 Post-tissue adhesive with BCL

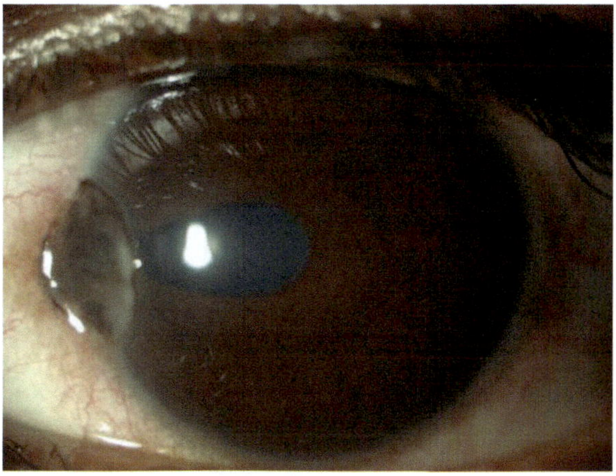

Image 18.3 The area of perforation is now epithelized (3 months after the episode)

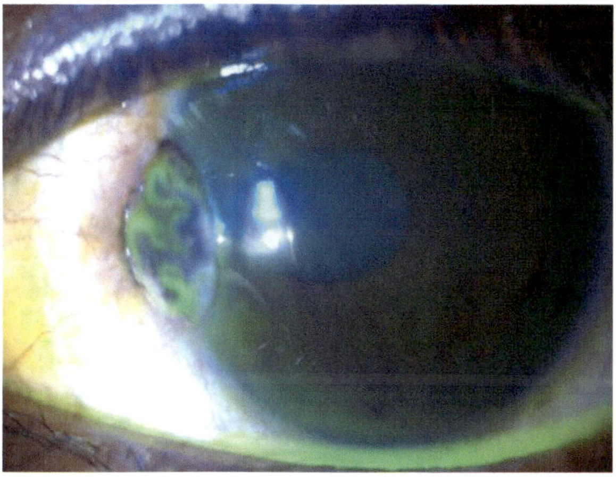

Image 18.4 Epithelized defect with pooling of fluorescein

18.3 Case 2

- Large circumferential area of corneal melt
- Managed with systemic medication
- Exacerbation after cataract surgery
- Raised c-ANCA

This is another case of a 55-year-old female who presented with pain, redness, and watering in one eye, with the other eye being essentially normal. She was being treated elsewhere for 1 month with topical antibiotics and lubricants, with a poor response. At presentation, she had a best corrected visual acuity of 20/200 in the affected eye (Image 18.5).

She was investigated thoroughly, and the blood investigations revealed significantly raised c-ANCA levels suggestive of Wegener's granulomatosis. She was kept

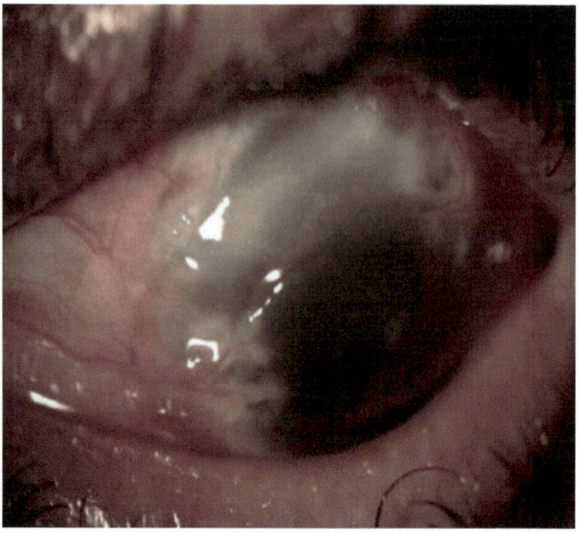

Image 18.5 At presentation, 360 degrees of circumferential thinning

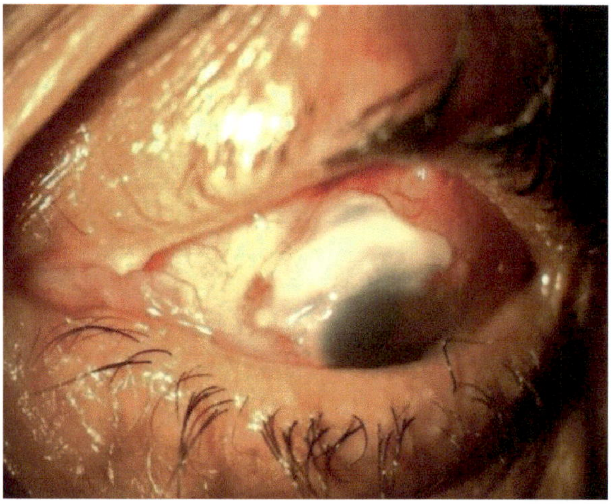

Image 18.6 Two months posttreatment with vascularization approaching the limbus

on a high dose of systemic steroids and methotrexate, and over a course of 2 months, the lesion resolved with vascularization (Image 18.6).

After 4 months on maintenance therapy, the lesion completely resolved, and she was posted for a cataract surgery under immunosuppressive cover, which was uneventful (Image 18.7).

At 2 months post-phacoemulsification, the patient presented with an area of scleral melt with uveal prolapse 2 mm behind the limbus (Image 18.8). The patient underwent a patch graft under aggressive systemic immunosuppression [8]. With this episode, the patient also developed respiratory symptoms secondary to Wegener's and was then lost to follow-up.

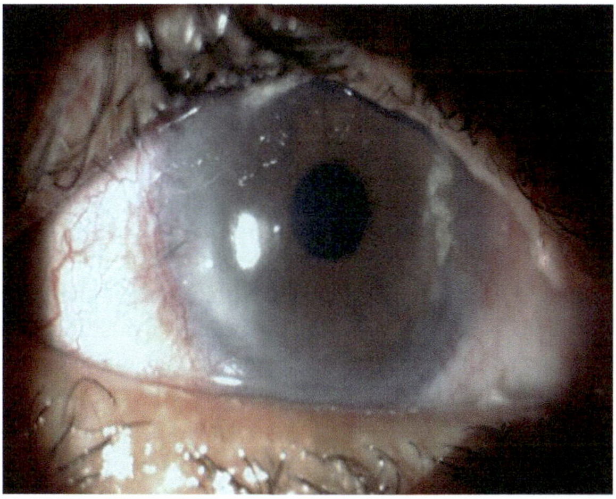

Image 18.7 Post-phacoemulsification the surface was stable with no surface inflammation, and the patient gained vision

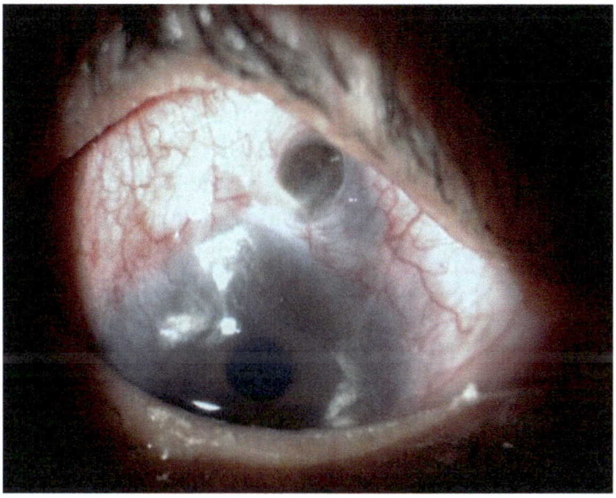

Image 18.8 Post-phacoemulsification at 2 months 2 × 2 mm of scleral melt noted 1 mm behind the limbus

This case highlights the need for a tailor-made approach to systemic immunosuppression in the management of PUK secondary to noninfectious systemic causes and the management of cataracts in such cases.

18.4 Case 3

- PUK secondary to herpes simplex keratitis
- Unilateral involvement
- Not responding to systemic management
- Role of patch graft in the management of PUK

A 50-year-old female presented with a history of redness, watering, and pain in the right eye for the past month. There was no history of ocular trauma or any similar episode in the past. She complained of joint pains for the past 3 months that were preceded by high-grade fever. The fever subsided after a few days, but the joint pains persisted. There was no associated history of weight loss, fatigue, skin changes, or systemic illness.

At presentation, visual acuity was hand movement close to face with accurate projection of rays and 20/80 in the right and the left eye, respectively. On slit lamp examination, the right eye showed a crescent-shaped defect in the cornea with iris prolapse, 4 × 2 mm in size, 5–7 o'clock position sparing the limbus by 2–3 mm (Image 18.9). There was surrounding stromal edema with Descemet's membrane folds extending up to the visual axis. The anterior chamber was shallow, and the pupil was peaked inferiorly. There was associated immature senile cataract, grade three as per the LOCS III grading. The left eye was essentially normal with immature senile cataract.

Based on the clinical ocular picture and a history of joint pains [9], a preliminary diagnosis of PUK was made. Laboratory tests were advised, which revealed a raised ESR. Rheumatoid factor and anti-cyclic citrullinated peptide antibodies were within normal limits.

After consulting a physician, to rule out any systemic conditions, a diagnosis of perforated PUK secondary to systemic autoimmune disorder was made, and the patient was advised right eye patch graft and systemic immunosuppression. Postoperatively, the patient was started on tablet prednisolone 50 mg daily, topical prednisolone hourly, eye drop carboxymethyl cellulose six times a day, and eye drop moxifloxacin (0.3%) four times a day.

Keeping in mind the underlying suspicion of rheumatoid arthritis (RA), a tablet methotrexate 10 mg weekly was started. On the postoperative follow-up, the patient was noted to have an epithelial defect on the patch graft (Image 18.10), which did

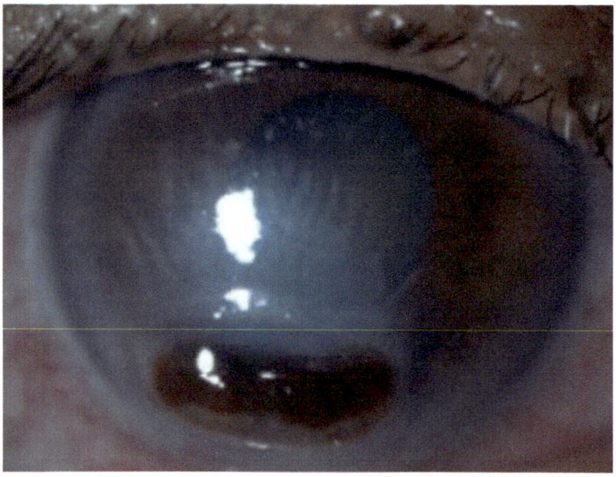

Image 18.9 At presentation, PUK-like picture with 4 × 2 mm defect with iris prolapse with surrounding corneal edema extending from 5–7 o'clock. A clear area of 2–3 mm present between the defect and the limbus. Sclera not involved. Inferior peaking of pupil and shallowing of anterior chamber seen

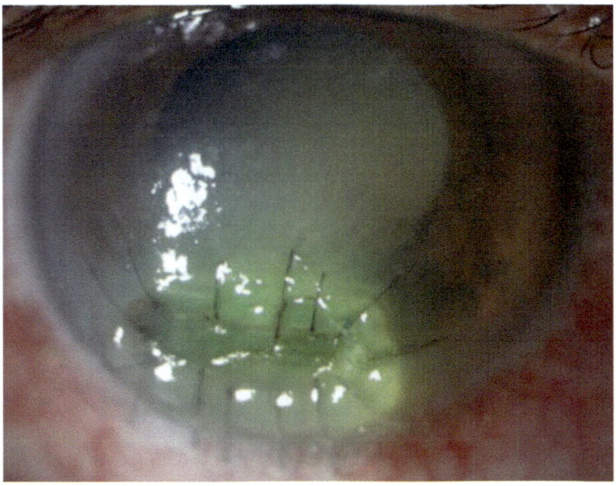

Image 18.10 Two weeks post-patch graft. Nonhealing epithelial defect present on the patch graft

not resolve with medications for 2 weeks. Considering it to be a nonhealing epithelial defect, a lateral permanent tarsorrhaphy was performed. Laboratory investigations were repeated, and ESR was found to have normalized. Two weeks later, an early graft melt was noted, and amniotic membrane grafting with a bandage contact lens was performed.

When the patient presented a month later for examination, two branching, linear lesions were seen on the fluorescein staining. Also noted were heaped-up epithelium and terminal bulbs. An associated history of fever and myalgia was also revealed on inquiring. A diagnosis of herpes simplex epithelial dendritic keratitis was made [10]. The patient was started on eye ointment acyclovir (3%) and tablet acyclovir (400 mg) five times a day, and the tear substitute was continued. A week after starting antiviral therapy, the dendritic lesions resolved, and the persistent epithelial defect on the patch graft dramatically healed. Following this, acyclovir eye ointment was discontinued, and tablet acyclovir was continued in a prophylactic dose twice daily. Tablet methotrexate was tapered and stopped [11].

Six months later, phacoemulsification with IOL placement was performed (Image 18.11) under a prophylactic dose of tablet acyclovir and tablet prednisolone. The patient regained a best corrected visual acuity (BCVA) of 20/25 postoperatively in the right eye and has maintained the vision since then. The left eye also underwent cataract surgery with a postoperative BCVA of 20/20. The patient is still under the prophylactic dose of tablet acyclovir. The kidney function tests are being routinely monitored. Recurrence has not been noted in the last 3 years.

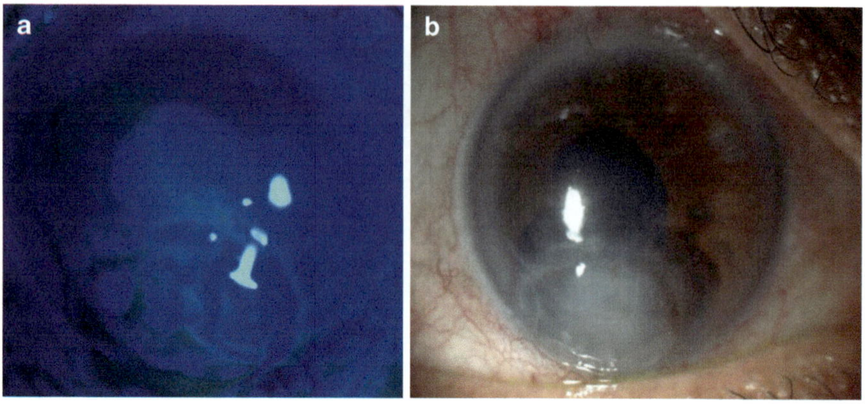

Image 18.11 (**a**) One month post-surgery. An incompletely healed epithelial defect on the patch graft, presence of two linear, branching, fluorescein-positive lesions with terminal bulbs noted on the host cornea. (**b**) One month follow-up picture after cataract surgery. Patient has a visual acuity of 6/9 and a clear visual axis. A patch graft is present inferiorly with stromal scarring

18.5 Case 4

- HSV
- Bilateral involvement
- Not responding to systemic management
- Role of amniotic membrane in the management of PUK

Another case highlights the herpes simplex virus (HSV) as an important causative agent in PUK, along with bilateral involvement.

A 49-year-old male patient with a known history of recurrent episodes of HSV keratouveitis [10] and trabeculitis in both eyes over the last 5 years presented this time with an active lesion of crescentic corneal melt with significant thinning, involving six clock hours, and sparing the limbus in the right eye (Image 18.12).

The left eye also had diffuse leucomatous scarring, with 360 degrees of peripheral vascularization. He had undergone a complete systemic evaluation and investigations ruling out any systemic involvement, and a diagnosis of PUK with HSV etiology was made. The patient was put on topical and systemic acyclovir and steroids and was regularly followed up. After day seven of the treatment, no significant response was noted, and the lesion was significantly thinned out [12]. At this point, the patient was advised an amniotic membrane grafting with fibrin glue [13] (Baxter, Tiseel). A six-clock-hour conjunctival peritomy was done, and the heaped-up epithelium at the edges was scraped off, after which a single-layer amniotic membrane was placed on the surface of the lesion and secured with fibrin glue and anchoring sutures (Image 18.13).

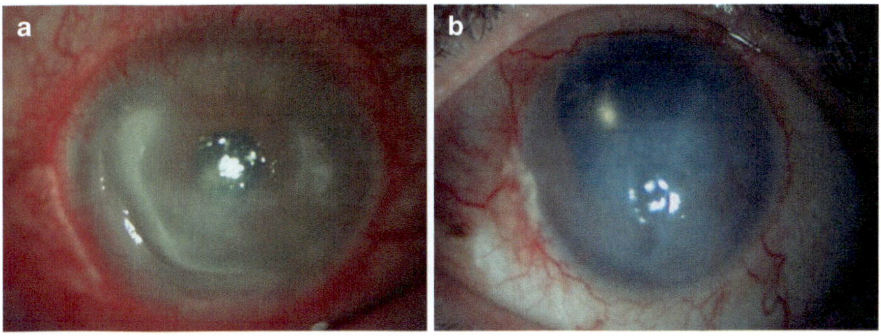

Image 18.12 (**a**) Right eye showing crescentic corneal melt with significant thinning, involving six clock hours, and sparing the limbus in the right eye. (**b**) Left eye showing diffuse scarring with the presence of peripheral vascularization

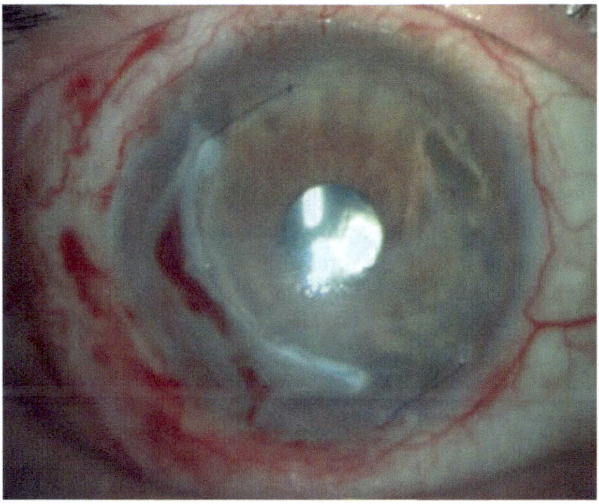

Image 18.13 Post-amniotic membrane application

The lesion scarred, the systemic steroids were slowly tapered, and the patient maintained a prophylactic dose of systemic acyclovir.

These two cases emphasize the role of HSV as a causative factor for PUK and show a unilateral and a bilateral involvement and the importance of a surgical intervention to prevent perforation.

18.6 Case 5

- Bilateral involvement
- Aggressive Mooren's ulcer
- Systemic management
- Patch graft

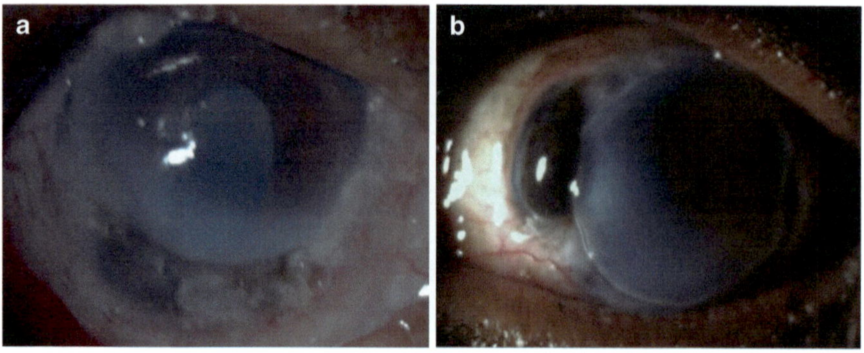

Image 18.14 (**a**) Right eye showed peripheral descemetocele with corneal ulceration extending for four clock hours. (**b**) Left eye showed peripheral descemetocele with corneal ulceration extending from 8 o'clock to 11 o'clock

A 63-year-old male patient from north India presented with pain and redness in both eyes, which gradually worsened over the last 6 months. The pain was accompanied by a diminution of vision, watering, and photophobia in both eyes. There was no history of ocular trauma, intraocular surgery, or systemic illness.

Ocular examination revealed uncorrected visual acuity (UCVA) of counting fingers at 1 m (with accurate projection of rays) in the right eye and hand motion close to face (with a precise projection of rays) in the left eye, which did not improve with refraction. Intraocular pressures could not be measured due to photophobia.

Slit-lamp examination (Haag-Streit BM 900) in the right eye showed peripheral descemetocele with corneal ulceration extending for four clock hours (Image 18.14a). The anterior chamber was quiet, and immature senile cataract was noted. A fundal glow was present, but the details of the posterior segment could not be appreciated. The left eye showed peripheral descemetocele with corneal ulceration extending from 8 o'clock to 11 o'clock (Image 18.14b). Anterior chamber examination showed a mature senile cataract with no view of the posterior segment [11, 14]. The conjunctival injection was present in both eyes, and the sclera remained uninvolved. The patient was taken up for emergency conjunctival resection and patch graft for both eyes under high-dose intravenous steroids (pulsed intravenous methylprednisolone 500 mg daily for 3 days). A freehand fashioned lamellar thickness crescentic customized corneal graft of therapeutic quality was used for both eyes. The patient was put on hourly topical steroids (1% prednisolone acetate), six hourly antibiotics (0.5% moxifloxacin), and cycloplegics (2% homatropine). The patient maintained a stable uncorrected vision of 20/200 in the right eye (Image 18.15a); however, the condition of his left eye deteriorated over the next 3 months (Image 18.15b). There was 360-degree peripheral involvement of the cornea, mature senile cataract, and shallow anterior chamber (Image 18.16a).

To control the aggressive corneal involvement [11] and to visually rehabilitate the patient, a triple procedure (penetrating keratoplasty, cataract extraction, and intraocular lens implantation) was planned for the left eye. This was combined with

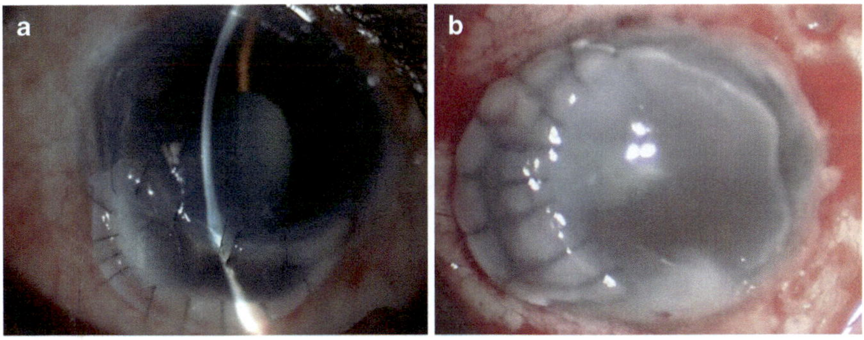

Image 18.15 (**a**) Post-patch graft right eye. (**b**) Post-patch graft left eye

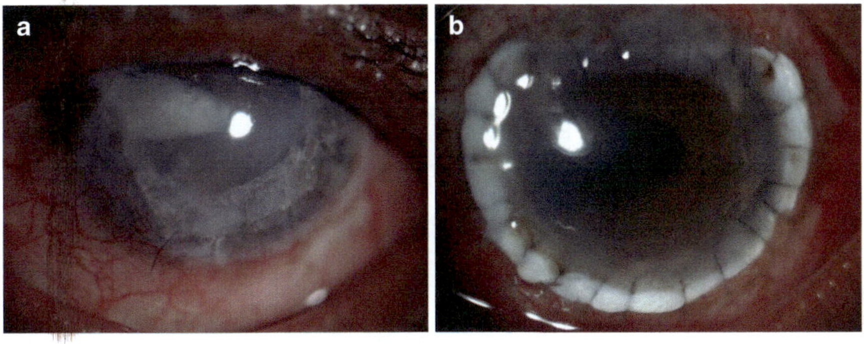

Image 18.16 (**a**) Left eye with 360-degree peripheral anterior synechiae, shallow anterior chamber, and total cataract. (**b**) Left eye post-penetrating keratoplasty

high dose intravenous cyclophosphamide (50 mg/kg) 1 day prior to the surgery and 1 day after the surgery. A final postoperative uncorrected visual acuity of 20/100 was achieved. The patient maintained a good ambulatory vision (Image 18.16b). He was kept on a long-term immunosuppressives [15], comprising oral azathioprine 50 mg twice a day.

18.7 Case 6

- Aggressive Mooren's ulcer in pediatric age group
- Difference in presentation in children
- Descemet's detachment in PUK
- Importance of visual rehabilitation post-interventions

A 15-year-old boy presented with a 1-month history of pain, redness, photophobia, and diminution of vision in the right eye. His BCVA in the right eye was finger counting at 1 m and in the left eye was 20/20.

Slit-lamp examination of the right eye showed peripheral corneal ulceration extending from 2 o'clock to 10 o'clock with cellular infiltration and a central overhanging edge. Iris incarceration with pseudocornea formation [16] was noted inferiorly in an area of 2 o'clock hours. Fundus was not visible in the right eye. Conjunctival resection, tissue adhesive (TISSEEL Kit from Baxter AG, Vienna, Austria), and bandage contact lens (PureconTM, size 18 mm) placement were performed. He was treated with systemic as well as hourly topical steroids.

One month later, he presented with acute-onset diminution of vision in the right eye. The BCVA dropped to perception of light (Image 18.17).

On slit-lamp examination, there was mild conjunctival congestion with marked corneal edema (central 5 mm) and peripheral cornea scarring as previously. A diagnosis of acute corneal hydrops (grade 2) in resolving Mooren's ulcer was made [17] (Image 18.18a). Intracameral injection of 0.1 ml of nonexpansile perfluoropropane (14% C3F8) gas was done through a 30-gauge needle under topical anesthesia. Seventy-five percent fill of the anterior chamber was achieved. On postoperative

Image 18.17 Right eye at 3 months

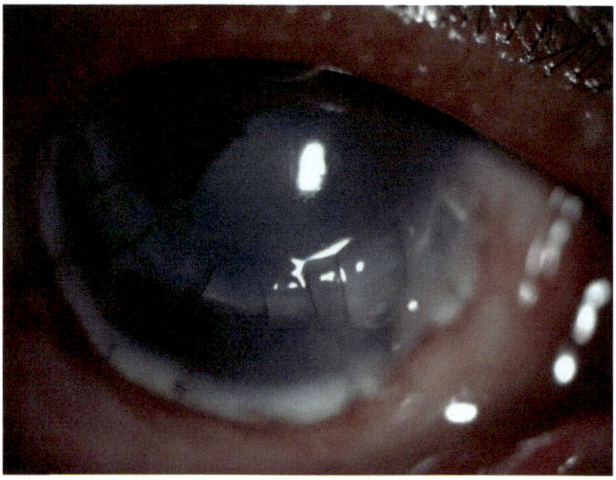

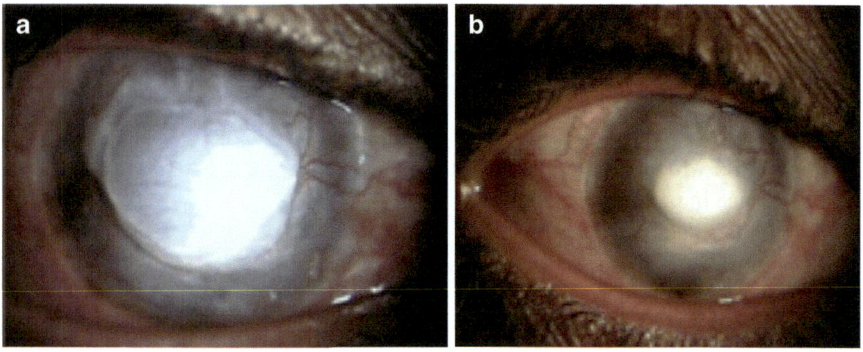

Image 18.18 (**a**) Right eye with Descemet's membrane detachment and hydrops. (**b**) Right eye post-descemetopexy

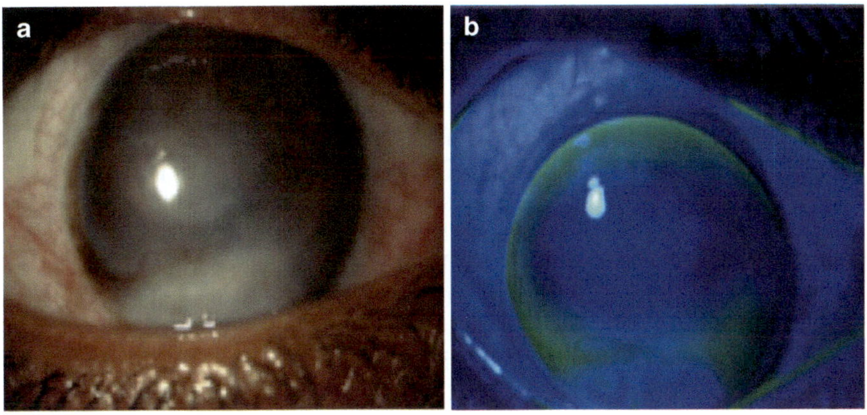

Image 18.19 (**a**) Right eye with central macular grade scarring. (**b**) Post-Rose-K IC fitting

examination, the central corneal edema started resolving after 1 week (Image 18.18b). Two months later, edema completely resolved, and there was central corneal scarring of macular grade (Image 18.19a). He was fitted with Rose-K IC (irregular cornea) contact lens in the right eye, and a BCVA of 20/80 was achieved [15] (Image 18.19b).

18.8 Immunopathogenesis of Peripheral Ulcerative Keratitis

Under normal conditions, the immune system is insensitive to self-antigens. However, in autoimmune diseases such as rheumatoid arthritis, Sjogren's syndrome, and systemic lupus erythematosus, among others, this mechanism breaks down [18]. Autoantibodies such as rheumatoid factor or anti-citrullinated antibodies bind to B cell receptors, triggering activation and subsequent differentiation of B cells into plasma cells. These rogue plasma cells produce autoantibodies triggering an immune response (Fig. 18.1c) [19, 20]. Complexed with autoantigens, these autoantibodies form immune complexes that are deposited in the peripheral cornea through the limbal vasculature (Fig. 18.1c). These immune complexes activate the complement pathway as well as resident immune cells in the limbus, which lead to the production of large amounts of pro-inflammatory cytokines (Fig. 18.1c) [21–23].

Systemic autoimmune conditions are correlated with increased numbers of CD4+ T cells [24], which differentiate into different types of T helper cells (e.g., T_H1, T_H2, and T_H17) [25]. These cells migrate to the limbal cornea in response to chemokines and further amplify the local concentration of pro-inflammatory cytokines [22] (Fig. 18.1c). T_H1 cells secrete interleukin 1 (IL-1) and tumor necrosis factor alpha (TNF-α); T_H2 cells secrete IL-4, IL-5, and IL-13 [26]; and T_H17 cells secrete IL-17 [27]. IL-17 is a key mediator of peripheral ulcerative keratitis (PUK), and tear concentration of IL-17 has been shown to be positively correlated with ocular degeneration [28]. IL-17 also stimulates the secretion of other cytokines such as IL-6, IL-8, and TNF-α [29, 30], all of which have been implicated as poor prognostic markers of PUK (Fig. 18.1c) [21–23].

The elasticity and structural integrity of the corneal stroma are regulated by a delicate balance of matrix metalloproteinases (MMPs) and tissue inhibitors of metalloproteinases (TIMPs) [31]. MMPs are a class of enzymes that degrade collagen and other extracellular matrix (ECM) components [32]. Any imbalance in the ratio of MMPs to TIMPs compromises the physical properties of the ECM [31]. MMP-1 and MMP-8 specifically dissolve types I, II, and III collagen [33], while MMP-2 and MMP-9 target type IV collagen [34]. Since the peripheral cornea primarily contains collagen I [2], MMP-1 and MMP-8 are known effectors of PUK [21–23]. In response to IL-6, IL-8, IL-17, and TNF-α, MMP-2 and MMP-9 are secreted by corneal and conjunctival epithelial cells and cells in the lacrimal glands and trigger the dissolution of collagen IV, which affects the integrity of the corneal basement membrane [1]. As a diagnostic marker, MMP-2, MMP-8, and MMP-9 levels have been found to be elevated in the tear film of patients with corneal ulcers [35, 36].

Understanding the immunopathogenesis of PUK has been crucial to the development of targeted therapeutics toward T cells (e.g., cyclophosphamide, cyclosporine A) [22, 23] and novel biologics against TNF-α (adalimumab, certolizumab, etanercept, golimumab, Infliximab) and against interleukins (anakinra, secukinumab, tocilizumab) [4, 22, 23].

References

1. Smith VA, Rishmawi H, Hussein H, Easty DL. Tear film MMP accumulation and corneal disease. Br J Ophthalmol. 2001;85(2):147–53.
2. Sridhar MS. Anatomy of cornea and ocular surface. Indian J Ophthalmol. 2018;66(2):190–4.
3. Messmer EM, Foster CS. Vasculitic peripheral ulcerative keratitis. Surv Ophthalmol. 1999;43(5):379–96.
4. Dominguez-Casas LC, Sanchez-Bilbao L, Calvo-Rio V, Maiz O, Blanco A, Beltran E, et al. Biologic therapy in severe and refractory peripheral ulcerative keratitis (PUK). Multicenter study of 34 patients. Semin Arthritis Rheum. 2020;50(4):608–15.
5. Sharma N, Sinha G, Shekhar H, Titiyal JS, Agarwal T, Chawla B, et al. Demographic profile, clinical features and outcome of peripheral ulcerative keratitis: a prospective study. Br J Ophthalmol. 2015;99(11):1503–8.
6. Timlin HM, Hall HN, Foot B, Koay P. Corneal perforation from peripheral ulcerative keratopathy in patients with rheumatoid arthritis: epidemiological findings of the British Ophthalmological Surveillance Unit. Br J Ophthalmol. 2018;102(9):1298–302.
7. Gupta N, Chawla B, Venkatesh P, Tandon R. Necrotizing scleritis and peripheral ulcerative keratitis in a case of Sweet's syndrome found culture-positive for mycobacterium tuberculosis. Ann Trop Med Parasitol. 2008;102(6):557–60.
8. Tarabishy AB, Schulte M, Papaliodis GN, Hoffman GS. Wegener's granulomatosis: clinical manifestations, differential diagnosis, and management of ocular and systemic disease. Surv Ophthalmol. 2010;55(5):429–44.
9. Ruiz-Lozano RE, Ramos-Davila EM, Garza-Garza LA, Gutierrez-Juarez K, Hernandez-Camarena JC, Rodriguez-Garcia A. Rheumatoid arthritis-associated peripheral ulcerative keratitis outcomes after early immunosuppressive therapy. Br J Ophthalmol. 2023;107(9):1246–52.

10. Chranioti A, Malamas A, Metallidis S, Mataftsi A, Chalvatzis N, Ziakas N. Bilateral herpes simplex virus-related peripheral ulcerative keratitis leading to corneal perforation in a patient with primary herpes simplex virus infection. J Ophthalmic Vis Res. 2019;14(1):93–6.
11. El Bahloul M, Lambarki O, Bennis A, Chraibi F, Abdellaoui M, Benatiya I. Severe chronic peripheral ulcerative keratitis: approach to diagnosis and treatment. J Fr Ophtalmol. 2021;44(4):e231–e3.
12. Gomes BF, Santhiago MR. Biology of peripheral ulcerative keratitis. Exp Eye Res. 2021;204:108458.
13. Eslami M, Benito-Pascual B, Goolam S, Trinh T, Moloney G. Case report: use of amniotic membrane for tectonic repair of peripheral ulcerative keratitis with corneal perforation. Front Med (Lausanne). 2022;9:836873.
14. Fu L, Jones S. Peripheral ulcerative keratitis. Treasure Island, FL: StatPearls; 2022.
15. Kasparova EA, Krasnolutskaya EI, Kruglova EM. Mooren's ulcer. Vestn oftalmol. 2020;136(5. Vyp. 2):241–7.
16. Ogra S, Sims JL, McGhee CNJ, Niederer RL. Ocular complications and mortality in peripheral ulcerative keratitis and necrotising scleritis: the role of systemic immunosuppression. Clin Experiment Ophthalmol. 2020;48(4):434–41.
17. Bonnet C, Debillon L, Al-Hashimi S, Hoogewoud F, Monnet D, Bourges JL, et al. Anterior segment optical coherence tomography imaging in peripheral ulcerative keratitis, a corneal structural description. BMC Ophthalmol. 2020;20(1):205.
18. Wang L, Wang FS, Gershwin ME. Human autoimmune diseases: a comprehensive update. J Intern Med. 2015;278(4):369–95.
19. Kondo N, Kuroda T, Kobayashi D. Cytokine networks in the pathogenesis of rheumatoid arthritis. Int J Mol Sci. 2021;22(20):10922.
20. Wu F, Gao J, Kang J, Wang X, Niu Q, Liu J, et al. B cells in rheumatoid arthritis: pathogenic mechanisms and treatment prospects. Front Immunol. 2021;12:750753.
21. Hassanpour K, ElSheikh RH, Arabi A, Frank CR, Elhusseiny AM, Eleiwa TK, Arami S, Djalilian AR, Kheirkhah A. Peripheral ulcerative keratitis: a review. J Ophthalmic Vis Res. 2022;17(2):252–75.
22. Cao Y, Zhang W, Wu J, Zhang H, Zhou H. Peripheral ulcerative keratitis associated with autoimmune disease: pathogenesis and treatment. J Ophthalmol. 2017;2017:7298026.
23. Gupta Y, Kishore A, Kumari P, Balakrishnan N, Lomi N, Gupta N, et al. Peripheral ulcerative keratitis. Surv Ophthalmol. 2021;66(6):977–98.
24. Rao DA, Gurish MF, Marshall JL, Slowikowski K, Fonseka CY, Liu Y, et al. Pathologically expanded peripheral T helper cell subset drives B cells in rheumatoid arthritis. Nature. 2017;542(7639):110–4.
25. Luckheeram RV, Zhou R, Verma AD, Xia B. CD4(+)T cells: differentiation and functions. Clin Dev Immunol. 2012;2012:925135.
26. Walker JA, McKenzie ANJ. TH2 cell development and function. Nat Rev Immunol. 2018;18(2):121–33.
27. Korn T, Bettelli E, Oukka M, Kuchroo VK. IL-17 and Th17 cells. Annu Rev Immunol. 2009;27:485–517.
28. Kang MH, Kim MK, Lee HJ, Lee HI, Wee WR, Lee JH. Interleukin-17 in various ocular surface inflammatory diseases. J Korean Med Sci. 2011;26(7):938–44.
29. Fossiez F, Djossou O, Chomarat P, Flores-Romo L, Ait-Yahia S, Maat C, et al. T cell interleukin-17 induces stromal cells to produce proinflammatory and hematopoietic cytokines. J Exp Med. 1996;183(6):2593–603.
30. Berry SPD, Dossou C, Kashif A, Sharifinejad N, Azizi G, Hamedifar H, et al. The role of IL-17 and anti-IL-17 agents in the immunopathogenesis and management of autoimmune and inflammatory diseases. Int Immunopharmacol. 2022;102:108402.
31. Cabral-Pacheco GA, Garza-Veloz I, Castruita-De la Rosa C, Ramirez-Acuna JM, Perez-Romero BA, Guerrero-Rodriguez JF, et al. The roles of matrix metalloproteinases and their inhibitors in human diseases. Int J Mol Sci. 2020;21(24):9739.

32. Iyer RP, Patterson NL, Fields GB, Lindsey ML. The history of matrix metalloproteinases: milestones, myths, and misperceptions. Am J Physiol Heart Circ Physiol. 2012;303(8):H919–30.
33. Van Doren SR. Matrix metalloproteinase interactions with collagen and elastin. Matrix Biol. 2015;44-46:224–31.
34. Zeng ZS, Cohen AM, Guillem JG. Loss of basement membrane type IV collagen is associated with increased expression of metalloproteinases 2 and 9 (MMP-2 and MMP-9) during human colorectal tumorigenesis. Carcinogenesis. 1999;20(5):749–55.
35. Sakimoto T, Sawa M. Metalloproteinases in corneal diseases: degradation and processing. Cornea. 2012;31(Suppl 1):S50–6.
36. Sakimoto T, Ohnishi T, Ishimori A. Simultaneous study of matrix metalloproteinases, proinflammatory cytokines, and soluble cytokine receptors in the tears of noninfectious corneal ulcer patients. Graefes Arch Clin Exp Ophthalmol. 2014;252(9):1451–6.

Mooren's Ulcer

19

S. Watson OAM

19.1 Introduction

Bowman in 1849 first described Mooren's ulcer of the cornea which has also been called chronic serpiginous ulcer and ulcer rodens [1]. Then, in 1867, Mooren provided details of cases of the condition in a publication that established Mooren's corneal ulcer as a distinct clinical entity [1]. Formal guidelines for the diagnosis of Mooren's ulcer have not been developed [2]. Amongst clinicians and in the literature, there is general agreement that the condition is characterised by a painful, relentless, chronic ulceration of the cornea that begins in the corneal periphery with progression circumferentially and centrally [3]. Mooren's ulcer has a variable presentation in terms of demographics, severity and disease progression. Medical and/or surgical management is required to heal the ulceration, to prevent vision loss from scarring and astigmatism and to avoid complications including corneal perforation, uveitis and infection.

Challenges remain in understanding the exact pathogenesis of Mooren's ulcer. At present, it is considered an autoimmune response to corneal antigens such as calgranulin C and the zinc-binding protein S100A12 [4]. The inflammatory nature of Mooren's ulcer has been supported by conjunctival biopsy specimens from affected patients which have revealed many different types of inflammatory cells, adhesion molecules and costimulatory molecules [5]. Helper T lymphocytes and macrophages have been found in the conjunctival submucosa adjacent to the corneal ulceration [6] as well as upregulated NLRP3 inflammasome components [7]. Proteomics have also suggested the activation of immune-associated pathways in

S. Watson OAM (✉)
Sydney Medical School, Faculty of Medicine and Health, The University of Sydney, Sydney, NSW, Australia
e-mail: stephanie.watson@sydney.edu.au

F. A. Woreta, R. B. Singh (eds.), *Cornea Casebook*, Current Practices in Ophthalmology, https://doi.org/10.1007/978-981-96-0495-1_19

Mooren's ulcer, with the top five upregulated protein pathways identified being lysosomes, antigen processing and presentation, platelet activation, oxidation phosphorylation and phagosomes [8]. B lymphocytes and NETS as well as PAD14-mediated citrullination have also been implicated in the pathogenesis [8] along with T cells (CD^{4+} and CD^{8+}) and macrophages [9].

Patients with Mooren's ulcer have been reported to have a recent history of trauma, surgery (including cataract surgery [10]) or infection involving the cornea [2, 3, 11–13]. It may be that the prior corneal incidents expose antigens that are normally hidden to antigen-presenting cells [4]. Cases have also been reported to occur in patients with systemic hepatitis C infection [14, 15], and it has been postulated that hepatitis C may be an underlying cause for Mooren's ulcer. In the past, hepatitis C may have been missed as an underlying cause due to the lack of serological tests and/or signs and symptoms of the condition [2]. Hookworm infestation of the intestine has also been associated with Mooren's ulcer first in Africa [16–18] and then in South India [19]. Interestingly, corneal calgranulin C has also been identified as a protein involved in the immune response to parasitic infections and is also in the corneal stroma [20, 21]. As such, it is likely that genetic and environmental factors may also have a role in pathogenesis [8]. In a recent report, it was postulated that a patient with lattice corneal dystrophy type 1 may have developed bilateral Mooren's ulcer due to repeated episodes of corneal epithelial breakdown inducing an autoimmune reaction to corneal antigens [22]. Further investigations are needed to determine the exact pathogenesis of the condition. The cases presented in this chapter demonstrate typical features of Mooren's ulcer and the difficulties in managing the condition.

19.2 Diagnosis

19.2.1 Key Points

- Mooren's ulcer is diagnosed based on history and examination and investigations to exclude any underlying cause (systemic or local).
- Investigations in Mooren's ulcer are used to exclude any underlying causes for inflammation.

19.2.2 History, Examination and Investigations

Mooren's ulcer is predominately a disease of adults and is considered a rare entity [2, 54]. Men are generally thought to be affected more than women [2, 3, 26, 54]. In Mooren's ulcer, the ulceration of the peripheral cornea may be extensive, but the sclera is not involved [46]. The ulceration may be partial or complete [2] and unilateral or bilateral [3] and may evolve in a typical pattern. For example, in a case series from India over 10 years, the ulceration was noted to affect the interpalpebral limbus first followed by the inferior and then superior zones [3]. Such ulceration of the peripheral cornea may also occur in the setting of systemic disease such as autoimmune disease (e.g. rheumatoid arthritis, Wegener's granulomatosis, systemic lupus erythematous, polyarteritis nodosa), dermatological disease, malignancy or from infection and local factors (e.g. exposure) [31, 55]. Indeed, infection has been found to be the second most common cause of peripheral ulcerative keratitis, occurring in up to around 20% of cases [56]. Mooren's ulcer though is "idiopathic" occurring without a causal underlying systemic disease or infection which may be local or systemic [2, 54].

Three types of Mooren's ulcer have been described in the literature [57]. In type 1, the corneal ulceration is unilateral and progressive, associated with ischaemia of the adjacent conjunctiva and limbus, and occurs in the elderly. The second type is distinguished by bilateral disease that is aggressive, seen in younger patients, and has neovascularisation of the ulcer demonstrated on angiography by proliferation and leakage of blood vessels. In the third type, there is bilateral corneal ulceration that is indolent and with less inflammation and vasculature that is relatively normal [57]. Cohorts of patients with Mooren's ulcer have been described across the globe with differing demographics and clinical characteristics [2, 3, 12, 13, 17–19, 26, 27, 58]. Race, gender and race cannot predict the severity or natural history of Mooren's ulcer [3]. As such, the three characteristic types of Mooren's ulcer have not been identified in all cohorts [26].

The diagnosis of Mooren's ulcer is by history, examination and investigations to exclude any underlying cause [31, 55]. Features on history include ocular symptoms such as pain, watering and photophobia which are progressive. The ocular pain can be severe and out of proportion to the signs on examination [54]. Vision can also be affected due to irregular astigmatism, central ulceration or secondary iritis. As the condition progresses, conjunctival hyperaemia usually accompanies the corneal changes. Patients with Mooren's ulcer may also present with complications of the condition such as microbial keratitis necessitating corneal scraping to identify a causal organism [59, 60]. A medical history looking for potential underlying causes should be taken. Signs of Mooren's ulcer include peripheral corneal thinning and melting with an overlying epithelial defect. At the onset, peripheral corneal stromal involvement may be patchy.

As Mooren's ulcer is idiopathic, investigations are typically performed to exclude infection such as herpes simplex keratitis and underlying systemic disease [31, 56]. As such, a diagnosis of Mooren's ulcer is only made after an underlying cause has been excluded [61]. To exclude Mooren's ulcer, the patient was investigated, and no underlying cause was found. Investigations are needed if the diagnosis cannot be established following history taking and examination and should be targeted towards likely causes and be correlated with the clinical feature [31]. Recently, anterior segment optical coherence tomography (AS-OCT) has been used to evaluate Mooren's ulcer [62]. Using AS-OCT, corneal ulceration, neovascularisation and fibrovascular membranes have been identified via hyperreflectivity and progression of stromal thinning monitored [62].

19.3 Case 1

19.3.1 Key Points

- Vision can remain reduced after resolution of the corneal ulceration due to scarring, ectasia and irregular astigmatism
- Surgical treatment can be used to repair ectatic cornea and restore vision following resolution of the inflammation
- Recurrence of the Mooren's ulceration can occur and may be induced by surgical interventions

19.3.2 Case History

A 41-year-old man presented with a history of Mooren's ulcer 18 years prior. He was complaining of poor vision, and his eyes were comfortable. At presentation he was otherwise well. On examination, vision was hand movements on the right and left, and there was no improvement with pinhole nor refraction in either eye. On slit lamp examination, the right cornea was scarred, vascularised and grossly ectatic from limbus to limbus. The left eye had a small inferiorly displaced penetrating keratoplasty with thin and scarred corneal host tissue.

Due to the poor vision from the corneal scarring and ectasia, a right limbal-sparing lamellar keratoplasty was performed [23–25]. This procedure alone may improve vision and reduce the risk of graft rejection as the patients' endothelium is retained. A penetrating keratoplasty was considered unsuitable due to the severe peripheral ectasia. Notably, Mooren's ulcer typically heals over 4–18 months leaving a vascularised and scarred cornea; vision in this case was reduced by scarring on the right and irregular astigmatism associated with the small graft and scarred peripheral host tissue on the left.

The right limbal-sparing lamellar keratoplasty was carried out by performing radial conjunctival incisions in each quadrant which were used to enable superficial dissection of the host limbal tissue. The flaps of host limbal tissue were then reflected onto the cornea, and epithelium was removed from the recipient bed via the application of ethanol 100% and superficial keratectomy. A scleral pocket was then created with a 0.3 mm step-knife peripheral to the limbus. A 15.0 mm lamellar corneoscleral donor button was cut freehand from a fresh donor whole eye after removal of the endothelium and Descemet's membrane with trypan blue (Vision Blue, DORC, the Netherlands). The donor button was sized to cover the entire cornea and limbus. The button had a rim of scleral tissue; the posterior aspect of the scleral tissue was trimmed with Vannas scissors to facilitate the fit of the graft onto the scleral bed. The anterior chamber was shallowed via a paracentesis to assist with fitting the graft. The graft was sutured in place with interrupted 9/0 nylon sutures with long bites placed in the scleral pocket. The host limbal flaps were then attached to the graft in the limbal position with 9/0 vicryl [24]. In Mooren's ulcer, the limbal pockets are fashioned from the conjunctival side compared to cases such as keratoglobus where the thinning occurs in the mid-periphery with the pockets created from the corneal side [24, 25].

Postoperatively, there was recurrence of the ulceration at the graft-host junction which led to melting of the lamellar graft. Postoperative ulceration can recur in around one in four cases and has generally been reported within the first 6 months after surgery [26]. Recurrence generally occurs at the site of a graft, such as in this case, and there is increased risk of perforation [27]. Ocular infection and corneal perforation have also been associated with recurrence [27]. Mooren's ulcer can be recurrent in up to 44% of patients, further complicating management of the condition [27]. Corneal perforation has been reported in around one in ten eyes [3, 26] at presentation and may be more common in those older than 60 years [3] and/or patients younger than 55 years [13]. Higher rates of perforation, of up to around one in nearly two have also been reported [13, 27–29]. In vivo confocal microscopy can be used to monitor dendritic cell density in lamellar grafts after Mooren's ulcer and may provide data for decision-making on topical and systemic immunosuppressive therapy [30].

Management of Mooren's ulcer can be complex as the condition may progress despite maximal therapy, recur and be complicated by severe anterior chamber inflammation, iritis, glaucoma and cataract and in at least one third there may be corneal perforation [26, 28, 31]. The aim of treatment is to epithelialise the cornea, control inflammation, prevent worsening of the ulceration and maintain the cornea's structural integrity [27]. Both medical and surgical options have been reported for Mooren's ulcer, but there have been no randomised clinical trials to determine the efficacy and safety of the different approaches [31, 32].

In our case, to manage the recurrence of the Mooren's ulcer, medical therapy with a step ladder approach utilising systemic immunosuppression was used [33], and oral prednisone was commenced with oral cyclosporine. In the management of Mooren's ulcer, the step ladder begins with oral cyclosporine for patients less than 60 years or methotrexate, then if insufficient response or intolerance stepping up to mycophenolate or azathioprine, then to cyclophosphamide and finally to biologicals, e.g. anti-tumour necrosis factor (anti-TNF) agents, rituximab or intravenous immunoglobulin [33, 34]. In the short term, high-dose prednisone is often given to achieve rapid control of inflammation [33]. It is important that the clinician determines the minimum treatment necessary including the duration of treatment to reduce the risks of side effects with immunosuppressive medication [33]. Systemic immunosuppressive agents such as cyclosporine cyclophosphamide have been used to control severe inflammation in the condition [35, 36]. Cases refractory to cyclophosphamide have been managed with TNF-alpha blockers, such as infliximab and adalimumab [37–40]; such therapy may not be effective for all patients [39]. Adalimumab may have advantages over infliximab as it has less propensity to hypersensitivity reactions and is given subcutaneously [41]. Infliximab is given intravenously and has a rapid onset such that it may be preferred in some cases with rapid progression [39]. Surgical management may be needed but can be temporising and palliative if the immune response is not controlled [38]. Campath-1H, a humanised lymphocytotoxic monoclonal antibody (mAb) that targets the CD52 antigen on

T lymphocytes, has been reported to reduce inflammation in Mooren's ulcer progression despite triple immunosuppression (prednisone, cyclosporine A, mycophenolate mofetil) and conjunctival resection [42]. Campath-1H can be considered for patients with progressive disease despite maximal therapy with close monitoring due to the risks of infection and malignancy [42].

Repeat limbal-sparing lamellar keratoplasty was performed 9 months later with a 14.0 mm corneoscleral graft. Systemic immunosuppression with oral prednisone and cyclophosphamide was used to prevent a recurrence of ulceration in the postoperative period. The limbus contains the limbal epithelial stem cells which are the source of the transient amplifying cells that differentiate to renew the corneal epithelium [43]. In Mooren's ulcer, sparing the limbus is important for preventing postoperative epithelial disturbance including epithelial defects which may expose corneal antigens predisposing to recurrence. The oral immunosuppression was maintained to prevent further recurrence. Postoperatively, there was an interface haemorrhage, and on resolution vision in the right eye was hand movements. At 7 months postoperatively, a penetrating keratoplasty along with extracapsular cataract extraction and posterior chamber intraocular lens implantation was performed. At 2 months following the penetrating keratoplasty, the patient experienced graft rejection which led to graft failure. Repeat penetrating keratoplasty was performed 6 months later with postoperative immunosuppression with azathioprine. On follow up at 2 years and following suture removal, the final postoperative visual acuity was 6/6 with a scleral contact lens and topical therapy was with g. cyclosporine and g. dexamethasone (Figs. 19.1 and 19.2). The systemic immunosuppression was then tapered and stopped.

In the acute management of Mooren's ulcer, a range of surgical tools may be needed including resection of the inflamed conjunctiva with the aim of reducing local inflammation and collagenases [18, 44, 45]. Tissue adhesive (TISSEEL Kit, Baxter AG, Vienna, Austria) has been used in conjunction with conjunctival resection [46], with the aim of promoting healing. Amniotic membrane has also been

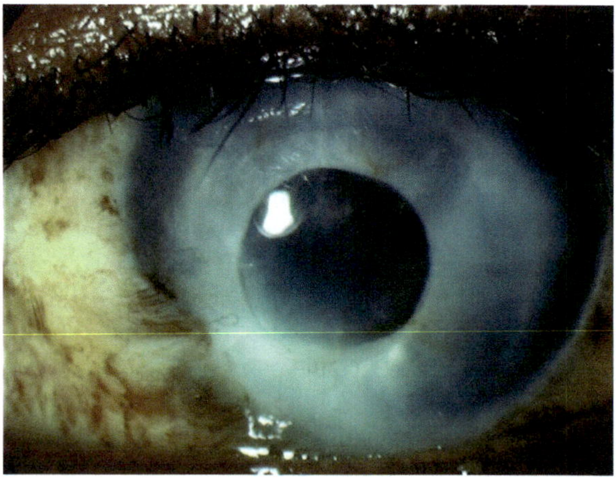

Fig. 19.1 Left eye with small penetrating keratoplasty and peripheral scarring following Mooren's corneal ulceration

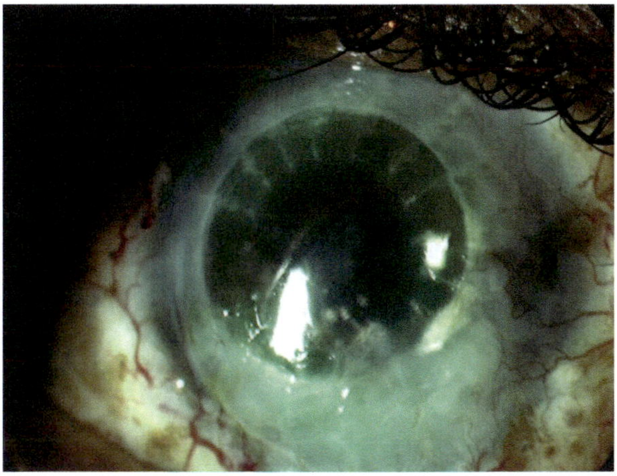

Fig. 19.2 Case 1 right eye with clear penetrating keratoplasty with limbal-sparing lamellar keratoplasty for visual rehabilitation in Mooren's corneal ulcer

used to promote healing of the cornea whilst the inflammation rescinds [44, 47, 48] and has been used in combination with autologous serum eye drops [47]. Amniotic membrane may be of use when immunosuppressive therapy is not available due to its anti-inflammatory effects [48]. In a comparative study patients having lamellar keratoplasty had greater improvement in vision and quicker healing than those treated with frozen amniotic membrane transplantation [49].

Keratoepithelioplasty with donor corneal lenticules sutured to the bare sclera near areas of corneal ulceration has also been used with success in cases of Mooren's ulcer and is thought to work by blocking the infiltrated conjunctival invasion [50]. Lamellar keratoplasty has been reported for the repair of melted corneal stroma [26] with AS-OCT used to assess the extent of the corneal thinning [26]. Success rates of lamellar keratoplasty surgery in Mooren's ulcer have been reported as around 90% and up to 96% with topical cyclosporine used postoperatively [26]. Lamellar keratoplasty has been hypothesised to remove corneal antigenic targets, to prevent immune reactions and to restore the corneal anatomy [26]. Postoperative topical therapy may include topical steroids and topical cyclosporine 1% [26]. A case of bullous keratopathy due to CMV corneal endotheliitis has been reported in a patient with Mooren's ulcer. This patient underwent successful Descemet's stripping automated keratoplasty [51], suggesting that this procedure can be considered if needed in patients with Mooren's ulcer and corneal endothelial decompensation. Finally, the use of bilateral Boston keratoprosthesis type I has been reported in Mooren's ulcer but with poor outcomes [52, 53].

References

1. Nettleship E. Chronic serpiginous ulcer of the cornea (Mooren's ulcer). Trans Ophthalmol Soc UK. 1902;98:383.
2. Zegans M, Srinivasan M, McHugh T, Whitcher J, Margolis T, Lietman T, et al. Mooren ulcer in South India: serology and clinical risk factors. Am J Ophthalmol. 1999;128(2):205–10.

3. Srinivasan M, Zegans ME, Zelefsky JR, Kundu A, Lietman T, Whitcher JP, et al. Clinical characteristics of Mooren's ulcer in South India. Br J Ophthalmol. 2007;91(5):570–5.
4. Gottsch J, Liu S, Minkovitz J, Goodman D, Srinivasan M, Stark W. Autoimmunity to a cornea-associated stromal antigen in patients with Mooren's ulcer. Invest Ophthalmol Vis Sci. 1995;36(8):1541–7.
5. Kafkala C, Choi J, Zafirakis P, Baltatzis S, Livir-Rallatos C, Rojas B, et al. Mooren ulcer: an immunopathologic study. Cornea. 2006;25(6):667–73.
6. Shinomiya K, Ueta M, Sotozono C, Inatomi T, Yokoi N, Koizumi N, et al. Immunohistochemical analysis of inflammatory limbal conjunctiva adjacent to Mooren's ulcer. Br J Ophthalmol. 2013;97(3):362–6.
7. Li Z, Wei C, Wang S, Liu T, Zhai H, Shi W. Upregulation of NLRP3 inflammasome components in Mooren's ulcer. Graefes Arch Clin Exp Ophthalmol. 2017;255(3):607–12.
8. Chi H, Hao W, Qi X, Zhang T, Dong Y, Gao H, et al. A proteomic approach towards understanding the pathogenesis of Mooren's ulcer. Exp Eye Res. 2021;205:108509.
9. Lee H, Kim M, Wee W, Oh J. Interplay of immune cells in Mooren ulcer. Cornea. 2015;34(9):1164–7.
10. Acharya N, Srinivasan M, Kundu A, Lietman T, Whitcher J, Cunningham E Jr. Mooren's ulcer following extracapsular cataract extraction. Eur J Ophthalmol. 2008;18(3):351–5.
11. Gottsch J, Liu S, Stark W. Mooren's ulcer and evidence of stromal graft rejection after penetrating keratoplasty. Am J Ophthalmol. 1992;113(4):412–7.
12. Wood T, Kaufman H. Mooren's ulcer. Am J Ophthalmol. 1971;71(1 Pt 2):417–22.
13. Kim D, Kim M, Wee W, Oh J. Mooren's ulcer in a cornea referral practice in Korea. Ocul Immunol Inflamm. 2016;24(1):55–9.
14. Wilson S, Lee W, Murakami C, Weng J, Moninger G. Mooren-type hepatitis C virus-associated corneal ulceration. Ophthalmology. 1994;101(4):736–45.
15. Moazami G, Auran J, Florakis G, Wilson S, Srinivasan D. Interferon treatment of Mooren's ulcers associated with hepatitis C. Am J Ophthalmol. 1995;119(3):365–6.
16. Kuriakose E. Mooren's ulcer. Etiology and treatment. Am J Ophthalmol. 1963;55:1064–9.
17. van der Gaag R, Abdillahi H, Stilma JS, Vetter JC. Circulating antibodies against corneal epithelium and hookworm in patients with Mooren's ulcer from Sierra Leone. Br J Ophthalmol. 1983;67(9):623–8.
18. Stilma JS. Conjunctival excision or lamellar scleral autograft in 38 Mooren's ulcers from Sierra Leone. Br J Ophthalmol. 1983;67(7):475–8.
19. Zelefsky J, Srinivasan M, Kundu A, Lietman T, Whitcher J, Wang K, et al. Hookworm infestation as a risk factor for Mooren's ulcer in South India. Ophthalmology. 2007;114(3):450–3.
20. Gottsch J, Li Q, Ashraf F, O'Brien T, Stark W, Liu S. Cytokine-induced calgranulin C expression in keratocytes. Clin Immunol. 1999;91(1):34–40.
21. Gottsch J, Liu S. Cloning and expression of human corneal calgranulin C (CO-Ag). Curr Eye Res. 1998;17(9):870–4.
22. Kayukawa K, Kitazawa K, Wakimasu K, Sotozono C, Kinoshita S. A case of lattice corneal dystrophy type 1 with bilateral Mooren's ulcer. Am J Ophthalmol Case Rep. 2023;29:101796.
23. Karimian F, Baradaran-Rafii A, Faramarzi A, Akbari M. Limbal stem cell-sparing lamellar keratoplasty for the management of advanced keratoglobus. Cornea. 2014;33(1):105–8.
24. Watson S, Rauz S, Dart J. Limbal-sparing lamellar keratoplasty. Br J Ophthalmol. 2005;89
25. Vajpayee RB, Bhartiya P, Sharma N. Central lamellar keratoplasty with peripheral intralamellar tuck: a new surgical technique for keratoglobus. Cornea. 2002;21(7):657–60.
26. Chen J, Xie H, Wang Z, Yang B, Liu Z, Chen L, et al. Mooren's ulcer in China: a study of clinical characteristics and treatment. Br J Ophthalmol. 2000;84(11):1244–9.
27. Yang L, Xiao J, Wang J, Zhang H. Clinical characteristics and risk factors of recurrent Mooren's ulcer. J Ophthalmol. 2017;2017:8978527.
28. Kietzman B. Mooren's ulcer in Nigeria. Am J Ophthalmol. 1968;65(5):679–83.
29. Zegans ME, Srinivasan M. Mooren's ulcer. Int Ophthalmol Clin. 1998;38(4):81–8.

30. Liu J, Shi W, Li S, Gao H, Wang T. Modified lamellar keratoplasty and immunosuppressive therapy guided by in vivo confocal microscopy for perforated Mooren's ulcer. Br J Ophthalmol. 2015;99(6):778–83.
31. Gupta Y, Kishore A, Kumari P, Balakrishnan N, Lomi N, Gupta N, et al. Peripheral ulcerative keratitis. Surv Ophthalmol. 2021;66(6):977–98.
32. Alhassan M, Rabiu M, Agbabiaka I. Interventions for Mooren's ulcer. Cochrane Database Syst Rev. 2014;2014(1):CD006131.
33. Saw V. Immunotherapy for corneal inflammatory disorders: stepping up and down the ladder. Br J Ophthalmol. 2013;97(11):1364–7.
34. Cunningham ET, Agarwal M, Smit DP, Tugal-Tutkun I, Thorne JE. Mooren's ulcer. Ocul Immunol Inflamm. 2023;31(4):673–4.
35. Foster C. Systemic immunosuppressive therapy for progressive bilateral Mooren's ulcer. Ophthalmology. 1985;92(10):1436–9.
36. Ashar J, Mathur A, Sangwan V. Immunosuppression for Mooren's ulcer: evaluation of the step-ladder approach—topical, oral and intravenous immunosuppressive agents. Br J Ophthalmol. 2013;97(11):1391–4.
37. Saw V, Cornelius N, Salama A, Pusey C, Lightman S. Infliximab therapy for aggressive Mooren ulceration. Arch Ophthalmol. 2008;126(5):734.
38. Cordero-Coma M, Benito M, Fuertes C, Antolin S, Garcia RJ. Adalimumab for Mooren's ulcer. Ophthalmology. 2009;116(8):1589, 1589.e1.
39. Xia A, Dietrich-Ntoukas T, Pleyer U. Effect of Anti-TNF Treatment on Mooren's Ulcer: A Case Series and Review of the Literature. Ocul Immunol Inflamm. 2023;31(4):675–81.
40. Cakmak AI, Akova Y, Yildirim N. The complete success in refractory Mooren's ulcer treated with infliximab. Ocul Immunol Inflamm. 2023;31(4):682–8.
41. Chilton F, Collett R. Treatment choices, preferences and decision-making by patients with rheumatoid arthritis. Musculoskeletal Care. 2008;6(1):1–14.
42. van der Hoek J, Azuara-Blanco A, Greiner K, Forrester JV. Mooren's ulcer resolved with campath-1H. Br J Ophthalmol. 2003;87(7):924–5.
43. Dua HS, Azuara-Blanco A. Limbal stem cells of the corneal epithelium. Surv Ophthalmol. 2000;44(5):415–25. https://doi.org/10.1016/s0039-6257(00)00109-0.
44. Lambiase A, Sacchetti M, Sgrulletta R, Coassin M, Bonini S. Amniotic membrane transplantation associated with conjunctival peritomy in the management of Mooren's ulcer: a case report. Eur J Ophthalmol. 2005;15(2):274–6.
45. Brown S. Mooren's ulcer. Treatment by conjunctival excision. Br J Ophthalmol. 1975;59(11):675–82.
46. Farooqui J, Acharya M, Jain S, Dave A. Aggressive Mooren's ulcer and challenges in its management: tale of three patients in pictures. Saudi J Ophthalmol. 2019;33(1):112–5.
47. Lavaju P, Sharma M, Sharma A, Chettri S. Use of amniotic membrane and autologous serum eye drops in Mooren's ulcer. Nepal J Ophthalmol. 2013;5(1):120–3.
48. Ngan ND, Chau HT. Amniotic membrane transplantation for Mooren's ulcer. Clin Experiment Ophthalmol. 2011;39(5):386–92.
49. Chen Y, Gao R, Gao M, Liu Q, Song L. Comparative study on the efficacy of frozen amniotic membrane transplantation and lamellar keratoplasty in the treatment of Mooren ulcer. J Craniofac Surg. 2021;32(2):637–41.
50. Kinoshita S, Ohashi Y, Ohji M, Manabe R. Long-term results of keratoepithelioplasty in Mooren's ulcer. Ophthalmology. 1991;98(4):438–45.
51. Ueda K, Ono T, Toyono T, Yoshida J, Kaburaki T, Miyai T. Descemet stripping endothelial keratoplasty after cytomegalovirus corneal endotheliitis and immunosuppression for Mooren's ulcer. Am J Ophthalmol Case Rep. 2021;22:101088.
52. Geoffrion D, Harissi-Dagher M. Comment on Bilateral Boston keratoprosthesis type 1 in a case of severe Mooren's ulcer. Eur J Ophthalmol. 2022;32(1):NP297–NP8.
53. Jerez-Pena M, Salvador-Culla B, de la Paz M, Barraquer R. Bilateral Boston keratoprosthesis type 1 in a case of severe Mooren's ulcer. Eur J Ophthalmol. 2021;31(2):NP33–NP8.
54. Chow C, Foster C. Mooren's ulcer. Int Ophthalmol Clin. 1996;36(1):1–13.

55. Tauber J, Sainz de la Maza M, Hoang-Xuan T, Foster C. An analysis of therapeutic decision making regarding immunosuppressive chemotherapy for peripheral ulcerative keratitis. Cornea. 1990;9(1):66–73.
56. Sharma N, Sinha G, Shekhar H, Titiyal J, Agarwal T, Chawla B, et al. Demographic profile, clinical features and outcome of peripheral ulcerative keratitis: a prospective study. Br J Ophthalmol. 2015;99(11):1503–8.
57. Watson P. Management of Mooren's ulceration. Eye (Lond). 1997;11(Pt 3):349–56.
58. Majekodunmi AA. Ecology of Mooren's ulcer in Nigeria. Doc Ophthalmol. 1980;49(2):211–9.
59. Cabrera-Aguas M, Khoo P, Watson S. Infectious keratitis: a review. Clin Experiment Ophthalmol. 2022;50(5):543–62.
60. Todokoro D, Miyakubo T, Komori A, Tamura T, Makimura K, Akiyama H. Successful management of fungal keratitis by Alternaria alternata complicating Mooren's ulcer. Case Rep Ophthalmol. 2023;14(1):153–8.
61. Bagheri N, Wajda B, Calvo C. The Wills eye manual: office and emergency room diagnosis. Philadelphia, PA: Lippincott Williams & Wilkins; 2017.
62. Lian X, Wang C, Yang S, Zhou S. Evaluation of Mooren's corneal ulcer by anterior segment optical coherence tomography. Photodiagn Photodyn Ther. 2023;44:103806.

Marginal Keratitis

20

Gabriele Gallo Afflitto, Katherine Leviste, Nicholas Reyes, and Sonia H. Yoo

20.1 Background

The term marginal keratitis or marginal catarrhal keratitis (MK) refers to a peripheral corneal disorder, of infectious, noninfectious, or immune-related etiology, that is generally self-limiting in nature [1, 2].

It is believed to result from a delayed (type IV) hypersensitivity reaction to both endogenous and exogenous antigens, with the deposition of immune complexes in the peripheral cornea, complement activation, and leukocytic infiltration [3–5].

As MK arises from hypersensitivity reactions, the origins of MK vary. While classically associated with long-standing staphylococcal blepharitis, conjunctivitis, or meibomitis [6], less commonly, MK has been reported as a postsurgical complication from ocular surgeries [7–10]. In addition, MK should be considered in the context of immune-mediated disorders [11] such as vasculitis [12], ocular rosacea [13], Behcet's [14], or a form of idiosyncratic drug reaction [15].

Marginal keratitis typically presents as unilateral multiple subepithelial marginal sterile infiltrates separated from the limbus by a clear zone of 1–2 mm, often associated with an adjacent area of conjunctival hyperemia [16, 17]. Concurrent epithelial defects will appear considerably smaller than the area of the infiltrate. Chronic blepharitis and dry eye are common findings in patients with MK, and punctate

G. G. Afflitto
Bascom Palmer Eye Institute, University of Miami Miller School of Medicine, Miami, FL, USA

Ophthalmology Unit, Department of Experimental Medicine, University of Rome "Tor Vergata", Rome, Italy

K. Leviste · N. Reyes · S. H. Yoo (✉)
Bascom Palmer Eye Institute, University of Miami Miller School of Medicine, Miami, FL, USA
e-mail: kdleviste@med.miami.edu; SYoo@med.miami.edu

F. A. Woreta, R. B. Singh (eds.), *Cornea Casebook*, Current Practices in Ophthalmology, https://doi.org/10.1007/978-981-96-0495-1_20

epitheliopathy is defined as an early manifestation of the disorder [16, 17]. Anterior chamber reaction and severe manifestations are uncommon findings [18], and the clinical scenario generally resolves within 4 weeks.

Concerning management, it is imperative to rule out any cause of infectious keratitis. Once a noninfectious process is suspected, marginal keratitis should be differentiated by other forms of peripheral inflammatory corneal disorders, including Terrien's marginal degeneration, peripheral ulcerative keratitis, Fuchs' superficial marginal keratitis, Mooren's ulcer, and contact lens-associated peripheral ulceration. Other ocular or systemic conditions should be investigated and co-managed with a multidisciplinary approach [19, 20].

Once infectious sources have been ruled out, ocular treatment includes the use of topical corticosteroids which are recommended as the first-line treatment of choice. A weak topical steroid drop (e.g., fluorometholone or loteprednol) should be instilled at least four times a day for 1–2 weeks until the complete resolution of the clinical scenario [19–21].

The reduction of the local antigenic burden is crucial in the management of MK. Blepharitis treatment should be considered in all MK patients, which include warm compresses and improved lid hygiene with frequent eyelid scrubs [4, 5, 16, 17]. Topical and/or systemic antibiotics might be considered in the acute setting of infection, with the oral antibiotic usually being a macrolide or a tetracycline [19–21].

In this chapter, we present three cases of MK associated with various ocular and systemic comorbidities. Clinical presentation, medical history, and specific management are analyzed to provide a comprehensive view of the variations and often subtle nature of MK.

20.2 Case 1

20.2.1 Summary

- Marginal keratitis is commonly associated with staphylococcal blepharitis.
- Proper management of staphylococcal blepharitis is necessary in the presence of marginal keratitis.
- Marginal keratitis can present in the form of an ulcer and may result in corneal scarring, pannus formation, and neovascularization.

A 64-year-old male presented to the ophthalmology clinic with a chief complaint of sandy sensation in the right eye with an accompanying white spot on his cornea since waking the prior morning. His past medical history was significant for type II diabetes mellitus and external hordeolum of the left eye. Of note, he was diagnosed with a corneal ulcer in his right eye 10 months prior which was treated with antibiotic drops, artificial tears, and discontinued use of contact lens for 1 week. For this episode, he denied the use of contact lens for months but endorsed wiping his sleeve across his right eye earlier that week while in the gym. His reported allergies include Keflex, Bactrim, and latex.

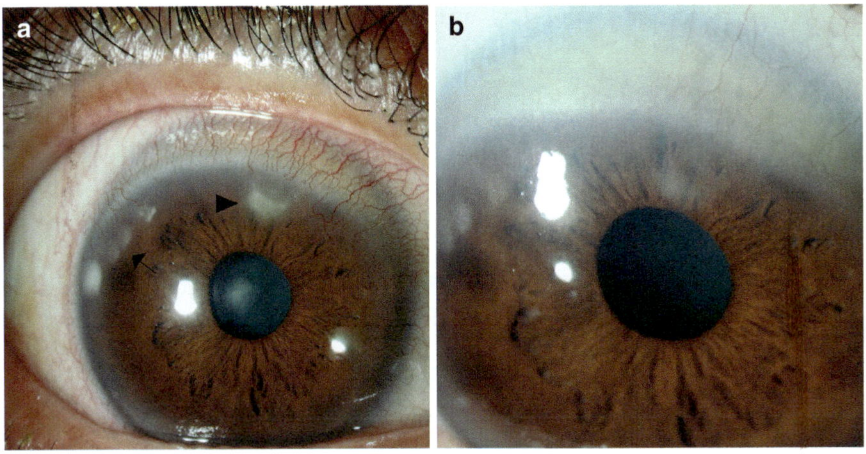

Fig. 20.1 Staphylococcal blepharitis pre- (**a**) and posttreatment (**b**). In A, extensive corneal neovascularization in the superior and nasal quadrant is observed, with corneal scarring (arrows), the presence of a new-onset marginal corneal ulcer with irregular borders, and a faint surrounding corneal haze (arrowhead). After treatment (**b**), resolution of the corneal neovascularization and corneal scarring at the site of the corneal ulcer is observed

At initial presentation, his best corrected visual acuity was 20/20 in the right eye (OD) and 20/20- in the left eye (OS), and intraocular pressure (IOP) measured 10 mmHg in both eyes (OU). Slit lamp exam revealed anterior blepharitis and conjunctival papillae OU, along with trace conjunctival injection OD. Corneal pannus OU with neovascularization was also visualized. His right eye displayed a 1 mm corneal ulcer with central staining noted in the superior quadrant with approximately 11 small, white lesions overlaying pannus neovascularization. Slit lamp photos were taken that day (Fig. 20.1). A differential of anterior blepharitis, neovascularization, papillae, and staphylococcal marginal keratitis was initially suspected. Lower on the differential, vernal keratoconjunctivitis was considered, however ruled out, as the observed papillae were small and not giant. Contact lens-related ulcers were also suspected, but he denied usage of the lenses for months. Management for the right eye included ciprofloxacin eye drops, erythromycin ointment, fluorometholone eye drops, discontinued contact lens use, and artificial tears.

Upon follow-up 5 days later, the patient reported no ocular discomfort and no change in visual acuity. The examination of his right eye revealed two areas of white opacities at 10 and 2 o'clock with healed epithelium as well as an area of scarring from 10 to 12 o'clock suggestive of prior staphylococcal marginal episodes. Slit lamp photos taken in this visit supported exam findings (Fig. 20.1). The patient was instructed to discontinue his antibiotic drops and ointment and begin a taper of the steroid drops over the course of 4 weeks. He was also advised of the potential for future episodes given his history and to return to clinic if he experienced symptoms such as red eyes, foreign body sensation, or ocular pain.

20.3 Case 2

20.3.1 Summary

- The onset of marginal keratitis can be subtle, with indistinct symptoms which may otherwise go unnoticed.
- A high level of suspicion for marginal keratitis must be considered in the presence of several ocular comorbidities, including blepharitis.
- The presence of systemic immune-mediated conditions, such as rheumatoid arthritis, may accompany and/or predispose the patient to develop marginal keratitis.
- Immediate recognition of local and systemic comorbidities is crucial for the proper and effective management of marginal keratitis.

A 59-year-old Caucasian female presented to the outpatient clinic with a chief complaint of foreign body sensation in the left eye starting 4 days prior. Her medical history was remarkable for rheumatoid arthritis (RA) and essential hypertension. Sicca syndrome-associated dry eye was the only reported ocular comorbidity, for which the patient had been treated with topical cyclosporine A and autologous serum eye drops.

Her best corrected visual acuity was 20/20 OU, and IOP was measured at 13 mmHg OU. Ophthalmic examination in the left eye revealed mild lower lid posterior blepharitis, mild, localized conjunctival injection, and diffuse punctate epitheliopathy. In addition, a 1 mm wide area of neovascularization with leading edge opacity was identified in the corneal infero-nasal quadrant, and no epithelial defect characterized (Fig. 20.3). Anterior segment and fundoscopic examinations were otherwise unremarkable.

The concomitant presence of a systemic inflammatory background (i.e., RA) and a new-onset peripheral corneal lesion inflammatory in nature suggested a diagnosis of noninfectious autoimmune etiology for marginal keratitis. The patient was prescribed with autologous serum eye drops for dry eye treatment OU, warm compresses, and eyelid hygiene for the management of blepharitis. A 4-week course of fluorometholone eye drops with taper was added to the therapeutic regimen to obtain a primary anti-inflammatory effect.

At the follow-up visit 1 month later, slit lamp examination of the left eye revealed a notable improvement of the conjunctival reaction with marked regression of corneal neovasculature. Residual faint stromal opacities with well-defined borders were still present relative to the original leading edge (Fig. 20.2). No steroid-induced ocular hypertension was detected. At this time, anterior segment optical coherence tomography (OCT) scan demonstrated the presence of a subepithelial hyperreflective lesion consistent with subepithelial fibrosis (Fig. 20.3). The patient was discontinued from topical steroids, and regular follow-up visits were scheduled over time.

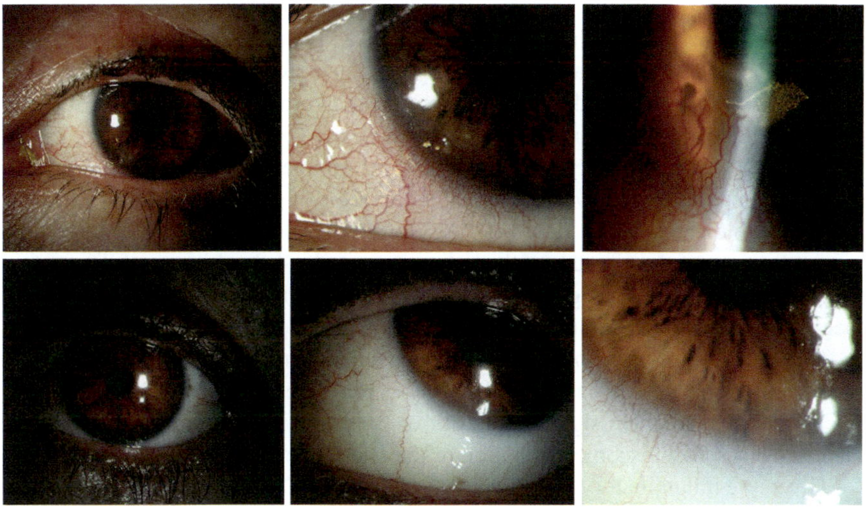

Fig. 20.2 Marginal keratitis can occur in the context of systemic immune-mediated disorder. At the top, an active inflammatory response presents with trace conjunctival injection, corneal neovascularization, and marginal keratitis with no associated epithelial defect. At the bottom line, full resolution of the clinical scenario can be observed after treatment, with only residual faint stromal opacities with well-defined borders at the original leading edge

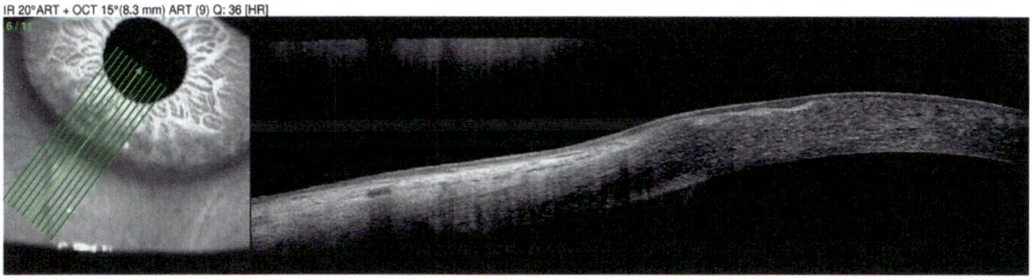

Fig. 20.3 Anterior segment OCT of the cornea demonstrates a subepithelial hyperreflective lesion consistent with subepithelial fibrosis in a patient with a recent history of marginal keratitis

20.4 Case 3

20.4.1 Summary

- MK can arise as a postoperative complication of refractive surgery.
- In selected cases, MK can present a chronic, long-term course.
- MK may have a profound impact on the quality of life of affected patients.
- A prolonged and intense immunosuppressive regimen may be indicated for effective management of MK.

A 38-year-old Caucasian female was referred to the outpatient clinic for a 1-year history of recurrent keratitis in the right eye, with the onset following bilateral myopic laser in situ keratomileusis (LASIK) procedure performed elsewhere. While responsive to topical high-dose steroids, the keratitis episodes were reported to recur upon tapering of anti-inflammatory therapy.

Her past medical history was significant for cutaneous rosacea with no ocular involvement. The family history and review of systems were otherwise unremarkable.

At the time of the encounter, the patient reported a 4-day history of discomfort, swelling, and pain in the right eye with no associated vision loss, for which she had been receiving a fixed combination of tobramycin and dexamethasone.

Slit lamp examination of the right eye revealed normal adnexa, white and quiet conjunctiva, and the presence of inflammatory infiltrate within the LASIK flap with no epithelial defect. No signs of anterior or posterior chamber inflammation were detected. Ophthalmoscopic evaluation of the contralateral eye was unremarkable.

Given the inflammatory nature of the infiltrate in OD and the history of recurrent keratitis, a diagnosis of marginal keratitis was made. A decision was made to stop the fixed combination of aminoglycosides and steroids. A punctum plug was placed in the right eye, and the patient was started on Medrol 4 mg and cyclosporine A eye drops. An 8-week tapering course of loteprednol eye drops and loteprednol gel at night was planned, and a follow-up visit was planned in 1 month.

One week later, due to a flare of the ocular condition with pain and inflammation in the right eye, the patient was shifted from loteprednol to prednisolone acetate, and she was prescribed oral doxycycline 100 mg once a day.

At the follow-up visit 3 weeks later, the patient reported a subjective improvement of symptoms. The corneal infiltrate was markedly reduced, and inflammatory precipitates appeared at the hinge of the flap. The patient was continued with the present therapeutic regimen, while a tapering plan for topical and systemic steroids was prescribed over the course of 6 weeks.

Five weeks later, a reactivation of the inflammatory process occurred. The patient came to the clinic complaining of unbearable pain. The slit lamp examination revealed conjunctival chemosis, worsening corneal infiltrate within the LASIK flap hinge, corneal haze, and diffuse corneal punctate staining (Fig. 20.4). No corneal epithelial defect was otherwise detected. Despite the inflammatory nature of the patient's corneal haze, corneal scraping was performed to exclude bacterial, mycobacterial, or fungal infections. In addition, blood tests were run to screen for systemic inflammatory disorders. The patient was started on azithromycin and a fixed combination of polymyxin B and trimethoprim. Tacrolimus ointment at night was prescribed, and prednisolone and cyclosporine A were continued. A subconjunctival triamcinolone injection was performed, and the patient was administered ibuprofen for pain control and for systemic anti-inflammatory coverage.

Within 1 week, the active signs of MK appeared to improve, with a marked reduction of conjunctival chemosis and the corneal infiltrate. At that time, the microbiological analysis and blood tests returned negative results, with the only exception of positive HSV1-IgG. For this reason, the topical antibiotic treatment

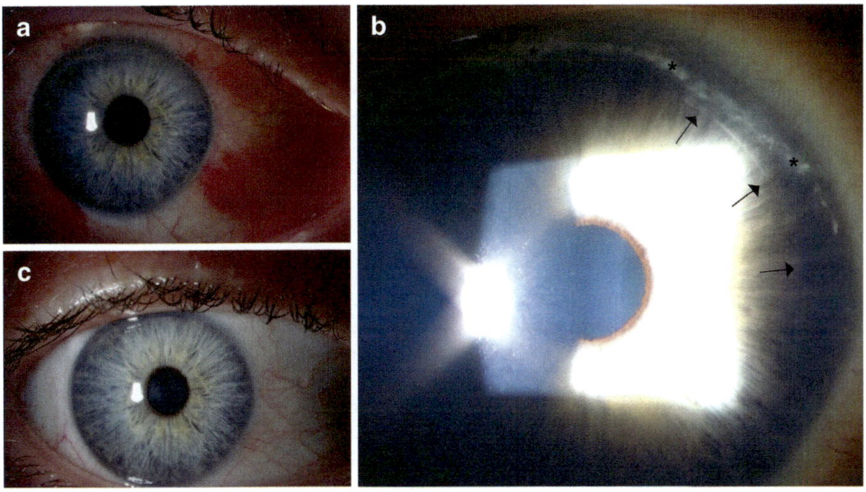

Fig. 20.4 Post-laser in situ keratomileusis marginal keratitis. In the active phase (**a** and **b**), the slit lamp examination revealed conjunctival injection and chemosis, corneal infiltrate within the LASIK flap hinge (arrow), corneal haze (asterisks), and diffuse corneal punctate staining with no associated epithelial defect. In (**c**), partial resolution of the clinical scenario

was stopped, and the anti-inflammatory regimen was tapered. Follow-up visits were then planned as needed.

At the last consultation, the patient reported to have experienced fluctuating pain ranging from moderate to excruciating over time (Fig. 20.4). Despite the amelioration of the clinical scenario, the intermittent pain significantly affected her quality of life. Accordingly, the patient was prescribed pregabalin 75 mg, and she was started on autologous serum eye drops 40%. Cyclosporine A eye drops were discontinued. Diclofenac epolamine cutaneous patch and systemic ibuprofen were indicated to control pain. The patient was referred to a pain specialist, and a psychiatric consultation for mood disorder was recommended.

References

1. Thygeson P. Complications of staphylococcic blepharitis. Am J Ophthalmol. 1969;68:446–9.
2. Ueta M, Sotozono C, Takahashi J, Kojima K, Kinoshita S. Examination of Staphylococcus aureus on the ocular surface of patients with catarrhal ulcers. Cornea. 2009;28:780–2.
3. Aiello F, Congliaro P, Malaspina C, Gallo Afflitto G, Nucci C. Peripheral ulcerative keratitis as the primary clinical manifestation of type 2 cryoglobulinemia. Can J Ophthalmol. 2021;56:e148–50.
4. Mondino BJ, Kowalski R, Ratajczak HV, Petes J, Cutler SB, Bronw SI. Rabbit model of phlyctenulosis and catarrhal infiltrates. Arch Ophthalmol. 1981;99:891–5.
5. Mondino BJ, Adamu SA, Pitchekian-Halabi H. Antibody studies in a rabbit model of corneal phlyctenulosis and catarrhal infiltrates related to Staphylococcus aureus. Invest Ophthalmol Vis Sci. 1991;32:1854–63.
6. Bernardes TF, Bonfioli AA. Blepharitis. Semin Ophthalmol. 2010;25:79–83.

7. Liu X, Ye X, Bi Y. Staphylococcus-associated marginal keratitis secondary to pterygium surgery: a case report. BMC Ophthalmol. 2021;21:157.
8. Moshirfar M, Somani SN, Tingey MT, Hastings JP, Shmunes KM, Hoopes PC. Marginal Keratitis with Secondary Diffuse Lamellar Keratitis after Small Incision Lenticule Extraction (SMILE) after Initiation of Continuous Positive Airway Pressure (CPAP) Therapy. Int Med Case Rep J. 2020;13:685–9.
9. Aslan Bayhan S, Bayhan HA, Adam M, Gurdal C. Marginal keratitis after intravitreal injection of ranibizumab. Cornea. 2014;33:1238–9.
10. Lifshitz T, Levy J, Mahler O, Levinger S. Peripheral sterile corneal infiltrates after refractive surgery. J Cataract Refract Surg. 2005;31:1392–5.
11. Dai E, Couriel D, Kim SK. Bilateral marginal keratitis associated with engraftment syndrome after hematopoietic stem cell transplantation. Cornea. 2007;26:756–8.
12. Keenan JD, Mandel MR, Margolis TP. Peripheral ulcerative keratitis associated with vasculitis manifesting asymmetrically as fuchs superficial marginal keratitis and terrien marginal degeneration. Cornea. 2011;30:825–7.
13. Tavassoli S, Wong N, Chan E. Ocular manifestations of rosacea: a clinical review. Clin Experiment Ophthalmol. 2021;49:104–17.
14. Glavici M, Glavici G. Marginal keratitis in Behcet's disease. Oftalmologia. 1997;41:224–7.
15. Taguri AH, Khan MA, Sanders R. Marginal keratitis: an uncommon form of topical dorzolamide allergy. Am J Ophthalmol. 2000;130:120–2.
16. Mondino BJ. Inflammatory diseases of the peripheral cornea. Ophthalmology. 1988;95:463–72.
17. Cohn H, Mondino BJ, Brown SI, Hall GD. Marginal corneal ulcers with acute beta streptococcal conjunctivitis and chronic dacryocystitis. Am J Ophthalmol. 1979;87:541–3.
18. Hoffman J, Hassan A. Severe staphylococcal marginal keratitis presenting with hypopyon. BMJ Case Rep. 2015;2015:bcr2015211979.
19. Yanoff M, Duker JS. Mosby; St. Louis MO. Ophthalmology. 5th ed; 2018.
20. Salmon J. Kanski's clinical ophthalmology. 9th ed. Elsevier; Amsterdam. 2020.
21. Mannis M, Holland E. Cornea. 5th ed. Elsevier; Amsterdam. 2021.

Interstitial Keratitis

21

Farida E. Hakim and Vishal Jhanji

21.1 Introduction

Interstitial keratitis is a non-ulcerating inflammation of the corneal stroma, characterized by neovascularization and cellular infiltration. The associated thinning and opacification of the corneal stroma ultimately leads to decreased vision, which can be permanent if left untreated. While the exact pathophysiology is not known and may vary depending on etiology, it is generally understood to be a T-cell-mediated immune response to antigens in the corneal stroma. Interstitial keratitis was classically categorized as syphilitic and non-syphilitic keratitis. However, over the twentieth century, syphilis dramatically declined as a cause of stromal keratitis, now accounting for less than 1% of cases [1]. In the United States, rates of congenital syphilis in the United States reached a low of 8.4 per 100,000 births in 2012. However, there has been an increase over the last several years, with over 2000 cases reported in 2020 [2, 3]. The rise of this preventable condition and cause of systemic and ocular morbidity is a grave public health concern. While congenital syphilis is considered the classic cause of interstitial keratitis, herpes simplex virus (HSV) has been found to be the most common etiology [4]. Other viral etiologies include varicella zoster virus (VZV) and Epstein-Barr virus (EBV), while bacterial and parasitic causes include tuberculosis, leprosy, Lyme disease, acanthamoeba, trypanosomiasis, leishmaniasis, and onchocerciasis. Interstitial keratitis in a patient with SARS-CoV-2 has also been reported [5]. Cogan's syndrome is a rare but established cause of interstitial keratitis, which typically presents bilaterally. It is associated with vestibular abnormalities such as tinnitus, ataxia, nausea, or nystagmus,

F. E. Hakim · V. Jhanji (✉)
Department of Ophthalmology, The University of Pittsburgh Medical Center, Pittsburgh, PA, USA
e-mail: hakimf@upmc.edu; jhanjiv@upmc.edu

F. A. Woreta, R. B. Singh (eds.), *Cornea Casebook*, Current Practices in Ophthalmology, https://doi.org/10.1007/978-981-96-0495-1_21

followed by progressive sensorineural hearing loss. Cogan's syndrome is a diagnosis of exclusion, and other known infectious and inflammatory entities must be ruled out. It is essential to promptly identify and treat patients with Cogan's syndrome as they can rapidly sustain irreversible hearing loss [6].

Patients with interstitial keratitis may present with symptoms of tearing, injection, photophobia, and decreased vision. Initial evaluation should include a thorough history and review of systems, visual acuity, intraocular pressure, and slit lamp biomicroscopy. In the acute phase, slit lamp biomicroscopy is essential for examining the cornea for stromal haze and infiltration of inflammatory cells and lack of epithelial or endothelial abnormalities. The presence of corneal neovascularization, including the depth and caliber of blood vessels and the proximity to the visual axis, should be noted. Upon recovery, patients may have residual corneal scarring in the area of infiltration and stromal lipid exudates adjacent to persistent corneal neovascularization (lipid keratopathy). Inactive or involuted vessels may be visible as faint lines on direct and retroillumination, dubbed "ghost vessels." Corneal scarring, lipid exudation, and ghost vessels can cause irregular astigmatism and decreased vision. Pediatric patients should be monitored closely for prevention and treatment of amblyopia from corneal scarring. Other corneal sequelae of syphilitic interstitial keratitis include retrocorneal fibrosis and Descemet's membrane scrolls, which form smooth, rounded "glassy" elevations on the posterior corneal surface that can form rods, branching lines, or weblike pattern on the posterior cornea [7–9].

Interstitial keratitis is primarily a clinical diagnosis. Laboratory testing for syphilis, tuberculosis, or other rare infectious etiologies is a useful adjunct when guided by pertinent details from the patient history and examination. No laboratory tests are specific for Cogan's syndrome, but inflammatory markers, such as the erythrocyte sedimentation rate, may be elevated, and associations with anti-neutrophil cytoplasmic antibodies (ANCA) have been reported [10]. Workup for systemic vasculitides may also be warranted in patients with systemic symptoms.

21.2 Case 1

- Clinical features of interstitial keratitis include corneal neovascularization and stromal haze that leads to significant vision loss.
- Close follow-up to monitor the extent of inflammation and adjust treatment is essential for the management of interstitial keratitis.
- Other systemic conditions may play a role in the recurrence and activity of interstitial keratitis.

21.2.1 Presentation

A 20-year-old female with no significant past medical history presented for a corneal evaluation. She reported the onset of redness and tearing 3–4 months prior to presentation and was started on topical moxifloxacin, topical prednisolone, and topical trifluridine. She denied any history of cold sores and had no recent vaccinations, international travel, or risk factors for tuberculosis exposure. Her visual acuity was 20/150 in the right eye and 20/20 in the left eye, with pinhole acuity of 20/50 in the right eye. Her intraocular pressure (IOP) was 10 mmHg in both eyes. Slit lamp examination was notable for a large area of central corneal edema with deep stromal neovascularization in the superior quadrant and pigmented keratic precipitates (Fig. 21.1). The left eye was unremarkable. Treatment with valacyclovir, ganciclovir ointment, and topical moxifloxacin to the right eye was initiated for presumed herpetic keratitis. At her 1-week follow-up, topical prednisolone acetate 1% was added, and valacyclovir was reduced to prophylactic dose. After 1 month, she was lost to follow-up and subsequently presented again 5 months after her initial visit. The extent and caliber of the superior stromal vessels had increased with new deposition of lipid in the central cornea (Fig. 21.2). She was offered needle diathermy for management and restarted on valacyclovir prophylaxis and topical prednisolone daily. She was again lost to follow-up for 11 months and did not undergo any procedure. At her next visit, approximately 18 months after her initial presentation, her vision was counting fingers at 3 feet with pinhole acuity of 20/100 in the right eye. On slit lamp examination, she had a large area of central corneal scarring with central and paracentral thinning and lipid deposition. Deep vessels in the superior quadrant appeared to be quiet (Fig. 21.3). At this visit, she was also noted to be in the first trimester of pregnancy. Over the next 6 months, her course was complicated by recurrent anterior uveitis for which she was treated with topical prednisolone.

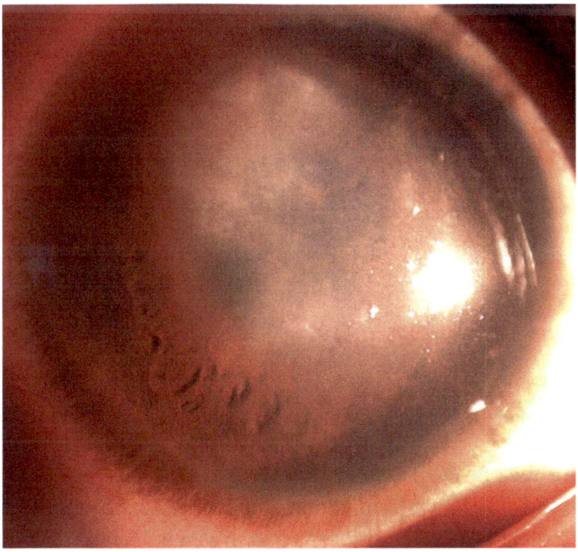

Fig. 21.1 Slit lamp photograph of the right eye notable for central corneal edema and deep corneal neovascularization superiorly

Fig. 21.2 Slit lamp photograph of the right eye demonstrating an increase in the extent and caliber of corneal vessels and deposition of lipid in the central stroma

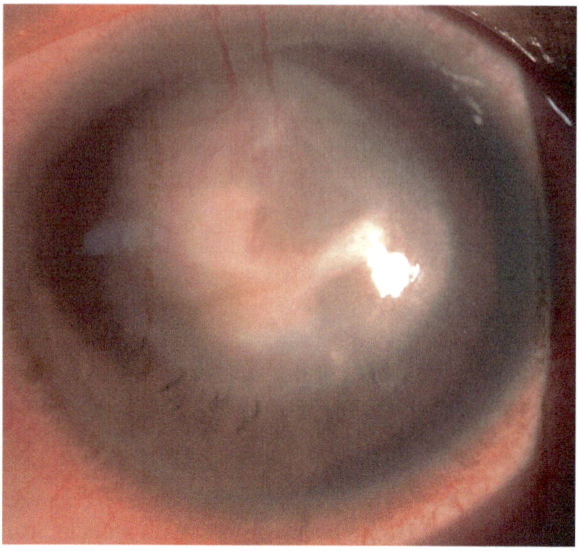

Fig. 21.3 Slit lamp photograph of the right eye demonstrating residual corneal scarring. The corneal clarity improved with topical treatment alone; superior vessels appear quiet

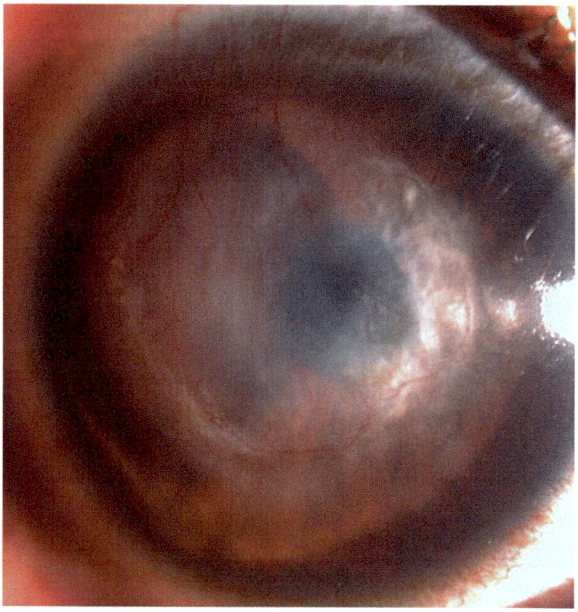

21.2.2 Discussion

In this case, the etiology of the patient's interstitial keratitis was presumed to be viral. The interstitial keratitis appears as a stromal haze with thinning and a characteristic crescentic leading edge. It is a non-ulcerative process and therefore the epithelium should be intact; one would not expect to see fluorescein staining on examination. The patient's condition progressed over the course of several months, with an increase in the size and caliber of neovascularization. Her case was complicated by periods of time without examination. Ultimately, she improved with topical steroids and without any surgical intervention.

As interstitial keratitis is understood to be an autoimmune response to antigens in the cornea, it is possible that changes in the immune system during pregnancy can impact the course of the disease. This patient experienced recurrent anterior uveitis during her pregnancy but did not have notable worsening of her interstitial keratitis. While there is little to no data specifically regarding recurrence of HSV interstitial keratitis in pregnancy, other conditions have been associated with flares of interstitial keratitis during pregnancy. For example, relapse of ocular disease in a patient with previously controlled Cogan's syndrome during the first trimester of pregnancy has been reported [11]. Further study is necessary to understand the impact of pregnancy on disease activity and progression in patients with interstitial keratitis.

21.3 Case 2

- Corneal neovascularization in interstitial keratitis may lead to lipid deposition within the corneal stroma, also termed lipid keratopathy.
- Corneal neovascularization that does not improve with topical steroids can be treated with needle diathermy and intrastromal or subconjunctival bevacizumab injection.
- Chronic steroid use can cause ocular hypertension, and patients must be monitored carefully for this side effect.

21.3.1 Presentation

A 68-year-old male with a past medical history notable for primary varicella infection, intermittent soft contact lens wear, and ocular rosacea presented for corneal evaluation. He reported multiple episodes of redness, irritation, and sensitivity to light in the left eye for which he was previously prescribed antibiotic eye drops. He denied a history of cold sores.

Visual acuity with correction was 20/20 in the right eye and 20/40 in the left eye. IOP was 17 mmHg in the right eye and 14 mmHg in the left eye. Corneal sensation was intact. Slit lamp examination was notable for mild ptosis in the left eye, bilateral lid margin telangiectasias, left eye conjunctival injection, a 4.0 mm × 4.5 mm area of corneal stromal haze with mild thinning, and deep large-caliber stromal corneal neovascularization (Fig. 21.4). The leading edge of the haze was adjacent to the temporal edge of the pupil, encroaching upon the visual axis (Fig. 21.5). The remainder of the anterior segment and posterior segment exam was normal.

The patient was started on topical prednisolone acetate 1% with plan for slow taper over several months and erythromycin ointment to the left eye at nighttime. Treatment with cyclosporine 0.05% in both eyes was initiated for findings of

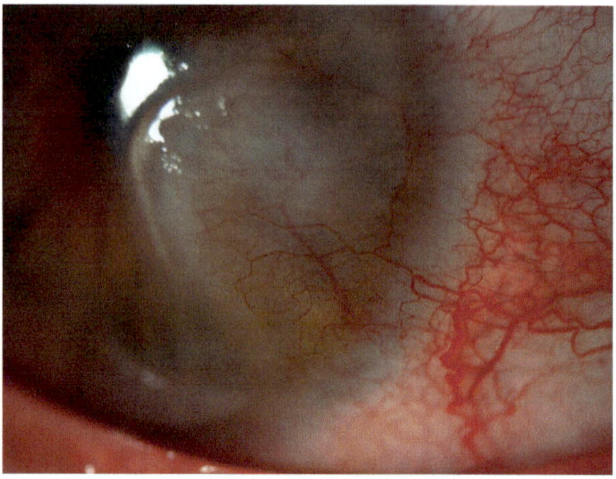

Fig. 21.4 Slit lamp photograph depicting interstitial keratitis and deep large-caliber stromal corneal neovascularization

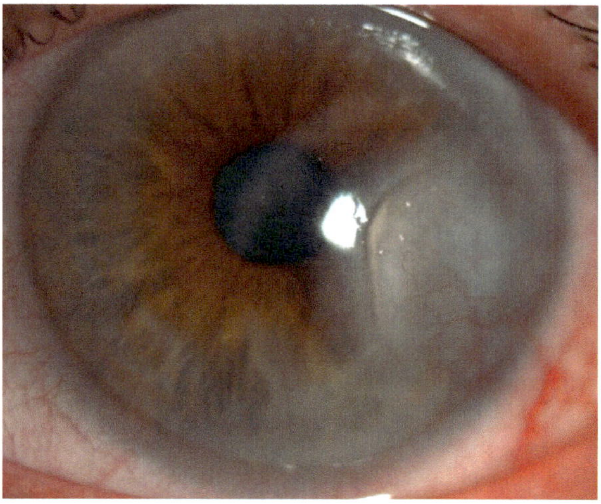

Fig. 21.5 Slit lamp photograph of the left eye demonstrating a characteristic crescentic leading edge with lipid deposition and adjacent haze abutting the visual axis

ocular rosacea. A conjunctival swab was sent for HSV and VZV PCR testing and was negative.

Two months later, the patient had partial improvement in corneal neovascularization. Intraocular pressure in the left eye was slightly elevated at 22 mmHg. Given that the patient would require a prolonged course of topical steroids, the decision was made to start IOP-lowering therapy with dorzolamide-timolol. The patient underwent needle diathermy and intrastromal bevacizumab injection 1 month later and again 6 months after initial presentation. Figure 21.6 demonstrates marked improvement and near complete regression of blood vessels. He continued a course of topical prednisolone with a 3-month taper and remained stable without recurrence off steroids. He was also able to discontinue the dorzolamide-timolol after cessation of steroids.

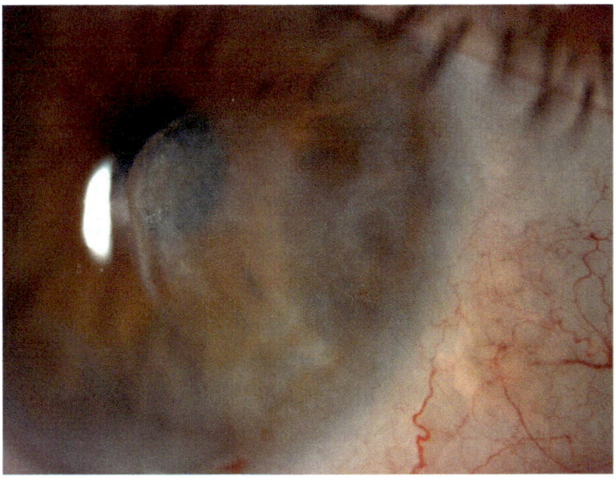

Fig. 21.6 Slit lamp photograph showing regression of corneal neovascularization following treatment with fine needle diathermy and intrastromal bevacizumab

21.3.2 Discussion

Steroids are a mainstay of initial therapy for interstitial keratitis and promote the regression of corneal neovascularization. Effort is made to taper the steroids to the lowest dose and frequency necessary to suppress inflammation. Prednisolone acetate is a common choice due to cost and availability; fluorometholone and loteprednol have a less potent ocular hypertensive effect due to reduced penetration into the anterior chamber. Children are at an especially high risk of experiencing steroid-induced ocular hypertension. Steroid-sparing immunosuppressive agents such as tacrolimus have been reported to be successful [12]. This patient developed signs of steroid-induced ocular hypertension; antihypertensive treatment was initiated before he experienced a severe increase in IOP. It is critical to monitor patients on long-term topical steroids (>1 month) for ocular hypertension and the development of steroid-induced glaucoma.

For corneal neovascularization that persists despite treatment with topical steroids, there are several surgical treatment options. In fine needle diathermy (FND), a 10-0 spatulated needle is passed into the corneal stroma at approximately 50% depth so that the tip of the needle is adjacent to the trunk of new abnormal blood vessels. A sterile electrode connected to electrocautery or a monopolar diathermy device is applied gently to the needle; the goal is to apply enough heat to cause occlusion and blanching of blood vessels without shrinkage of collagen. This procedure can be repeated in other areas, with vessels targeted individually or collectively. It is effective for treatment of established blood vessels, as opposed to new or growing blood vessels. Complications include corneal perforation, intracorneal hemorrhage, crystalline deposits, and corneal striae. Corneal perforation is the most severe adverse event [13]. In a retrospective review examining long-term outcomes and efficacy of FND, 68% of cases had regression of blood vessels after one treatment and 89% with two or fewer treatments [14].

Treatment with anti-VEGF compound bevacizumab (off-label use) has also been described and can be administered as an intrastromal or subconjunctival injection. Intrastromal injection may provide a more durable regression of neovascularization due to a longer duration of action compared to a subconjunctival route [15]. Anti-VEGF injections may be used in conjunction with FND, and this combination has also been shown to be successful in children [16]. However, stromal thinning and corneal melting have also been reported with bevacizumab [17, 18]. Further investigation is necessary to elucidate the ideal timing, dose, and route of administration of this treatment.

Mitomycin C (MMC) intravascular chemoembolization (MICE) is another technique that has been reported to be successful for the treatment of corneal neovascularization and lipid keratopathy [19]. In this procedure, MMC is injected directly into a corneal blood vessel with a 33-gauge needle. MMC is thought to inhibit vascular endothelial cell proliferation. Further investigation is needed to evaluate the efficacy and safety of this treatment on a large scale.

Penetrating keratoplasty can be considered in cases of interstitial keratitis with scarring or lipid keratopathy that is large or obstructing the visual axis. Preexisting corneal neovascularization increases the risk of graft rejection. Thus, treatment of corneal neovascularization prior to surgery is recommended.

21.4 Summary

Interstitial keratitis is a non-ulcerative inflammation of the corneal stroma that can occur secondary to numerous infectious etiologies and is also associated with Cogan's syndrome. Visual impairment results from corneal neovascularization, lipid deposition, and scarring. Topical steroids are a mainstay of treatment. Fine needle diathermy, bevacizumab, and MICE are possible treatment strategies for persistent corneal neovascularization.

References

1. Wilhelmus KR. Syphilitic keratitis. In: Mannis MJ, Holland EJ, editors. Cornea. Amsterdam: Elsevier; 2022. p. 917–26.
2. STD facts—congenital syphilis [Internet]. 2022 [cited 2022 Nov 12]. Available from: https://www.cdc.gov/std/syphilis/stdfact-congenital-syphilis.htm.
3. Increase in incidence of congenital syphilis—United States, 2012–2014 [Internet]. 2015 [cited 2022 Nov 12]. Available from: https://www.cdc.gov/mmwr/preview/mmwrhtml/mm6444a3.htm.
4. Schwartz GS, Harrison AR, Holland EJ. Etiology of immune stromal (interstitial) keratitis. Cornea. 1998;17:278–81.
5. Cano-Ortiz A, Leiva-Gea I, Ventosa ÁS, González-Cruces T, Sánchez-González J-M, Morales P, et al. Stromal interstitial keratitis in a patient with COVID-19. J Fr Ophtalmol. 2022;45:e175–7.
6. Espinoza GM, Wheeler J, Temprano KK, Keller AP. Cogan's syndrome: clinical presentations and update on treatment. Curr Allergy Asthma Rep. 2020;20:46.

7. Jin Y-Q, Hu Y-P, Dai Q, Wu S-Q. Bilateral retrocorneal hyaline scrolls secondary to asymptomatic congenital syphilis: a case report. World J Clin Cases. 2021;9:2274–80.
8. Kasetsuwan N, Reinprayoon U, Chantaren P. Descemet's scroll in syphilitic interstitial keratitis: a case report with anterior segment evaluation and a literature review. Int Med Case Rep J. 2015;8:219–23.
9. Dzhaber D, Shah AP, Dubovy S, Patel U, Koo EH. Descemet membrane endothelial keratoplasty for corneal edema and visually significant Descemet membrane scrolls due to syphilitic keratitis. Cornea. 2022;41:769–71.
10. D'Aguanno V, Ralli M, de Vincentiis M, Greco A. Optimal management of Cogan's syndrome: a multidisciplinary approach. J Multidiscip Healthc. 2018;11:1–11.
11. Deliveliotou A, Moustakarias T, Argeitis J, Vaggos G, Vitoratos N, Hassiakos D. Successful full-term pregnancy in a woman with Cogan's syndrome: a case report. Clin Rheumatol. 2007;26:2181–3.
12. Martin J, Kopplin L, Costakos D. Syphilitic interstitial keratitis treated with topical tacrolimus. Am J Ophthalmol Case Rep. 2021;23:101175.
13. Faraj LA, Elalfy MS, Said DG, Dua HS. Fine needle diathermy occlusion of corneal vessels. Br J Ophthalmol. 2014;98:1287–90.
14. Trikha S, Parikh S, Osmond C, Anderson DF, Hossain PN. Long-term outcomes of Fine Needle Diathermy for established corneal neovascularisation. Br J Ophthalmol. 2014;98:454–8.
15. Gupta AA, Mammo DA, Page MA. Intrastromal bevacizumab in the management of corneal neovascularization: a retrospective review. Graefes Arch Clin Exp Ophthalmol. 2020;258:167–73.
16. Elbaz U, Mireskandari K, Shen C, Ali A. Corneal fine needle diathermy with adjuvant bevacizumab to treat corneal neovascularization in children. Cornea. 2015;34:773–7.
17. Bhasin P, Gujar P, Bhasin P. A case of recipient bed melt and wound dehiscence after penetrating keratoplasty and subconjunctival injection of bevacizumab. Cornea. 2012;31:1342–3.
18. Sun KJ, Jun AS, Bohm K, Daroszewski D, Jabbour S. Corneal thinning following bevacizumab intrastromal injection for the treatment of idiopathic lipid keratopathy. Am J Ophthalmol Case Rep. 2022;27:101618.
19. Mimouni M, Ouano D. Initial outcomes of mitomycin intravascular chemoembolization (MICE) for corneal neovascularization. Int Ophthalmol. 2022;42:2407–16.

Atopic and Vernal Keratoconjunctivitis 22

Zala Lužnik Marzidovšek, Miha Marzidovšek,
and Petra Schollmayer

22.1 Introduction

Allergy occurs when a person develops hypersensitivity reactions to substances (allergens) in the environment that are harmless to most people [1]. Atopy is an exaggerated immunoglobulin (Ig) E-mediated immune response, which develops in persons with hereditary (genetic) tendency to develop allergic disease [1]. Some of the most common atopic conditions include atopic dermatitis (eczema), asthma and allergic rhinitis. Atopic conditions affect 28–32% of the population [2] with children and young adults being most commonly affected [3]. Allergic eye diseases include seasonal and perennial allergic conjunctivitis (AC), vernal keratoconjunctivitis (VKC), atopic keratoconjunctivitis (AKC), giant papillary conjunctivitis (GPC) and contact dermatoconjunctivitis [3]. VKC and AKC are similar yet distinct chronic allergic eye entities that can cause significant ocular surface complications and lead to vision loss due to corneal scarring [1, 2]. Type I and type IV (delayed, cell-mediated) hypersensitivity reactions play important pathophysiologic roles, with mast cell activation being implicated in both diseases [2, 4]; however, inflammatory cell-mediated immunopathologic changes with activation and migration of helper T cells likely drive the development of vision loss [2, 4]. Early diagnosis and appropriate treatment is essential to avoid sight-threatening complications, to reduce relapses and to enhance patient self-care [3].

This chapter provides guidance in a case-based approach on recognising the two most severe forms of allergic eye diseases and on their management.

Z. Lužnik Marzidovšek (✉) · M. Marzidovšek · P. Schollmayer
Eye Hospital, University Medical Centre, Ljubljana, Slovenia
e-mail: zala.luznik@kclj.si; miha.marzidovsek@kclj.si

F. A. Woreta, R. B. Singh (eds.), *Cornea Casebook*, Current Practices in Ophthalmology, https://doi.org/10.1007/978-981-96-0495-1_22

22.2 Case Presentation: Vernal Keratoconjunctivitis

22.2.1 Key Points

- VKC most commonly affects young males and has a seasonal pattern.
- The diagnosis is usually made based on a typical history of ocular surface inflammation characterised by severe itching, ocular redness, mucus discharge and photophobia and the presence of a papillary reaction on the upper tarsal conjunctiva (giant or cobblestone papillae) and at the limbus called Horner–Trantas dots.
- Although considered a severe chronic ocular allergic disease, many patients have no familial or personal history of atopic disease and have negative standard allergic test results.
- Education of patients and their parents on the natural course of the disease (which is chronic with seasonal exacerbations, but it usually tends to diminish until puberty) is crucial for good compliance and better treatment outcomes.

A 9-year-old healthy Caucasian boy with a negative family and personal history for atopy and with a negative skin prick tests for common environmental allergens presented to the Eye Hospital Emergency Department. He complained of red eyes and itching sensation and was treated with preserved olopatadine 0.1% for 30 days without success. He stopped therapy 2 days before presentation, which increased itching sensation. A physical examination showed a best corrected visual acuity (BCVA) of 20/20 in both eyes and normal intraocular pressure (IOP). Biomicroscopy of the right (RE) and left eye (LE) revealed the presence of fine papillary reaction of tarsal conjunctiva, small gelatinous Horner–Trantas dots of the superior limbus and clear corneas with no superficial punctuate keratopathy. Fundoscopy was unremarkable in both eyes. He was diagnosed with vernal keratoconjunctivitis. He was started on preservative-free (PF) dexamethasone 0.1% with a fast taper (six times daily for 3 days and then tapered in 1 week), PF ketotifen 0.025% twice daily, PF cyclosporine 0.1% twice daily and PF artificial tears as needed. At first, the prescribed therapy alleviated his symptoms, but later they got worse, and he consequently stopped all prescribed medical therapy and used alternative medicine treatment instead.

He was lost to follow-up for 5 months, when he presented again to our Eye Hospital Children's Department. Physical examination revealed stable BCVA (20/20) in OU and IOP in normal ranges. However, biomicroscopy of both eyes showed giant papillary reaction on the upper tarsal conjunctivas (Fig. 22.1a), low-grade bulbar conjunctival hyperaemia and Horner–Trantas dots with a superior paralimbal corneal scar on the LE (Fig. 22.1b); otherwise, the corneas were clear. He was again started on a short course with topical steroid eye drops (PF dexamethasone 0.1%) and put on topical maintenance therapy with anti-allergic eye drops and cyclosporine. With this topical therapy, he was relatively stable with mild flare-ups in the spring season.

At the age of 12 years, his symptoms again worsened. He reported severe itching and red eyes with some mucus discharge. Visual acuity was stable (20/20 in OU); however, biomicroscopy revealed Horner–Trantas dots 360 degrees around limbus

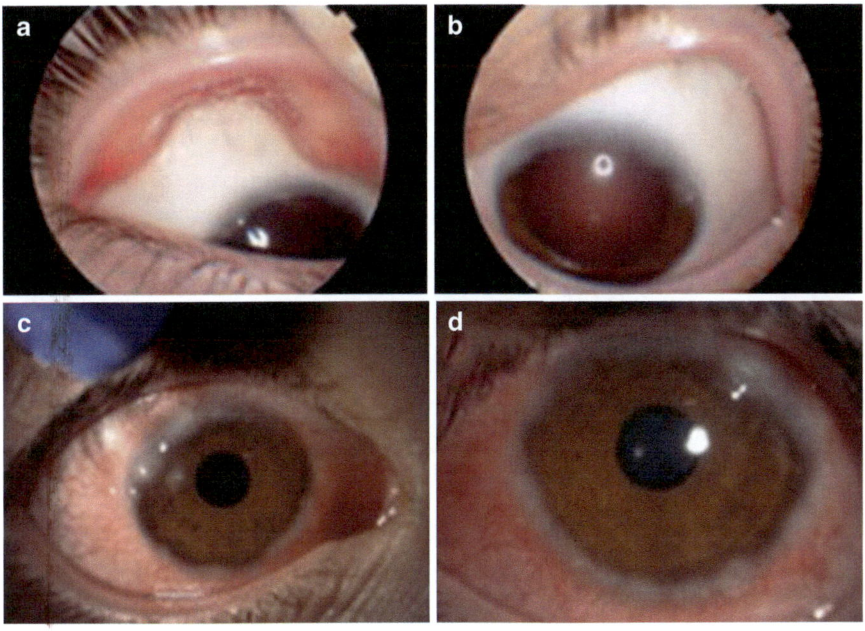

Fig. 22.1 Clinical course of vernal keratoconjunctivitis in a young boy. At 9 years of age, he presented with typical upper tarsal giant papillae (**a**) and Horner–Trantas dots with a superior paralimbal corneal scar on the left eye (**b**). At the age of 12 years, the disease worsened, with Horner–Trantas dots 360 degrees around limbus in the right (**c**) and left (**d**) eye

in both eyes (Fig. 22.1c, d). Due to superficial punctate epithelial corneal erosions and exacerbation of inflammation, conjunctival swabs were taken to exclude microbial superinfection (herpes simplex virus [HSV] 1 and 2, *Chlamydia trachomatis*, bacteria and fungus, which were all negative) before starting a new pulse of topical steroid therapy (PF dexamethasone 0.1% every hour for 1 day and then tapered fast in 1 week to three times daily) and increasing PF cyclosporine 0.1% eye drops to three times daily. He was also started on a systemic non-sedating antihistamine desloratadine (5 mg) and continued topical anti-allergic eye drops. However, despite taking all the prescribed medication, conjunctival inflammation did not improve; therefore, a short hospital admission for strict therapy control was suggested (as noncompliance was suspected). In addition to his already prescribed therapy, PF cyclosporine 1.0% twice daily and tacrolimus 0.03% ointment for eyelid margin application once daily were added. With this regimen and strict application control, he showed symptomatic and clinical improvement with regression of tarsal (Fig. 22.2a, b) and bulbar papillary reaction, Horner–Trantas dots remaining visible only on the superior limbus (Fig. 22.2c, d). Corticosteroid eye drops were slowly tapered over weeks and were changed for lower potency corticosteroid (PF hydrocortisone sodium phosphate 0.335%) to avoid steroid side effects when inflammation was under control. Commercially available cyclosporine 0.1% was prescribed to at least two to four times per day regularly depending on exacerbations and level

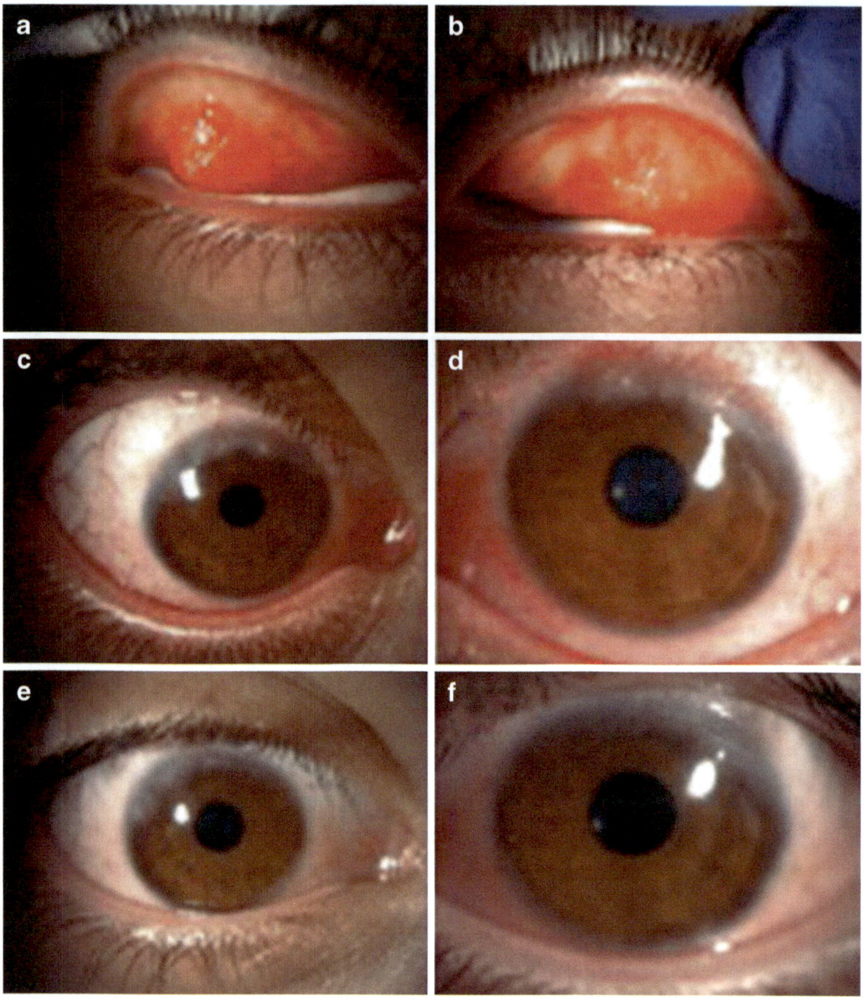

Fig. 22.2 After therapy, clinical improvement was noticed with regression of the right (**a**) and left (**b**) tarsal papillae and bulbar Horner–Trantas dots remaining visible only on the superior limbus in the right (**c**) and (**d**) left eye. On the last visit, Horner–Trantas dots resolved with faint superficial corneal neovascularisation and scarring at the superior limbus of the right (**e**) and left (**f**) eye

of inflammation. His regular therapy remained preservative-free ketotifen twice daily, tacrolimus 0.03% ointment externally on eyelid skin once daily and PF artificial tears several times per day. On the last visit, Horner–Trantas dots resolved with faint superficial corneal neovascularisation and scarring at the superior limbus (Fig. 22.2e, f), with less prominent tarsal papillary reaction.

22.3 Case Presentation 2: Atopic Keratoconjunctivitis

22.3.1 Key Points

- AKC is a severe form of allergic eye disease that occurs in the second through fifth decade of life in patients with a positive family or personal history for atopic disease and has a chronic natural course.
- AKC most commonly presents with severe itching and, in addition to conjunctival and corneal signs similar to VKC, also has eyelid involvement.
- Patients with AKC can, especially if not treated properly, have sight-threatening complications such as corneal infections or conjunctival or corneal scarring.

A 21-year-old Caucasian man with a history of hay fever was referred to the cornea department due to chronic ocular allergy in both eyes and reduced visual acuity. He complained of itching, ocular redness, burning sensation and blurry vision that lasted for 3 weeks. His BCVA was 20/100 in OU. He was using PF ketotifen 0.025% twice daily without symptom relief. Biomicroscopy revealed bilaterally anterior blepharitis and dry eyelid skin (Fig. 22.3a), upper tarsal conjunctival fibrosis (Fig. 22.3b), moderate bulbar conjunctival hyperaemia and corneal neovascularisation 360 degrees, especially across upper limbus affecting one third of the cornea (Fig. 22.3c), diffuse punctate epithelial erosions and multiple small subepithelial infiltrates, otherwise clear anterior chamber and unremarkable fundoscopy. Conjunctival swabs for bacterial, viral (adenovirus, herpes simplex virus (HSV) type 1 and type 2, varicella zoster virus), fungal and *Chlamydia trachomatis* infection were taken. The Schirmer test was in normal range. He received instructions for proper lid hygiene and was started on empirical topical antibiotic treatment with chloramphenicol 1% ointment twice daily for 2 weeks, which he should apply on eyelid margin after cleaning the eyelids; moxifloxacin 0.5% eye drops four times daily for 2 weeks; dexamethasone 0.1% once daily; and preservative-free artificial tears four times daily. Microbiology results revealed the presence of *Staphylococcus capitis* and *S. epidermidis*, both sensitive to prescribed topical antibiotic therapy. We scheduled an appointment in 2 weeks, which he did not attend, and neither did he visit any other ophthalmologist. After 3 months, he presented to the emergency department again due to worsening of symptoms not taking any topical eye therapy. He reported severe pain and decreased visual acuity with epiphora especially in the RE. Visual acuity was 20/120 in RE and 20/30 in LE, with normal IOP in OU. Biomicroscopy revealed, along other ocular pathology described above, eyelid oedema, meibomitis, a watery discharge, severe conjunctival hyperaemia and a newly formed small central round-shaped infiltrate in the anterior corneal stroma of the RE with epithelial defect (Fig. 22.3d). He was diagnosed with AKC with presumed microbial keratitis in his RE. After obtaining corneal scrapings for microbiology evaluation, he was immediately started on topical antibiotic therapy according to the protocol for presumed bacterial keratitis with moxifloxacin hourly for day and night for the first 2 days, then hourly for 3 days and after improvement to four times daily. In addition, PF artificial tears six times daily and systemic doxycycline

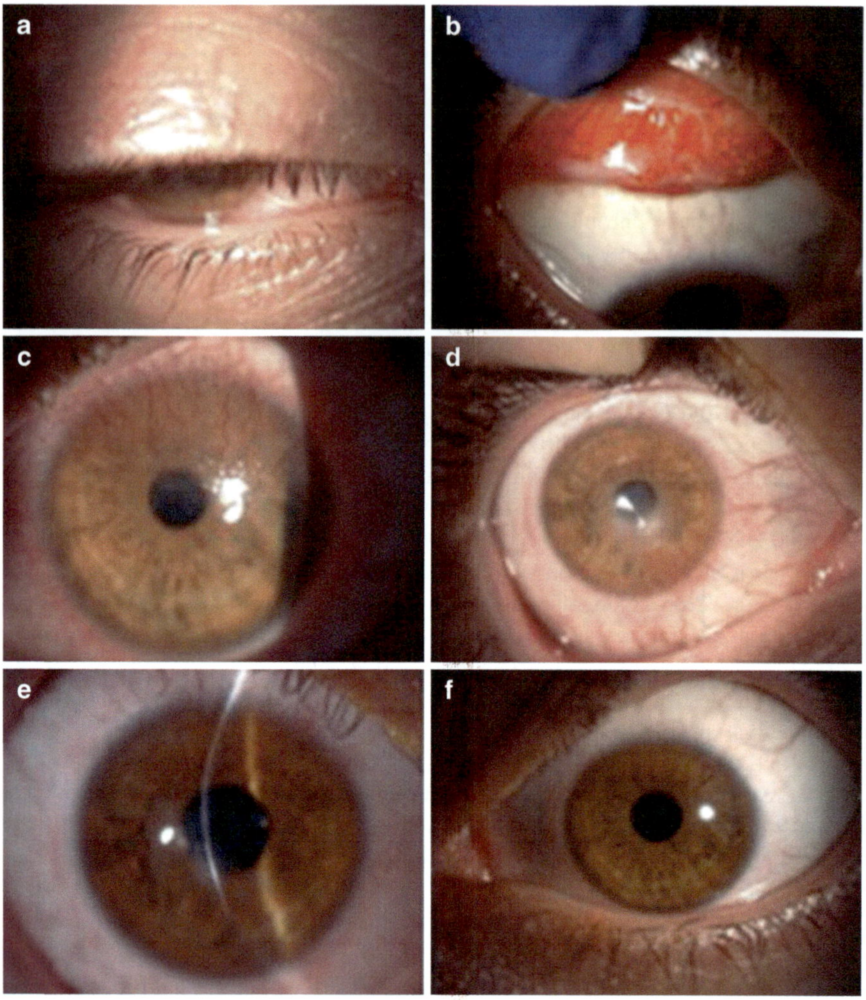

Fig. 22.3 Clinical course of atopic keratoconjunctivitis in a 21-year-old man. At presentation, biomicroscopy revealed anterior blepharitis and dry eyelid skin (**a**), upper tarsal conjunctival fibrosis (**b**), moderate bulbar conjunctival hyperaemia and corneal neovascularisation 360 degrees, especially across upper limbus affecting one third of the cornea (**c**). Severe conjunctival hyperaemia and a newly formed small central round-shaped infiltrate in the anterior corneal stroma of the right eye with epithelial defect (**d**). After treatment, a faint corneal scar remained in the right eye (**e**); however, corneal neovascularisation regressed and the ocular surface stabilised in the right (**e**) and left (**f**) eye

100 mg twice a day were started. After clinical improvement was noticed, PF dexamethasone 0.1% four times daily and cyclosporine 0.1% twice daily were added. Dexamethasone was tapered and finally switched to a soft steroid (PF hydrocortisone sodium phosphate 0.335%).

On follow-up visits, the corneal infiltrate slowly resorbed with faint corneal scarring (Fig. 22.3e). A fine papillary reaction with subepithelial fibrosis remained on upper tarsal conjunctivas. Corneal neovascularisation especially on upper limbus slowly regressed, diffuse punctate epithelial erosions healed and the ocular surface stabilised (Fig. 22.3e, f). On the last follow-up, BCVA of the RE remained poor 20/100 due to corneal scarring and irregular astigmatism, and on the LE BCVA was 20/20. IOP OU was normal. He remained on topical therapy with PF ketotifen 0.025% twice daily, cyclosporine 0.1% once daily and PF artificial tears four times daily. In case of flare-ups of ocular surface inflammation, he is prescribed a short course with topical fluorometholone 0.1% eye drops.

22.4 Definition

VKC and AKC are chronic bilateral allergic inflammatory diseases of the ocular surface (Table 22.1). VKC involves tarsal and/or bulbar conjunctival inflammation, with seasonal exacerbations; however, patients can have symptoms year-round [2]. In AKC patients, chronic allergic inflammation not only affects the conjunctiva (tarsal and bulbar) but also the eyelids, most commonly associated with eyelid eczema or blepharitis [1, 5]. VKC is most commonly found in children and young adults with an atopic background; however, a large proportion of patients have no family or personal history of atopic disease and test negative on the standard allergic diagnostic tests [2, 6]. One half of VKC patients have multiple atopic diseases, most commonly asthma [2, 7]. The disease onset starts usually before the age of 10 years with a male preponderance, lasts between 4 and 8 years and resolves spontaneously after puberty [8]. VKC is relatively rare in North America and Western Europe with the greatest prevalence in the Mediterranean and West Africa areas [2]. On the other hand, AKC usually presents in the second through fifth decade of life in patients with a known atopic disease (e.g. atopic dermatitis, asthma, hay fever, etc.) with no racial or geographic predilection and is chronic [1, 9, 10].

22.5 Symptoms and Signs

VKC presents with severe pruritus, conjunctival hyperaemia, ptosis, photophobia and tearing with thick mucus discharge characteristic for VKC [2]. Eyelid skin and fornices are usually normal (e.g. no foreshortening or symblepharon formation in contrast to AKC) [2]. Classically, it presents with conjunctival papillary response, especially of the upper tarsus and limbus. Based on the predominant involvement, VKC can be divided into palpebral, bulbar (limbal) or mixed forms, with limbal forms being prevalent in non-White patients [2]. Tarsal papillae have flattened tops and are large (giant) in diameter (>1 mm)—the cobblestone papillae. Limbal papillae are gelatinous and confluent yellow-white spots, known as Horner–Trantas dots, and are collections of degenerated eosinophils and epithelial cells [2]. Pain, foreign body sensation and photophobia are symptoms that are caused by corneal

Table 22.1 Comparison of vernal keratoconjunctivitis (VKC) and atopic keratoconjunctivitis (AKC) [3]

	VKC	AKC
Natural history	Onset in childhood/adolescence Predominantly males Chronic, bilateral, usually seasonal exacerbations Tends to resolve after puberty	Onset in late adolescence/ middle age Chronic bilateral with exacerbations, no spontaneous resolution
History of atopy	Possible	Always
Symptoms	Itching, ocular redness, photophobia and mucus discharge	Itching, watering, mucus discharge, ocular redness, blurring of vision, photophobia and pain
Clinical signs	No eyelid involvement Giant papillae of upper lid conjunctiva (tarsal form), limbal papillae or Horner–Trantas dots (bulbar form), conjunctival redness and watery and mucoid discharge SPK, corneal erosions, shield ulcer, corneal scars and NV	Eyelid involvement: Atopic dermatitis (eyelid eczema), blepharitis, meibomitis, eyelid oedema. Conjunctival tarsal and limbal papillae and hyperaemia SPK, corneal erosions, scars and NV
Complications	Corneal ulcers, corneal NV and pseudogerontoxon formation and corneal scars	Fornix foreshortening, symblepharon formation and eyelid margin keratinisation Persistent corneal epithelial defects, NV and scarring Limbal stem cell deficiency Early-onset cataract. Retinal detachment

SPK superficial punctate keratopathy, *NV* neovascularisation

involvement, which can be sight-threatening. Corneal changes include punctate epithelial keratitis; frank corneal epithelial erosions, with a fibrin and mucous plaque formation; oval-shaped shield ulcers in the upper half of the visual axis, which can leave a subepithelial ring-like scar; late corneal neovascularisation; and pseudogerontoxon formation [2].

The major symptom of AKC is pruritus (severe itching of eyelids), followed by watering, mucus discharge, redness, blurring of vision, photophobia and pain; the symptoms can be seasonal or perennial and most commonly exacerbate in the presence of fur-bearing animals [1]. AKC can affect the skin, lid margin, conjunctiva and cornea and produce lens changes. In 80% of AKC patients, the lids are involved and can present clinically with lid eczema, anterior blepharitis, meibomitis, maceration at the inner or outer canthi, punctual ectropion, cicatricial ectropion, lagophthalmos or madarosis [1]. In severe forms, lid margin keratinisation, fornix foreshortening and symblepharon formation can be seen (Fig. 22.4). Conjunctival signs include bulbar hyperaemia, in some patients also Horner–Trantas dots and chemosis. Tarsal conjunctiva can present with (macro)papillary reaction, with

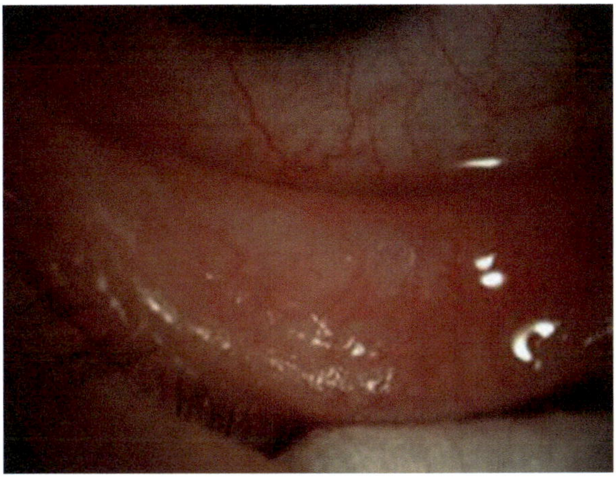

Fig. 22.4 Lower lid margin keratinisation due to severe atopic keratoconjunctivitis

reticular scarring or subepithelial fibrosis, with pale white oedema. Corneal signs include punctate epithelial keratopathy and intraepithelial microcyst formation, peripheral corneal neovascularisation that favours the superior corneal area, but can also be circumferential, and remaining anterior stromal scars after healed corneal ulcerations. In around 10% of AKC patients, keratoconus can be identified [1]. Typical AKC cataract is an anterior subcapsular lens opacification; retinal detachment is reported to be more common in AKC patients with or without previous cataract operation [1, 4]. Severe chronic AKC can progress to limbal stem cell deficiency and severe dry eye [1].

22.6 Pathophysiology

In AKC and VKC, mast cells, eosinophils and activated helper T cells (CD4) are the main cytokine-producing cell types infiltrating the conjunctiva during chronic allergic eye diseases [2, 4]. Conventionally, they were considered as a merely type 1 hypersensitivity reaction. However, IgE-mast-cell-mediated immunological reactions (type 1) are not enough, and the clear abundance of helper T cells and their cytokines (Th2 and Th1 cytokines) in tears and serum confirms the important role of the delayed-type hypersensitivity reaction (type 4) in the onset and the chronic inflammatory phases observed in VKC and especially in AKC patients [2, 4].

22.7 Diagnosis and Treatment

Diagnosis is based on the history and clinical findings; additional measurements such as tear fluid and plasma IgE level evaluation, cytology (e.g. conjunctival scraping to detect eosinophils) or conjunctival biopsy are rarely needed [11]. Microbiology testing is performed if microbial superinfection is suspected.

Patient management includes (a) preventive measures with patient education and (b) pharmacological and in severe cases (c) surgical therapy.

Education of patients and/or their parents is extremely important for good compliance and better outcomes of treatment. As in other atopic diseases, avoidance of allergen exposure is advised, however not always possible. Moreover, not all VKC patients have identifiable allergen sensitisation [12]. Although allergen immunotherapy has its limitations, subcutaneous immunotherapy showed effectiveness in reducing symptoms and serum IgE levels compared with topical treatment alone in some VKC patients [13, 14]. In addition, exposure to non-specific ocular surface irritants such as strong wind, sun, etc., should also be avoided with the use of protective eyewear. Acute relief from symptoms such as pruritus can be achieved with application of cold compresses and the regular use of artificial tears without preservatives (direct removal and dilution of allergens) [6].

Pharmacological and surgical treatment with risk assessment for vision loss in VKC patients can be guided by the clinical grading system introduced by Sacchetti et al., summarised in Table 22.2 [11].

For severe seasonal exacerbations in VKC or AKC patients including photophobia, diffuse SPK or corneal ulceration, a short-term, high-dose pulsed regimen of topical steroids brings fast relief (e.g. four to six times daily for 3 days, tapered over 1 week or eight times daily for 1 week using dexamethasone 0.1%, prednisolone phosphate 1% or 0.05% difluprednate) [11]. The use of steroids should be limited and used as little as needed to avoid cataract and elevated intraocular pressure formation.

Mast cell stabilisers and histamine (H)-1 receptor blockers should be used as first-line therapy at the onset of allergic season and should be used continuously [2]. Mast cell stabilisers, such as sodium cromoglicate, lodoxamide and nedocromil sodium, inhibit mast cell degranulation and require four times daily instillation, which can result in poor compliance and can take several weeks to take effect. Dual-acting second-generation topical antihistamines such as epinastine, azelastine, ketotifen or olopatadine with antihistamine and secondary mast cell stabilising properties are well tolerated and ideal for acute and chronic symptom relief; they are applied two times daily [3].

Table 22.2 Clinical grading of vernal keratoconjunctivitis and treatment [11]

Grade	Symptoms and signs Presence of symptoms with:	Treatment
1—mild	+ no corneal involvement	Anti-allergic eye drops occasionally
2—moderate	+ associated with photophobia with no corneal involvement	Anti-allergic eye drops daily
3—severe	+ associated with photophobia and mild to moderate SPK	Anti-allergic eye drops daily associated with pulsed low-dose topical steroid
4—very severe	+ associated with photophobia and diffuse SPK or corneal ulcer	Pulsed high-dose topical steroid eventually associated with surgical removal of corneal plaque

SPK superficial punctate keratopathy

Oral medications include steroids, antihistamines and nonsteroidal anti-inflammatory agents. Oral non-sedating antihistamines can be used when allergy also involves nose or pharynx; however, if allergy is limited to the eyes, topical treatment has superior effect [2]. Oral steroids are very rarely used for the treatment of VKC; in AKC, it is used only in sight-threatening conditions with uncontrolled dermatitis [2]. Immunomodulators that inhibit calcineurin, such as cyclosporine A (CsA) (topical 0.05–2.0%) and tacrolimus 0.03%, have been shown to be very effective in managing VKC and AKC [15–20]. In VKC, corneal shield ulcers with a transparent base (grade 1) can be managed with intensive topical therapy alone; however, if the ulcer base includes opaque deposits (grade 2) or an elevated plaque (grade 3), surgical debridement with or without amniotic membrane transplantation (AMT) and intensive pharmacological therapy is required to ensure epithelial closure [21, 22]. Some authors reported effective reduction of tarsal papillae size by injecting a short- or long-acting steroid subtarsally [2, 23] or with surgical removal (with/without mitomycin C application) and combined with amniotic membrane or buccal mucosal transplantation to treat recalcitrant corneal SPK or shield ulcers [24].

Persistent epithelial corneal defects are also hard to treat in AKC patients; topical lubrication and surgical approaches using AMT have been used successfully (Fig. 22.5).

VKC and AKC patients are prone to bacterial or viral infections such as bacterial or HSV microbial keratitis. *Staphylococcus aureus* can often be isolated from the lids of AKC patients [1]. Any staphylococcal blepharitis should receive adequate antibiotic treatment. Lid or ocular surface HSV infection should be treated with oral over topical antivirals due to epithelial toxicity. If frequent recurrent episodes of epithelial HSV keratitis occur, one may consider oral prophylaxis.

In AKC patient, oculoplastic referral is indicated if trichiasis or lid position abnormalities contribute to corneal disease, which must be corrected. Uncorrected lid and chronic ocular surface inflammation may contribute to the development of limbal stem cell deficiency [25].

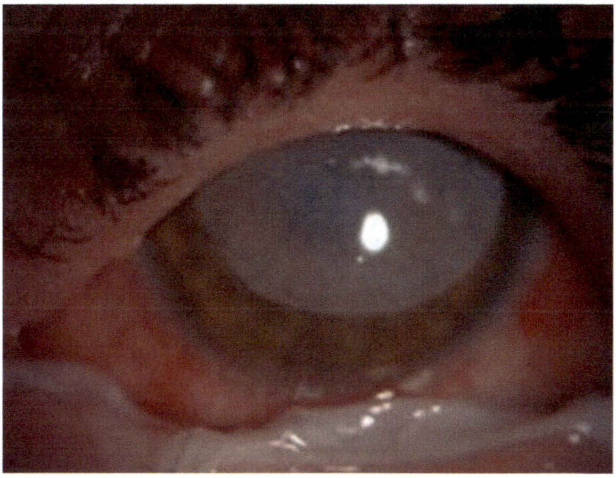

Fig. 22.5 Persistent epithelial corneal defect treatment with amniotic membrane transplantation in a patient with severe atopic keratoconjunctivitis

In 2017, FDA-approved injectable dupilumab, a human monoclonal antibody against interleukin-4 (IL-4) receptor, for the treatment of adults with moderate-to-severe atopic dermatitis whose disease is not adequately controlled with standard topical therapies or when those therapies are not advisable [26]. A dupilumab-induced ocular surface disease is not uncommon, including conjunctivitis, severe ocular redness and rarely even corneal ulceration [27]. In addition, dry eye disease increased in atopic dermatitis patients treated with dupilumab after 6 months [28]. With timely ophthalmology referral and appropriate treatment, these ocular side effects could be managed without dupilumab discontinuation [27].

Conflict of Interest Statement There is no conflict to disclose.

Financial Support or Funding Support None.

Patients have provided written informed consent for publication of clinical reports and pictures.

References

1. Tuft SJ, Kemeny DM, Dart JKG, Buckley RJ. Clinical features of atopic keratoconjunctivitis. Ophthalmology. 1991;98(2):150–8. https://doi.org/10.1016/S0161-6420(91)32322-4.
2. Kumar S. Vernal keratoconjunctivitis: a major review. Acta Ophthalmol. 2009;87(2):133–47. https://doi.org/10.1111/j.1755-3768.2008.01347.x.
3. Patel DS, Arunakirinathan M, Stuart A, Angunawela R. Allergic eye disease. BMJ. 2017;359:j4706. https://doi.org/10.1136/bmj.j4706.
4. Foster CS, Rice BA, Dutt JE. Immunopathology of atopic keratoconjunctivitis. Ophthalmology. 1991;98(8):1190–6. https://doi.org/10.1016/S0161-6420(91)32154-7.
5. Hogan MJ. Atopic keratoconjunctivitis. Am J Ophthalmol. 1953;36:937–47. PMID:13065376
6. Leonardi A. Vernal keratoconjunctivitis: pathogenesis and treatment. Prog Retin Eye Res. 2002;21(3):319–39. https://doi.org/10.1016/S1350-9462(02)00006-X.
7. Bonini S, Coassin M, Aronni S, Lambiase A. Vernal keratoconjunctivitis. Eye. 2004;18(4):345–51. https://doi.org/10.1038/sj.eye.6700675.
8. Leonardi A, Lazzarini D, Motterle L, et al. Vernal keratoconjunctivitis-like disease in adults. Am J Ophthalmol. 2013;155(5):796–803. https://doi.org/10.1016/j.ajo.2012.11.018.
9. Power WJ, Tugal-Tutkun I, Foster CS. Long-term follow-up of patients with atopic keratoconjunctivitis. Ophthalmology. 1998;105(4):637–42. https://doi.org/10.1016/S0161-6420(98)94017-9.
10. Thyssen JP, Heegaard S, Ivert L, et al. Management of ocular manifestations of atopic dermatitis: a consensus meeting using a modified delphi process. Acta Derm Venereol. 2020;100(16):1–6. https://doi.org/10.2340/00015555-3629.
11. Sacchetti M, Lambiase A, Mantelli F, Deligianni V, Leonardi A, Bonini S. Tailored approach to the treatment of vernal keratoconjunctivitis. Ophthalmology. 2010;117(7):1294–9. https://doi.org/10.1016/j.ophtha.2009.11.043.
12. Leonardi A, Brun P, Di Stefano A, Motterle L, Abatangelo G. Matrix metalloproteases in vernal keratoconjunctivitis, nasal polyps and allergic asthma. Clin Exp Allergy. 2007;37(6):872–9. https://doi.org/10.1111/j.1365-2222.2007.02732.x.
13. Dogan CU, Tuzer C, Turker IC, Alkan AA, Culha D, Demir S. Topical cyclosporine versus allergen specific immunotherapy in perennial allergic conjunctivitis. Int Ophthalmol. 2022;43(7):2161–9. https://doi.org/10.1007/s10792-022-02612-y.

14. Rahman Mahdy RA, Nada WM, Marei AA. Subcutaneous allergen-specific immunotherapy versus topical treatment in vernal keratoconjunctivitis. Cornea. 2012;31(5):525–8. https://doi.org/10.1097/ICO.0b013e3181eae270.
15. Vichyanond P, Kosrirukvongs P. Use of cyclosporine a and tacrolimus in treatment of vernal keratoconjunctivitis. Curr Allergy Asthma Rep. 2013;13(3):308–14. https://doi.org/10.1007/s11882-013-0345-0.
16. Bruschi G, Ghiglioni DG, Cozzi L, Osnaghi S, Viola F, Marchisio P. Vernal keratoconjunctivitis: a systematic review. Clin Rev Allergy Immunol. 2023;65(2):277–329. https://doi.org/10.1007/s12016-023-08970-4.
17. Leonardi A, Doan S, Aragona P, et al. Topical cyclosporine A cationic ophthalmic emulsion in paediatric vernal keratoconjunctivitis: pooled analysis of randomised NOVATIVE and VEKTIS trials. Eye (Lond). 2022;37(11):2320–6. https://doi.org/10.1038/s41433-022-02342-6.
18. Bourcier T, Dory A, Dormegny L, Alcazar J, Gaucher D, Sauer A. Efficacy and safety of 0.1% cyclosporine versus 2% cyclosporine in the treatment of severe vernal keratoconjunctivitis in children. Clin Ophthalmol. 2022;16(October):3589–96. https://doi.org/10.2147/OPTH.S370414.
19. Hirota A, Shoji J, Inada N, Shiraki Y, Yamagami S. Evaluation of clinical efficacy and safety of prolonged treatment of vernal and atopic keratoconjunctivitis using topical tacrolimus. Cornea. 2022;41(1):23–30. https://doi.org/10.1097/ICO.0000000000002692.
20. Rikkers SM, Holland GN, Drayton GE, Michel FK, Torres MF, Takahashi S. Topical tacrolimus treatment of atopic eyelid disease. Am J Ophthalmol. 2003;135(3):297–302. https://doi.org/10.1016/S0002-9394(02)01982-7.
21. Cameron JA. Shield ulcers and plaques of the cornea in vernal keratoconjunctivitis. Ophthalmology. 1995;102(6):985–93. https://doi.org/10.1016/S0161-6420(95)30925-6.
22. Stock RA, Stock RA, Lazzari SLT, Martins IP, Bonamigo EL. Surgical debridement of corneal shield ulcers in pediatric patients: two case reports and a review of the literature. J Med Case Rep. 2020;14(1):1–7. https://doi.org/10.1186/s13256-020-02407-8.
23. Holsclaw DS, Whitcher JP, Wong IG, Margolis TP. Supratarsal injection of corticosteroid in the treatment of refractory vernal keratoconjunctivitis. Am J Ophthalmol. 1996;121(3):243–9. https://doi.org/10.1016/S0002-9394(14)70271-5.
24. Tanaka M, Takano Y, Dogru M, et al. A comparative evaluation of the efficacy of intraoperative mitomycin C use after the excision of cobblestone-like papillae in severe atopic and vernal keratoconjunctivitis. Cornea. 2004;23(4):326–9. PMID: 15097124
25. Ang AY, Chan CC, Biber JM, Holland EJ. Ocular surface stem cell transplantation rejection: incidence, characteristics, and outcomes. Cornea. 2013;32(3):229–36. https://doi.org/10.1097/ICO.0b013e318255eac4.
26. D'Ippolito D, Pisano M. Dupilumab (Dupixent): an interleukin-4 receptor antagonist for atopic dermatitis. P T. 2018;43(9):532–5.
27. Pradhan SP, Sadiq SN, Cartes C, et al. Dupilumab induced ocular surface disease: a prospective case series. Eur J Ophthalmol. 2024;34(3):691–9. https://doi.org/10.1177/11206721231199155.
28. Marolo P, Ribero S, Caselgrandi P, Ghilardi A, de Sanctis U, Parisi G, Fallico M, Borrelli E, Ortoncelli M, Gelato F, Mastorino L, Tibaldi T, Roccuzzo G, Quaglino P, Reibaldi M. Ocular surface disease in patients with atopic dermatitis treated with dupilumab: a prospective case-control study. Cornea. 2024;43(2):221–7. https://doi.org/10.1097/ICO.0000000000003341.

Ocular Graft Versus Host Disease

23

M. Ogawa, Y. Ogawa, F. Yang, and K. Negishi

23.1 Introduction

Immune reaction and fibroinflammatory processes are characteristic features of chronic ocular graft-versus-host disease (GVHD) after hematopoietic stem cell transplantation (HSCT) for hematological and non-hematological malignancies [1, 2]. Ocular GVHD is a major complication that can affect the recipients' quality of vision, activity of daily living, and return to social life after successful HSCT and can lead to vision-threatening condition [3, 4].

Ocular GVHD-related fibrosis, one of the main complications of this disease, can be an early sign of the onset and also affects the later stage for the long term for many recipients as irreversible consequences after HSCT including bone marrow transplantation (BMT), peripheral blood stem cell transplantation (PBSCT), and cord blood cell transplantation (CBT) [5]. Pathogenic fibrosis by interacting between immune cells and mesenchymal cells leads to ocular surface deterioration including cornea, conjunctiva, meibomian glands, and lacrimal glands, resulting in a special subtype of severe and intractable dry eye disease. There are no approved topical medications for severe immune-mediated fibrosis on the ocular surface at present time. We report two cases of various patterns on ocular surface fibrosis with ocular GVHD after long-term follow-up after subsiding systemic chronic GVHD.

M. Ogawa · Y. Ogawa (✉) · K. Negishi
Department of Ophthalmology, Keio University School of Medicine, Tokyo, Japan
e-mail: yoko.z7@keio.jp

F. Yang
Department of Ophthalmology, Keio University School of Medicine, Tokyo, Japan

Department of Ophthalmology, Sun Yat-sen Memorial Hospital, Sun Yat-sen University, Guangzhou, China

F. A. Woreta, R. B. Singh (eds.), *Cornea Casebook*, Current Practices in Ophthalmology, https://doi.org/10.1007/978-981-96-0495-1_23

23.2 Case 1

A 52-year-old male underwent a related BMT for follicular lymphoma in August 2003. He was diagnosed as having a new onset of dry eye disease 12 months after BMT. Rapidly progressive, extensive, severe fibrovascular tissue developed on the upper tarsal conjunctiva of both eyes just 3 months after the onset of dry eye disease following BMT (Fig. 23.1).

Complete remission was achieved in systemic condition with no active GVHD in other organs 2 years after HSCT. However, his severe dry eye condition has been persisting and gradually worsened for the long term for 18 years until the present time. In addition to rapidly progressive tarsal conjunctival fibrosis, eyelid fibrosis with poliosis (Fig. 23.1), hypervascularity in the eyelid (Fig. 23.2) , and irregularity of the lid margin (Fig. 23.3) were recognized.

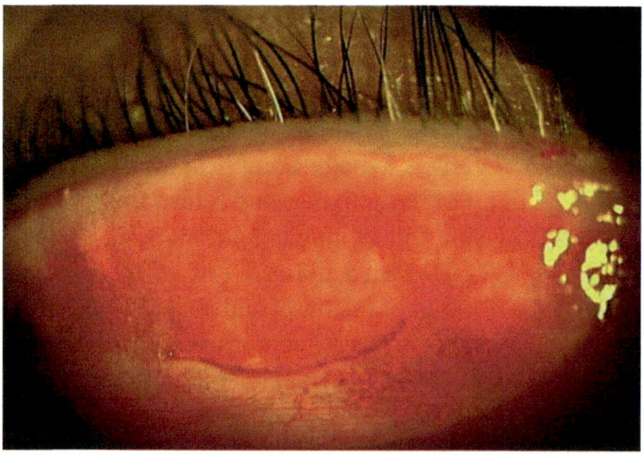

Fig. 23.1 Rapidly progressive fibrovascular tissue on upper tarsal conjunctiva just after the onset of dry eye disease after BMT. Slit lamp biomicroscopic findings. Tarsal conjunctiva on the right eye in case 1

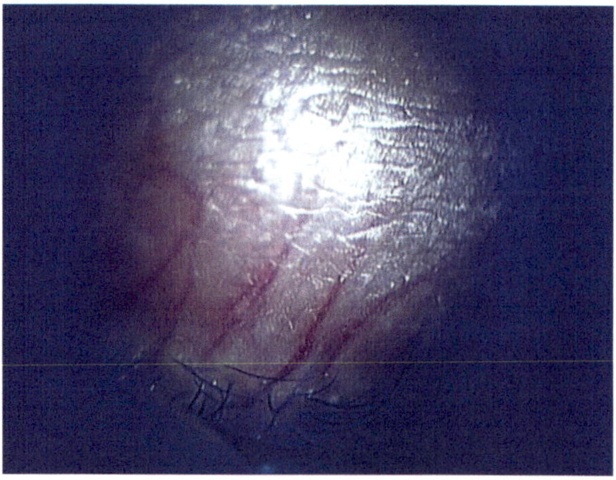

Fig. 23.2 Hypervascularity on the upper eyelid. An increased number of vessels with dilatation and irregularity in the eye lid. Slit lamp examination of the left eye in case 1

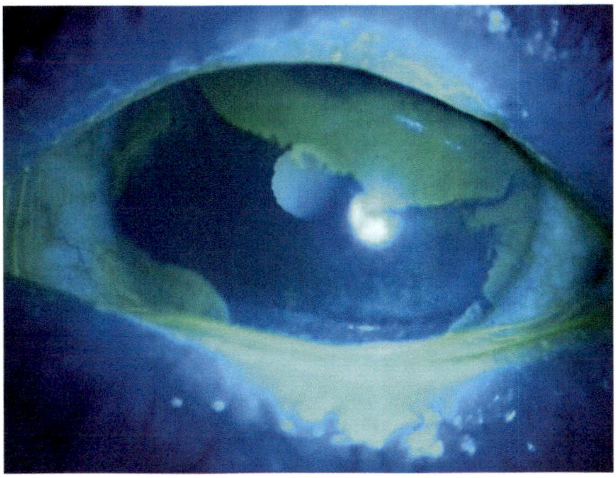

Fig. 23.3 Irregularity of lid margin and conjunctivalization from the limbal region. Chronic diffuse abnormality accompanied with fibrotic changes seen in meibomian glands in the eyelids. Conjunctivalization derived from multiple locations of the limbal region on the left eye in case 1

At present time, the diagnosis of ocular GVHD by the International Chronic Ocular GVHD Consensus Group (ICCGVHD) is definite ocular GVHD, while the National Institute of Health (NIH) is non GVHD because the presence of systemic GVHD is mandatory to diagnose ocular GVHD by the NIH criteria. The progression of the tarsal conjunctival fibrovascular region subsided gradually in recent 2 years because of controlling dry eye disease with the best available treatments including lubricants and anti-inflammatory medicines. During follow-up period of 18 years, corneal limbal stem cell deficiency with extremely thin conjunctivalization which can be detected by fluorescein staining on his left eye develops in covering the pupillary area (Fig. 23.3). Functional visual acuity (FVA) was obviously decreased in his left eye to 1.00 on LogMAR scale during FVA examination, while initial visual acuity was 0.05 in the same eye (left eye). FVA on his right eye was fluctuated from −0.10 to 0.20 on LogMAR scale throughout the same FVA examination (right eye). FVA system measures the change in visual acuity over time automatically [6, 7]. The results of FVA measure are recorded as a list of timewise visual acuity with decimal notations and logMAR conversion [7].

Confocal microscopic observation in the cornea under the conjunctivalization of the left eye revealed marked inflammatory cell infiltration compared to the right eye (Fig. 23.4a) compared to the left eye (Fig. 23.4b). Besides inflammation and fibrosis, he had been suffering from herpes labialis in 2012 and dacryocystitis for 2 years from 2017 to 2019, both of which were treated successfully by oral valacyclovir and by dacryocystorhinostomy operation with antibiotics, respectively. Although systemic GVHD had not existed, ocular GVHD exhibited multiple fibrotic changes probably due to limbal stem cell deficiency which was irreversible damage to maintain a corneal healthy condition.

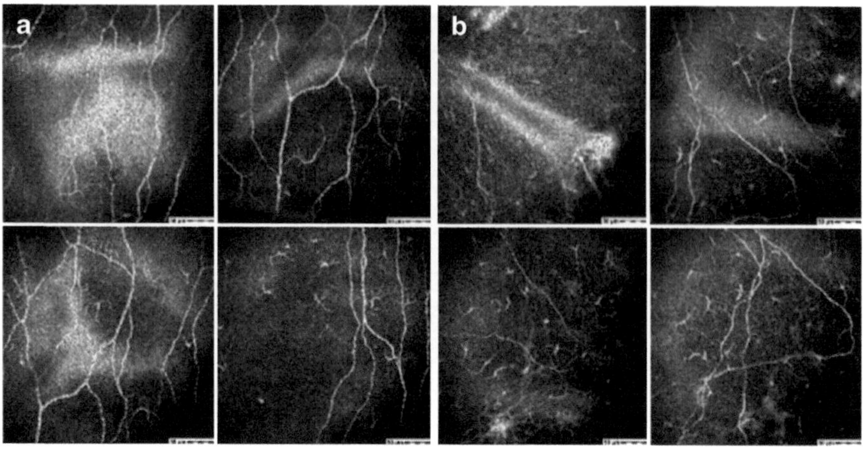

Fig. 23.4 Inflammatory cell infiltration under the conjunctivalization observed by confocal microscopy in the left eye. Scarce inflammatory cell infiltration with no conjunctivalization in his right cornea (**a**). An increased number in inflammatory cell infiltration with conjunctivalization from multiple sites of corneal limbus in his left cornea (**b**)

23.3 Case 2

A 53-year-old man was performed a related PBSCT for acute myeloid leukemia in Dec 2008 when the underlying disease was incomplete remission. Eight months after PBSCT, he developed severe dry eye disease with limbal stem cell deficiency associated with chronic GVHD in both eyes. Because PBSCT was performed when the acute myeloid leukemia was incomplete remission, GVHD occurred higher than usual based on the treatment protocol for the underlying disease. Complete remission was achieved in systemic condition at the early course after PBSCT. However, severe dry eye disease developed rapidly 8 months after PBSCT and was referred to Dry Eye Clinic at Keio University Hospital. Even after complete remission in systemic condition after PBSCT, ocular fibrosis in chronic GVHD including spontaneous lacrimal punctal occlusion, symblepharon, and squamous metaplasia of tarsal conjunctiva was observed at the first visit to our clinic (Fig. 23.5).

Corneal neovascularization, an increased number and dilatation in vessels in the eyelids (Fig. 23.6), meibomian gland dysfunction with irregularity of lid margin, and severe superficial limbal keratitis due to tarsal conjunctival fibrosis (Fig. 23.7) occurred as a severe form of ocular fibrosis at the first visit to our clinic 8 months after PBSCT.

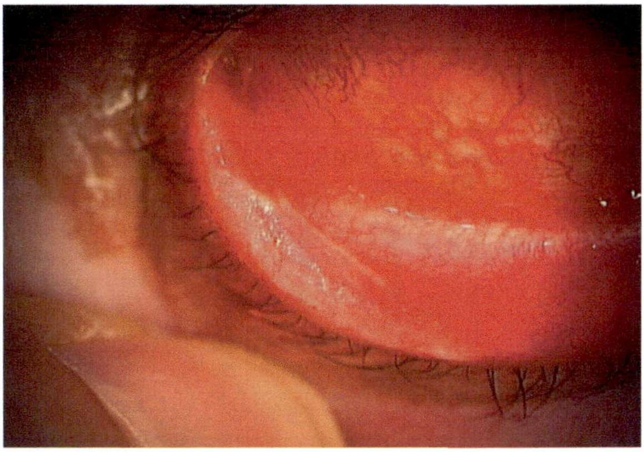

Fig. 23.5 Squamous metaplasia in lower tarsal conjunctiva. Right eye. Case 2

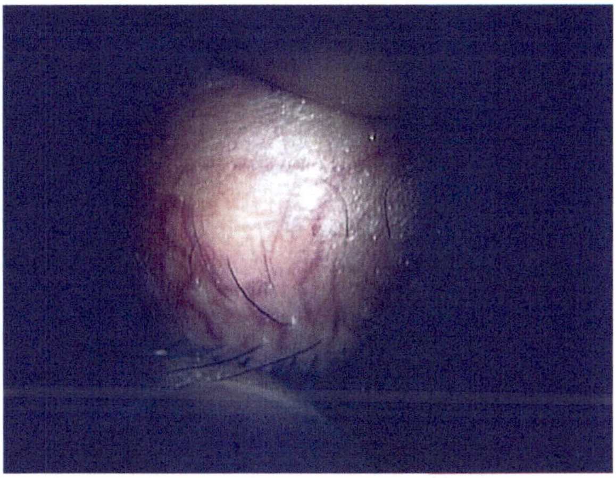

Fig. 23.6 Hypervascularity and dilated vessels seen in the upper eyelid. An increased number of vessels with dilatation and tortuosity in upper eyelid. Right eye. Case 2

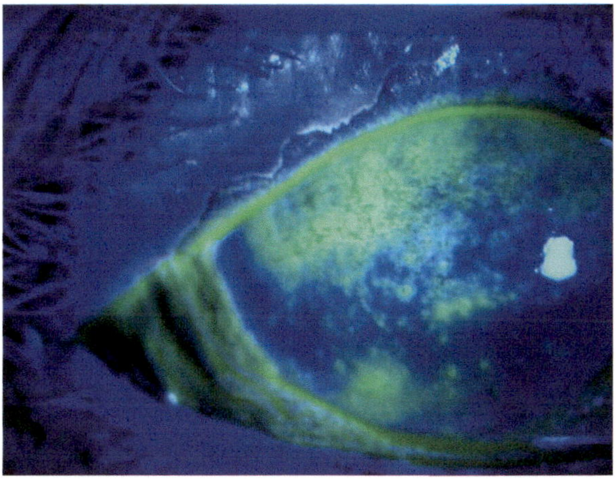

Fig. 23.7 Severe ocular GVHD. Lid margin irregularity and superficial punctate epitheliopathy are observed. Corneal fluorescein staining image. Right eye in case 2

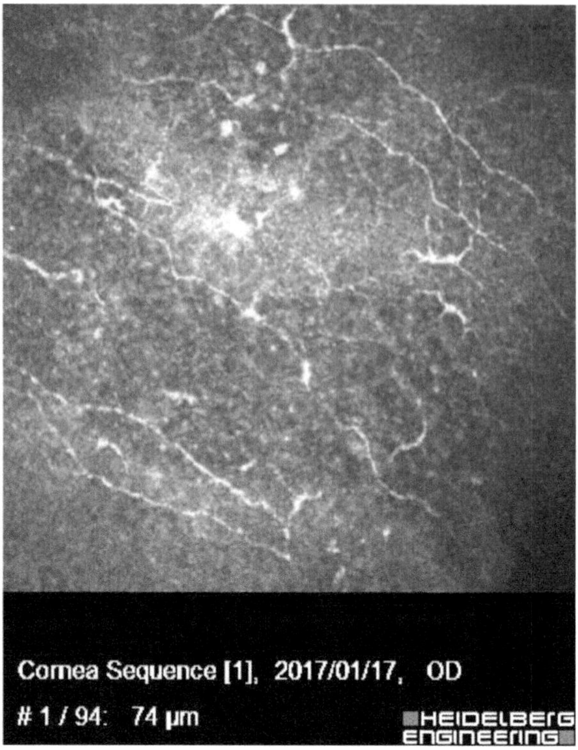

Fig. 23.8 Confocal microscopic findings. Branching and tortuosity of subbasal nerve plexus in the central cornea with ocular fibrosis associated with chronic GVHD. Right eye in case 2

Confocal microscopic observation revealed tortuosity and branching of subepithelial nerves (Fig. 23.8). Only ocular region was aggressive, severe, and irreversible during 14 years after PBSCT. He developed a diffuse filamentary keratitis and fornix shortening by active fibrotic condition. Minimum visual acuity was decreased until 1.00 on his right eye and 0.50 on his left eye on LogMAR scale during 60 second examination of FVA although initial visual acuity was 0.15 on his right eye and 0.05 on his left eye (Fig. 23.9). His systemic condition is stable after complete remission in recent 14 years for a long time. At present time, the diagnosis of ocular GVHD by the ICCGVHD is definite ocular GVHD, while the NIH is no GVHD.

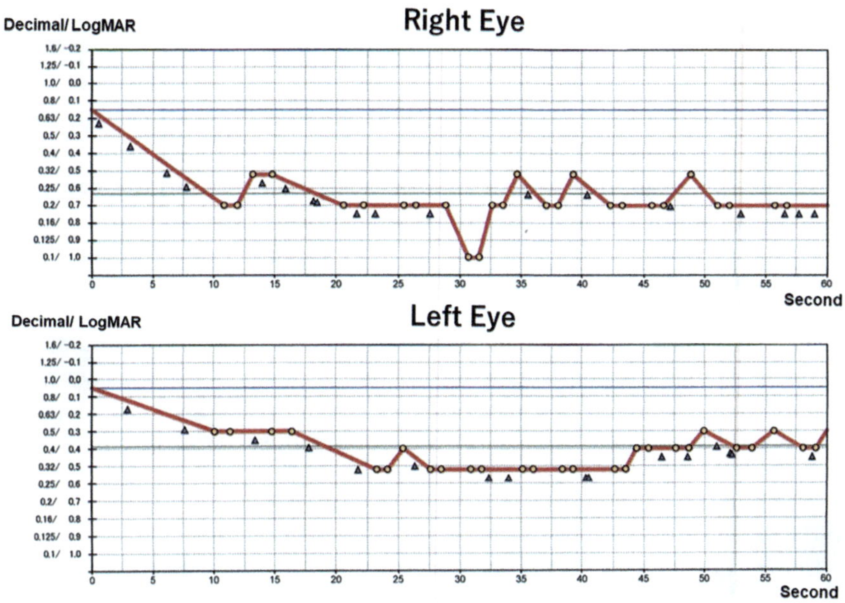

Fig. 23.9 Functional visual acuity (FVA) in case 2. A decreased FVA (0.65 on his right eye and 0.4 on his left eye on LogMar scale) was observed although initial visual acuity was 0.15 and 0.05 on his right and left eye, respectively. FVA measured during a 60-second interval with the eye in a natural blinking state. Triangle (Δ) indicates the timing of spontaneous blinking. Red line, visual acuity change with time; purple line, starting visual acuity score; green line, functional visual acuity (The avarage of visual acuity during 60 seconds)

23.4 Discussion

The characteristic feature of ocular fibrosis in GVHD is conjunctival fibrosis [8, 9] including tarsal conjunctival fibrovascular tissue, lacrimal gland duct obstruction, spontaneous lacrimal punctal occlusion [10], nasolacrimal duct obstruction, fornix shortening, symblepharon, ankyloblepharon, and conjunctivalization and/or neovascularization with limbal stem cell deficiency. Other fibrotic findings associated with ocular GVHD are meibomian gland fibrosis resulting in meibomian gland Mark line irregularity and atrophy [2], lacrimal gland fibrosis [2, 5], and eyelid fibrosis with trichiasis and dilated vessels [11]. The majority of ocular GVHD is associated with a significant reduction of quality of vision as shown in FVA in both cases, in part due to their irreversible and pathogenic fibrosis and significant long-term impact on the quality of vision [12]. The representative two cases associated with ocular GVHD in these case reports have been suffering from various types of ocular fibrosis for a long time even after systemic GVHD has been subsided in the early course after HSCT. Progress in the prevention of long-term severe morbidity associated with chronic GVHD is limited by a complex and partly unknown pathophysiology. Treatment advances for these highly morbid manifestations are limited due to the difficulty in conducting clinical trials in a heterogeneous disease with small patient numbers [5].

The fibrotic process is accelerated, and the resultant excessive fibrosis plays a main role in functional dysfnction in the ocular surface, including the lacrimal glands, cornea, conjunctiva, and meibomian glands during GVHD. One of the possibilities is that donor-derived mesenchymal stromal/stem cells may be involved in this pathogenic process [13, 14]. It has been reported that, in HSCT recipients, tissue damage caused by acute GVHD and/or a conditioning regimen promotes the homing of circulating stem cells and their differentiation into target tissues under the homing signals of the local microenvironment. Therefore, it is likely that the persistent fibrotic environment in chronic inflammatory lesions facilitates the recruitment of donor-derived mesenchymal cell progenitors, which may have growth potential or may be contineously supplied from the peripheral blood in chronic GVHD. Those processes may be related to rapidly progressive fibrovascular tissue in the tarsal conjunctiva only 3 months just after the onset of dry eye after HSCT as seen in case 1.

Corneal limbal stem cell deficiency was seen in both cases. There is a possibility that corneal limbal stem cells are targeted by immune competent cells in the early course of acute GVHD [15], resulting in severe conjunctivalization and neovascularization. Vascular fibrosis and its associated vascular tortuosity may be important indicators for GVHD to distinguish it from other types of MGD as the previous study reports the histology of hypervascularity of the eyelid in an animal model of chronic ocular GVHD [11].

Shared findings in both cases are that complete remission for systemic GVHD was achieved in the early course even though the ocular finding progressed rapidly after the onset of ocular GVHD and persisted for the long term for 18 years in case 1 and 14 years in case 2. In only ocular region, the progressed severe condition has been remained severe for long term. At the same time, this condition may be recognized as non-ocular GVHD according to the NIH definition as there is no systemic GVHD for both cases at present time. The ICCGVHD can diagnose ocular GVHD for this severe condition without systemic GVHD [16]. We have reported other two cases of continued progression of chronic ocular GVHD without concurrent systemic comorbidities treated by amniotic membrane transplantation [17]. Those two cases with the other two cases in this study suggest the ocular surface especially corneal limbal stem cells or basal epithelia of lacrimal gland, conjunctiva or meibomian gland in these four cases had been subclinically damaged and targeted during acute GVHD before subsiding of systemic GVHD, and then manifested as severe chronic ocular GVHD after the cessation of systemic anti-inflammatory treatment [17]. Once corneal limbal stem cell regions and/or basement membrane of conjunctival epithelia, meibomian gland epithelia, and/or lacrimal gland epithelia is targeted and/or disrupted, the fibrotic process might be accelerated and irreversible.

If corneal limbal stem cells have already been targeted by immune competent cells or the basement membrane of the lacrimal gland and conjunctival and meibomian gland epithelia early in the course of ocular GVHD, the condition may lead to irreversible fibrosis, i.e., immune-mediated fibrosis with specific features of chronic inflammation. Especially in corneal surface, abnormal epithelial regeneration may occur.

Besides ocular fibrosis, the importance of neurotrophic keratopathy in ocular GVHD has been reported that may cause corneal perforation in GVHD [18, 19]. Because corneal ulcer frequently regenerates abnormally in ocular GVHD, leading to corneal opacity, those conditions must be paid attention as important signs of disease progression to prevent permanent visual loss. Abnormal corneal regeneration seen in both cases might be affected by neurotrophic keratopathy.

In ocular GVHD patients, it has been reported the quality of vision is decreased [12, 20, 21]. In cases 1 and 2 in this case report, conventional visual testing in both cases is normal on both eyes. However, FVA dramatically decreased during examination in those ocular GVHD patients, suggesting that this subtype of dry eye patient's tear film stability is severely damaged due to ocular fibrosis. Mucin-producing goblet cells and ocular surface epithelium are reported to be severely affected by immune reaction and fibrosis [22, 23], partly resulting in decreased FVA.

Developing new approaches for early identification and treatment of ocular GVHD, by starting aggressive topical corticosteroids, immunosuppressants, biologically targeted treatments, and anti-fibrotic agents from the early course of ocular GVHD, is recommended, with a special focus on the prevention of devastating fibrotic changes [5].

At basic study, there are several studies on anti-fibrotic reagents including tranilast [24], heavy chain-hyaluronan/pentraxin 3 from the amniotic membrane [25], ABT-263 as an antiaging strategy [26], 4-phenyl butyric acid [27], angiotensin type I receptor inhibitor [28], and siRNA for heat shock protein 47 [29]. A randomized placebo-controlled phase 2 trial for patients with advanced hepatic fibrosis is ongoing and shows an improvement in the 90 mg group compared to the placebo group [30]. Topical application for ocular GVHD fibrosis is beneficial for avoiding systemic side effects. Translational studies from bench to bedside will eagerly be required to apply in clinical settings.

Acknowledgments We thank Drs. Masatoshi Hirayama, Yuichi Uchino, Miki Uchino, Mizka Kamoi, Yukako Tatematsu, Yumiko Saijyo, Saori Yaguchi, Masaki Fukui, Mio Yamane, Shinri Sato, Eisuke Shimizu, He Jingliang, Kazuki Asai and Isami Hayashi for imputing the insight and discussion for these cases.

Informed Consent Informed consent was obtained from these two patients. Ethical committee at Keio University School of Medicine approved this study (Approval number: 20170350).

Conflicts of Interests K.N. has a patent application number 2023-213755. Y.O. has patent numbers 6967260, 6936946, and 7279890. Y.O. has patent application numbers 2024-090577, 2023-121228, 2023-216626, and 2023-213755.

A Two- to Four-Bullet-Point Summary

1. Case 1 has ocular fibrosis including rapidly progressive fibrovascular tissue on the tarsal conjunctiva, an increased number of blood vessels in the eyelid, and conjunctivalization with limbal stem cell deficiency. Other complication was infection including dacryocystitis and herpetic labialis.
2. Case 2 has spontaneous lacrimal punctal occlusion, symblepharon, corneal neovascularization, fornix shortening, and conjunctivalization with limbal stem cell deficiency, squamous metaplasia on the tarsal conjunctiva, and an increasing number of blood vessels in the eyelid.
3. Both cases had severe progressive ocular GVHD, fibrotic changes, and decreased visual function even after complete remission of systemic GVHD.

References

1. Carreno-Galeano JT, Dohlman TH, Kim S, Yin J, Dana R. A review of ocular graft-versus-host disease: pathophysiology, clinical presentation and management. Ocul Immunol Inflamm. 2021;29(6):1190–9.
2. Ogawa Y, Kawakami Y, Tsubota K. Cascade of inflammatory, fibrotic processes, and stress-induced senescence in chronic GVHD-related dry eye disease. Int J Mol Sci. 2021;22(11):6114.
3. Nair S, Vanathi M, Mukhija R, Tandon R, Jain S, Ogawa Y. Update on ocular graft-versus-host disease. Indian J Ophthalmol. 2021;69:1038–50.
4. Kitko CL, Pidala J, Schoemans HM, Lawitschka A, Flowers ME, Cowen EW, et al. National Institutes of Health consensus development project on criteria for clinical trials in chronic graft-versus-host disease: IIa. The 2020 clinical implementation and early diagnosis working group report. Transplant Cell Ther. 2021;27:545–57.
5. Wolff D, Radojcic V, Lafyatis R, Cinar R, Rosenstein RK, Cowen EW, et al. National Institutes of Health consensus development project on criteria for clinical trials in chronic graft-versus-host disease: IV. The 2020 highly morbid forms report. Transplant Cell Ther. 2021;27(10):817–35.
6. Ishida R, Kojima T, Dogru M, Kaido M, Matsumoto Y, Tanaka M, et al. The application of a new continuous functional visual acuity measurement system in dry eye syndromes. Am J Ophthalmol. 2005;139:253–8.
7. Kaido M. Functional visual acuity. Invest Ophthalmol Vis Sci. 2018;59:DES29–35.
8. Kheirkhah A, Coco G, Satitpitakul V, Dana R. Subtarsal fibrosis is associated with ocular surface epitheliopathy in graft-versus-host disease. Am J Ophthalmol. 2018;189:102–10.
9. Kusne Y, Temkit M, Khera N, Patel DR, Shen JF. Conjunctival subepithelial fibrosis and meibomian gland atrophy in ocular graft-versus-host disease. Ocul Surf. 2017;15:784–8.
10. Kamoi M, Ogawa Y, Dogru M, Uchino M, Kawashima M, Goto E, et al. Spontaneous lacrimal punctal occlusion associated with ocular chronic graft-versus-host disease. Curr Eye Res. 2007;32:837–42.
11. Yang F, Hayashi I, Sato S, Saijo-Ban Y, Yamane M, Fukui M, et al. Eyelid blood vessel and meibomian gland changes in a sclerodermatous chronic GVHD mouse model. Ocul Surf. 2021;26:328–41.
12. Saboo US, Amparo F, Abud TB, Schaumberg DA, Dana R. Vision-related quality of life in patients with ocular graft-versus-host disease. Ophthalmology. 2015;122:1669–74.

13. Ogawa Y, Kodama H, Kameyama K, Yamazaki K, Yasuoka H, Okamoto S, et al. Donor fibroblast chimerism in the pathogenic fibrotic lesion of human chronic graft-versus-host disease. Invest Ophthalmol Vis Sci. 2005;46:4519–27.
14. Ogawa Y, Morikawa S, Okano H, Mabuchi Y, Suzuki S, Yaguchi T, et al. MHC-compatible bone marrow stromal/stem cells trigger fibrosis by activating host T cells in a scleroderma mouse model. elife. 2016;5:e09394.
15. He J, Ogawa Y, Mukai S, Saijo-Ban Y, Kamoi M, Uchino M, et al. In vivo confocal microscopy evaluation of ocular surface with graft-versus-host disease-related dry eye disease. Sci Rep. 2017;7:10720.
16. Ogawa Y, Kim SK, Dana R, Clayton J, Jain S, Rosenblatt MI, et al. International chronic ocular Graft-vs-Host-Disease (GVHD) consensus group: proposed diagnostic criteria for chronic GVHD (part I). Sci Rep. 2013;3:3419.
17. Ikarashi H, Aketa N, Shimizu E, Takano Y, Kawakita T, Uchino Y, et al. Two case reports of continued progression of chronic ocular graft-versus-host disease without concurrent systemic comorbidities treated by amniotic membrane transplantation. BMC Ophthalmol. 2021;21:164.
18. Wang S, Singh RB, Yuksel E, Musayeva A, Sinha S, Taketani Y, et al. Ocular pain in ocular graft-versus-host disease patients with neurotrophic keratopathy. Ocul Surf. 2022;26:142–7.
19. Singh RB, Yuksel E, Sinha S, Wang S, Taketani Y, Luznik Z, et al. Prevalence of neurotrophic keratopathy in patients with chronic ocular graft-versus-host disease. Ocul Surf. 2022;26:13–8.
20. Pezzotta S, Rossi GC, Scudeller L, Antoniazzi E, Bianchi PE, Perotti C, et al. A cross-sectional study on vision-related quality of life in patients with ocular GvHD. Bone Marrow Transplant. 2015;50:1224–6.
21. Shimizu E, Aketa N, Yazu H, Uchino M, Kamoi M, Sato Y, et al. Corneal higher-order aberrations in eyes with chronic ocular graft-versus-host disease. Ocul Surf. 2020;18:98–107.
22. Tatematsu Y, Ogawa Y, Shimmura S, Dogru M, Yaguchi S, Nagai T, et al. Mucosal microvilli in dry eye patients with chronic GVHD. Bone Marrow Transplant. 2012;47:416–25.
23. Ogawa Y, Shimmura S, Kawakita T, Yoshida S, Kawakami Y, Tsubota K. Epithelial mesenchymal transition in human ocular chronic graft-versus-host disease. Am J Pathol. 2009;175:2372–81.
24. Mukai S, Ogawa Y, Saya H, Kawakami Y, Tsubota K. Therapeutic potential of tranilast for the treatment of chronic graft-versus-host disease in mice. PLoS One. 2018;13:e0203742.
25. Ogawa Y, He H, Mukai S, Imada T, Nakamura S, Su CW, et al. Heavy chain-Hyaluronan/Pentraxin 3 from amniotic membrane suppresses inflammation and scarring in murine lacrimal gland and conjunctiva of chronic graft-versus-host disease. Sci Rep. 2017;7:42195.
26. Yamane M, Sato S, Shimizu E, Shibata S, Hayano M, Yaguchi T, et al. Senescence-associated secretory phenotype promotes chronic ocular graft-vs-host disease in mice and humans. FASEB J. 2020;34:10778–800.
27. Mukai S, Ogawa Y, Urano F, Kudo-Saito C, Kawakami Y, Tsubota K. Novel treatment of chronic graft-versus-host disease in mice using the ER stress reducer 4-phenylbutyric acid. Sci Rep. 2017;7:41939.
28. Yaguchi S, Ogawa Y, Shimmura S, Kawakita T, Hatou S, Satofuka S, et al. Angiotensin II type 1 receptor antagonist attenuates lacrimal gland, lung, and liver fibrosis in a murine model of chronic graft-versus-host disease. PLoS One. 2013;8:e64724.
29. Ohigashi H, Hashimoto D, Hayase E, Takahashi S, Ara T, Yamakawa T, et al. Ocular instillation of vitamin A-coupled liposomes containing HSP47 siRNA ameliorates dry eye syndrome in chronic GVHD. Blood Adv. 2019;3:1003–10.
30. Alexander KA, Flynn R, Lineburg KE, Kuns RD, Teal BE, Olver SD, et al. CSF-1–dependant donor-derived macrophages mediate chronic graft-versus-host disease. J Clin Invest. 2014;124:4266–80.

Part VI

Miscellaneous

Ocular Surface Squamous Neoplasia 24

Neha Ghose and Swathi Kaliki

24.1 Case 1

24.1.1 Case Highlights

- Ocular surface squamous neoplasia can be treated with medical therapy.
- Medical treatment options include interferon alpha 2b, 5-fluorouracil, and mitomycin C. Herein, we share a case treated with 5-fluorouracil.

24.1.2 Case Details

An 84-year-old woman presented to us with complaints of a mass lesion on the left eye since 6 months. Her left eye had a papilliform lesion between 6 and 9 clock hours of 8 mm × 5 mm × 3 mm dimensions, with intrinsic vascularity and an area of pigmentation. No keratin was noted but feeder vessels were present. Anterior segment optical coherence tomography (AS-OCT) showed an abrupt transition from normal to abnormal epithelium with epithelial hyperreflectivity, thickening and back-shadowing. She had no regional lymphadenopathy. Her viral screening was negative, and she had no other systemic diseases. A diagnosis of OSSN was made, and she was started on 5-FU drops four times a day for 1 week in the left eye followed by a drug holiday of 3 weeks. Simultaneous lubricants were prescribed four times a day for 1 month.

N. Ghose · S. Kaliki (✉)
Operation Eyesight Universal Institute for Eye Cancer, L V Prasad Eye Institute, Hyderabad, Telangana, India

F. A. Woreta, R. B. Singh (eds.), *Cornea Casebook*, Current Practices in Ophthalmology, https://doi.org/10.1007/978-981-96-0495-1_24

At 1-month follow-up, the tumor had completely resolved with an area of mild subepithelial thickening at the nasal limbus, confirmed on AS-OCT. There was patchy conjunctival pigmentation at 8 o'clock with some areas of corneal epithelial irregularity.

She was prescribed one more cycle of 5-fluorouracil with the same regimen. At the end of the second cycle, no evidence of tumor was observed—this was confirmed both clinically and on AS-OCT. The patient was followed up thereafter every 3 months for a year. The ocular surface was stable at all follow-up visits.

24.1.3 Discussion

Wide excisional biopsy with adjuvant cryotherapy is considered the gold standard for diagnosis and treatment of OSSN. However, the use of high-resolution AS-OCT [1] provides an optical biopsy of the lesion which also aids in diagnosis and allows for medical management and follow-up. Comparable outcomes have been found with medical and surgical treatment of OSSN [2]. Topical medications used in the medical management of OSSN include interferon alpha 2b, 5-fluorouracil, and mitomycin C (Table 24.1).

In a large series of 438 cases of OSSN in India, excisional biopsy was the most common (65%) treatment modality [14]. In this same series, interferon alpha 2b was the most commonly used topical medication for medical management of OSSN (28%).

A "no touch technique" as described by Shields et al. [15] involving wide excision biopsy of the tumor with cryotherapy to the conjunctival edges and application of an amniotic membrane graft over the defect is the appropriate technique to surgically excise OSSN. Risk factors which are associated with tumor recurrence following excisional biopsy are [16] tarsal tumor location, positive surgical margins, and higher grade lesions. Positive surgical margins should be treated with postoperative adjuvant chemotherapy to reduce the risk of tumor recurrence (Fig. 24.1).

24.2 Surgery vs Medical Treatment of OSSN

A literature-based decision analysis by Siedlecki et al. [11] found that the optimal approach for minimizing the likelihood of disease persistence or recurrence is surgical excision followed by topical IFN-a2b for cases with positive surgical margins. However, a case-control study of 98 patients of OSSN showed no statistically significant difference in the tumor recurrence rates between cases treated with surgery or topical interferon alpha 2b alone [2]. A study by Kaliki et al. [3] of 30 patients found that when IFN-α2b was advised for immunoreduction, it served as immunotherapy with 100% tumor regression in 92% of cases. With increasing evidence, medical treatment for OSSN has become popular and often the first choice of treatment in suitable cases (Fig. 24.2).

Table 24.1 Differentiating features of interferon alpha 2b, mitomycin C, and 5-fluorouracil

Name	Interferon alpha 2b (IFN)	Mitomycin C (MMC)	5-Fluorouracil (5-FU)
Type of therapy	Immunotherapy	Chemotherapy	Chemotherapy
Route	Topical and subconjunctival	Topical	Topical
Mode of action	Naturally occurring glycoproteins which are released from immune cells Antiangiogenic, antiproliferative, and cytotoxic effects, enhancement of host antitumor surveillance mechanism	Converted in tissues into an alkylating agent—DNA alkylation in all phases of cell cycle RNA, protein synthesis inhibition, and free radical generation also occur	Pyrimidine analogue which blocks DNA synthesis—inhibits cells in the S phase of cell cycle. Also inhibits RNA synthesis
Dose	1 MIU drops given four times/day [3] Perilesional IFN can be used in concentrations and doses of 5 MIU/cc once a month [3], 3 MIU/0.5 cc one to three times a week [4–6], or 10 MIU/cc once a month till clinical resolution of conjunctival tumor [7–9]	0.04% daily for 4 days/week for 4 weeks followed by 2 weeks of drug holiday or 0.02% week-on/week-off basis [10]	1% 5-FU four times/day for 1 week followed by 3 weeks of drug holiday
Time to resolution	Shortest with intralesional IFN and MMC [11] No statistical difference from 5-FU [12]	Shortest along with intralesional IFN [10]	No statistical difference from IFN alpha 2b [12]
Side effects	Flu-like symptoms with the injectable variant No serious side effects [12]	Allergic reaction and punctual stenosis are the main side effects. Long-term studies are needed to indicate whether limbal stem cell failure is a potential complication [13]	Pain and eyelid edema more than IFN. No limbal stem cell deficiency [12]
Cost	Expensive	Not expensive	Not expensive

24.3 Chemotherapy vs Immunotherapy

Venkateswaran et al. [12] studied 346 patients who were treated with either IFN alpha 2b or 5-fluorouracil as primary therapies for OSSN. They found that of the lesions that resolved completely with 5-FU and IFN therapy, there was no statistically significant difference in the time to resolution between the two agents (Fig. 24.3).

In a study of 51 eyes of 50 patients with OSSN by Kusumesh et al. [17], complete response was achieved in 89% and 92% of eyes with topical IFN-a2b and MMC, respectively ($p = 0.67$). The median time to lesion resolution was

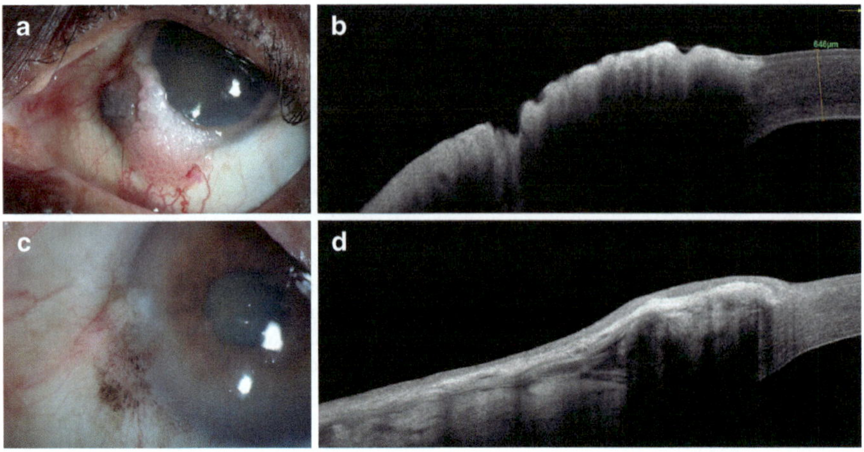

Fig. 24.1 Left eye limbal ocular surface squamous neoplasia treated with medical therapy. (**a**) Clinical photograph showing papilliform lesion between 6 and 9 clock hours of 8 mm × 5 mm × 3 mm dimensions, with intrinsic vascularity and an area of pigmentation at the nasal edge. Feeder vessels present at the inferior aspect of the lesion. (**b**) Anterior segment optical coherence tomography (AS-OCT) through the lesion showing an abrupt transition from normal to abnormal epithelium with epithelial hyperreflectivity, thickening, and back-shadowing. (**c**) Clinical photograph of the left eye after one cycle of 5-fluorouracil (5-FU) showing no evidence of tumor residue. Patchy conjunctival pigmentation noted at 8 o'clock with some areas of corneal epithelial irregularity. (**d**) AS-OCT after one cycle of 5-FU showing normal thickness and reflectivity of the epithelium with subepithelial thickening at the nasal limbus

significantly different between the groups (median 3.5 months in the IFN-a2b group and 1.5 months in the MMC group) with an average difference of 1.7 months ($p < 0.005$).

24.4 Adverse Effects

Venkateswaran et al. [12] found that tearing (5-FU 22.2% vs IFN 4.3%, $p = 0.02$) and eyelid edema (5-FU 9.3% vs IFN 0%, $p = 0.04$) were more common in the 5-FU group than the IFN group. There was no eyelid edema or keratopathy in the IFN group. Limbal stem cell deficiency was not seen in either group.

Khong et al. [13] studied the adverse effects of mitomycin C in a group of 100 patients with OSSN. They found allergic reaction to the drug to be the most common complication (34%) and epiphora secondary to punctal stenosis to be the second most common complication (14%). Kusumesh et al. [17] found that adverse effects occurred in 12% of patients using IFN-a2b and 88% of patients using MMC ($p < 0.005$). Based on the published reports, IFN alpha 2b, MMC, and 5-FU seem to be equally effective topical monotherapies. Despite a prolonged time to lesion resolution, IFN-a2b has a better safety and tolerance profile in comparison to MMC and 5-FU.

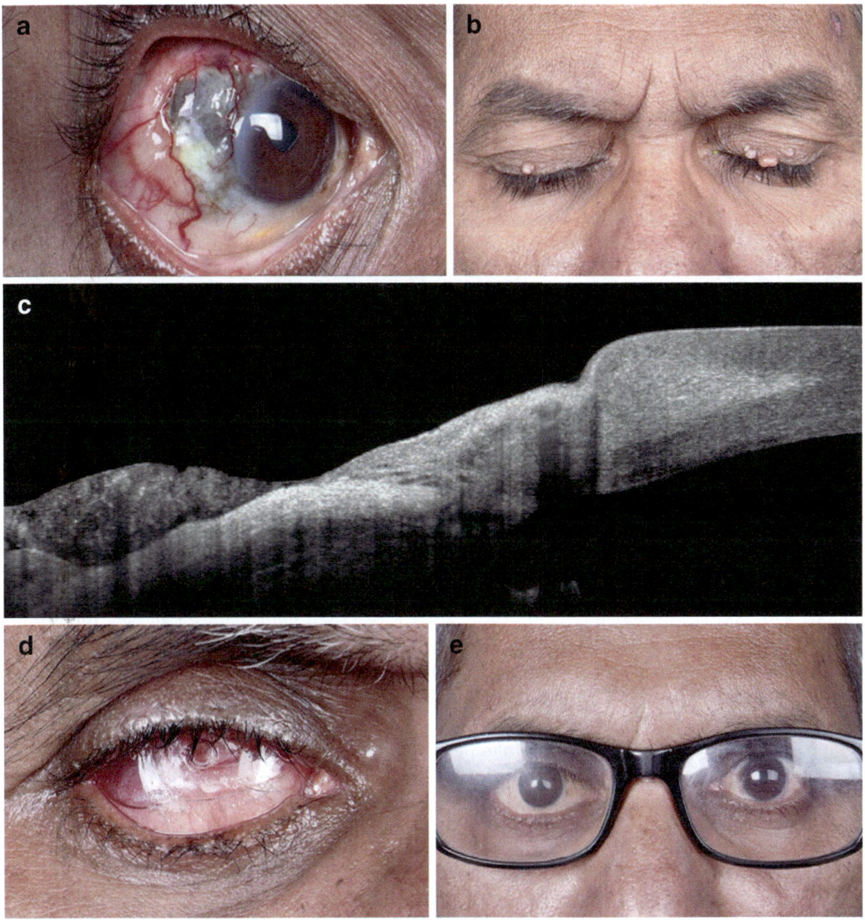

Fig. 24.2 Nodulo-ulcerative ocular surface squamous neoplasia. (**a**) Clinical photograph showing elevated pigmented lesion in the right eye extending from 8 to 11 clock hours of 12 mm × 5 mm × 2 mm dimensions with scleral thinning. Boggy conjunctival thickening around the lesion and corneal haze temporally adjacent to it is seen. Prominent feeder vessels and surface keratin are present. (**b**) Clinical photograph of both upper eyelids showing nodular umbilicated lesions. (**c**) Anterior segment optical coherence tomography (AS-OCT) of the right eye at presentation showing irregular hyperreflective epithelium with no distinct zone of separation from the subepithelial tissues and a tongue-shaped haze in the adjacent corneal stroma. (**d**) Clinical photograph of a healthy right socket with conformer in situ followed by a (**e**) customized ocular prosthesis with good cosmesis

24.5 Case 2

24.5.1 Case Highlights

- Nodulo-ulcerative variant of OSSN is rare.

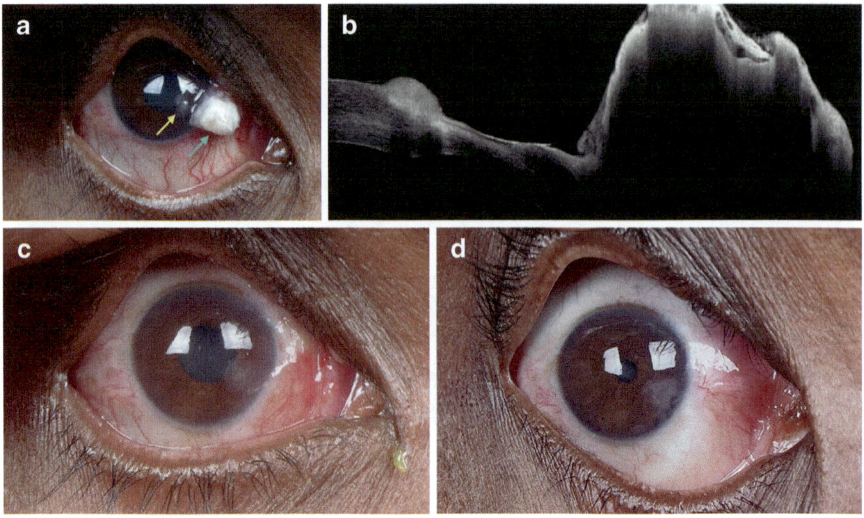

Fig. 24.3 Coexisting microbial keratitis and ocular surface squamous neoplasia. (**a**) Clinical photograph of the right eye showing a nodular lesion of 4 mm × 4 mm × 4 mm dimensions at the nasal limbus with feeder vessels and keratin (blue arrow). Adjacent cornea shows an anterior stromal infiltrate of 2 mm × 2 mm size (yellow arrow). (**b**) Anterior segment optical coherence tomography (AS-OCT) through the lesion showing epithelial thickening, abrupt transition, hyperreflectivity, and back-shadowing suggestive of ocular surface squamous neoplasia. AS-OCT through the corneal infiltrate shows a hyperreflective lesion extending from the epithelium to the anterior stroma with back-shadowing. (**c**) Clinical photograph of the right eye 2 weeks after the surgery showing nasal conjunctival congestion. (**d**) Clinical photograph of the right eye 2 months after the surgery showing a nebular grade corneal scar without evidence of residual/recurrent tumor

- It has characteristic features of scleral ulceration surrounded by scleral thickening, boggy conjunctiva, and corneal haze adjacent to the tumor.
- Nodulo-ulcerative variant of OSSN has high chances of intraocular tumor extension and thus should be treated aggressively.

24.5.2 Case Details

A 53-year-old man presented with a 6-month history of a mass lesion in the right eye. There was no history of trauma or previous surgery. There was an elevated, pigmented lesion in the right eye, measuring 12 mm × 5 mm × 2 mm, extending from the 8 to 11 o'clock positions. There was boggy conjunctival thickening around the lesion and corneal haze adjacent to the lesion. Prominent feeder vessels and surface keratin were present. There were also multiple nodular lesions with central umbilications on both upper eyelids. Both eyes had perilimbal racial melanosis. A diagnosis of right eye nodulo-ulcerative OSSN and both eyelid molluscum contagiosum was made. The patient was advised viral screening and tested positive for HIV. An incisional biopsy was performed from the conjunctival lesion to confirm the diagnosis of OSSN. The patient was simultaneously started on highly active antiretroviral therapy (HAART). Histopathology confirmed the diagnosis of OSSN.

The patient underwent extended enucleation of the right eye, along with cryotherapy to the edges, amniotic membrane grafting, and insertion of a polymethyl methacrylate implant. At the same sitting, he underwent excisional biopsies of the eyelid lesions. The histopathology report of the enucleated globe showed moderately differentiated squamous cell carcinoma with intraocular tumor extension. The conjunctival resected margins were free of tumor. The eyelid lesions were suggestive of molluscum contagiosum. At 6 weeks following enucleation, the patient received a customized ocular prosthesis (COP). The patient was followed up for a period of 2 years, and on every visit, he had a healthy socket with no tumor recurrence and a COP with good cosmesis.

24.5.3 Discussion

The risk factors for intraocular extension of OSSN include aggressive histopathological variants such as spindle-cell, mucoepidermoid, and adenoid squamous variants and other risk factors such as immunodeficiency, recurrent OSSN with a history of surgical intervention, and nodulo-ulcerative OSSN [18, 19].

The mechanisms of intraocular extension of OSSN include direct invasion of tumor through sclera, tumor inoculation via intraocular surgery incision, and along the tract of the anterior ciliary vessels [20].

Nodulo-ulcerative OSSN is a rare presentation of OSSN and was first described by Kaliki et al. [19]. It has characteristic clinical features of an ulcerated lesion with scleral thinning, surrounding conjunctival and scleral thickening, and an adjacent corneal haze.

The risk of intraocular extension of OSSN is higher in the nodulo-ulcerative variant of OSSN, especially those resembling sclerokeratitis or necrotizing keratitis. Nodulo-ulcerative OSSN is managed by extended enucleation or, rarely, with plaque brachytherapy if there is no evidence of intraocular extension.

Surrogate markers of invasive OSSN on AS-OCT as described by Singh et al. [21] include increased thickness and no visible plane of demarcation between tumor and subepithelial tissue. Invasive OSSN indicates tumor which has breached the basement membrane and not necessarily intraocular extension.

Ultrasound biomicroscopy is the investigation of choice to determine if there is intraocular extension of OSSN. The features suggestive of intraocular extension include hyperechoic tumor surface and hypoechoic stroma, blunting of anterior chamber angle, and uveal thickening.

Tumors with features of intraocular extension, even if not nodulo-ulcerative OSSN, are to be preferably treated with extended enucleation [20]. Those with orbital extension require orbital exenteration (total or subtotal exenteration) and, if surgically unresectable, need systemic chemotherapy [22].

24.6 Case 3

24.6.1 Case Highlights

- Two pathologies can coexist and may be interrelated.
- Ocular surface squamous neoplasia may be associated with microbial keratitis.
- Both conditions should be treated appropriately to achieve tumor and infection control.

24.6.2 Case Details

A 46-year-old woman presented with a mass on the right eye since 2 months, which increased in size over a 20-day period. On examination, the right eye had a nodular lesion, measuring 4 mm × 4 mm × 4 mm, at the nasal limbus with feeder vessels, keratin, and intrinsic vascularity. The adjacent cornea had an infiltrate with an epithelial defect. The fellow eye was normal. She had no regional lymphadenopathy. AS-OCT at the level of the limbal nodule showed epithelial thickening, abrupt transition, hyperreflectivity, and back-shadowing suggestive of OSSN. The AS-OCT at the level of the corneal infiltrate showed a hyperreflective lesion extending from the epithelium to the anterior stroma with back-shadowing. A diagnosis of right eye nasal OSSN with coexisting microbial keratitis was made.

The infiltrate was scraped, and the smear examined on the same day which revealed septate, hyaline fungal filaments. Thus, the patient was started on topical natamycin 5% eye drops hourly and atropine (1%) eye drops thrice a day and called for follow-up in 3 days. The culture report from the scraping taken at the first visit revealed significant growth of fungus after 2 days which was identified as the organism *Exserohilum rostratum*. At 3-day follow-up visit, the density of the infiltrate had reduced, and the nodular lesion was status remained unchanged. Two weeks later, she underwent a wide excisional biopsy of the nodule with cryotherapy to the conjunctival margins and amniotic membrane grafting, while topical antifungal drops were continued. Postoperatively, she did well with mild nasal conjunctival congestion, no evidence of residual tumor, and a nasal corneal anterior stromal scar secondary to healed keratitis. There was no infiltrate or epithelial defect. Histopathological assessment of the excised tissue confirmed OSSN, and the margins were free of atypia or dysplasia. Two months following the surgery, the patient is doing well with no tumor recurrence and with a nebular grade corneal scar.

24.6.3 Discussion

Kapoor et al. [23] described a case series of 20 cases of OSSN with coexistent microbial keratitis in which a management protocol was proposed for such cases. If there is orbital extension of OSSN, then orbital exenteration is advocated. In intraocular extension of OSSN without orbital extension, an extended enucleation is done. In OSSN restricted to the ocular surface, corneal integrity is assessed. If there is corneal perforation due to the microbial keratitis, visual potential is assessed. If there is no visual potential, extended enucleation is carried out. If the eye has visual potential, a wide excision biopsy with conjunctival edge cryotherapy is done, followed by tissue adhesive and bandage contact lens (TA-BCL) insertion or a therapeutic penetrating keratoplasty (TPK), as deemed appropriate by the treating cornea team, at the same sitting. If there is no corneal perforation, then the microbial keratitis is managed medically. If the keratitis is responding to medical therapy, the OSSN can be treated either with wide surgical excision or with topical immunotherapy or chemotherapy. If it is noted that the microbial keratitis is refractory to treatment, then visual potential is assessed, and surgical management is undertaken as per the algorithm described above, i.e., excision biopsy with TA-BCL/TPK in the eyes with visual potential or extended enucleation in the eyes without visual potential.

Microbial keratitis can occur concurrently with OSSN due to multiple reasons. The possible causes hypothesized include the presence of dellen, corneal invasion by tumor cells, and tumor cells at the limbus causing limbal stem cell destruction and partial limbal stem cell deficiency. Systemic and local immunosuppression may also play a role in the coexistence of these conditions. The HIV seropositivity rate in the cases with coexisting OSSN and microbial keratitis was found to be higher than the controls with only OSSN in their series [23].

References

1. Thomas BJ, Galor A, Nanji AA, El Sayyad F, Wang J, Dubovy SR, Joag MG, Karp CL. Ultra high-resolution anterior segment optical coherence tomography in the diagnosis and management of ocular surface squamous neoplasia. Ocul Surf. 2014;12(1):46–58.
2. Nanji AA, Moon CS, Galor A, Sein J, Oellers P, Karp CL. Surgical versus medical treatment of ocular surface squamous neoplasia: a comparison of recurrences and complications. Ophthalmology. 2014;121(5):994–1000.
3. Kaliki S, Singh S, Iram S, Tripuraneni D. Recombinant interferon alpha 2b for ocular surface squamous neoplasia: an efficient and cost-effective treatment modality in Asian Indian patients. Indian J Ophthalmol. 2016;64(10):702–9.
4. Nemet AY, Sharma V, Benger R. Interferon alpha 2b treatment for residual ocular surface squamous neoplasia unresponsive to excision, cryotherapy and mitomycin-C. Clin Experiment Ophthalmol. 2006;34(4):375–7.
5. Vann RR, Karp CL. Perilesional and topical interferon alfa-2b for conjunctival and corneal neoplasia. Ophthalmology. 1999;106(1):91–7.
6. Karp CL, Galor A, Chhabra S, Barnes SD, Alfonso EC. Subconjunctival/perilesional recombinant interferon α2b for ocular surface squamous neoplasia: a 10-year review. Ophthalmology. 2010;117(12):2241–6.
7. Kim HJ, Shields CL, Shah SU, Kaliki S, Lally SE. Giant ocular surface squamous neoplasia managed with interferon alpha-2b as immunotherapy or immunoreduction. Ophthalmology. 2012;119(5):938–44.
8. Shields CL, Kancherla S, Bianciotto CG, Lally SE, Shields JA. Ocular surface squamous neoplasia (squamous cell carcinoma) of the socket: management of extensive tumors with interferon. Ophthalmic Plast Reconstr Surg. 2011;27(4):247–50.

9. Shields CL, Kaliki S, Kim HJ, Al-Dahmash S, Shah SU, Lally SE, Shields JA. Interferon for ocular surface squamous neoplasia in 81 cases: outcomes based on the American Joint Committee on Cancer classification. Cornea. 2013;32(3):248–56.
10. Nanji AA, Sayyad FE, Karp CL. Topical chemotherapy for ocular surface squamous neoplasia. Curr Opin Ophthalmol. 2013;24(4):336–42.
11. Siedlecki AN, Tapp S, Tosteson AN, Larson RJ, Karp CL, Lietman T, Zegans ME. Surgery versus interferon alpha-2b treatment strategies for ocular surface squamous neoplasia: a literature-based decision analysis. Cornea. 2016;35(5):613–8.
12. Venkateswaran N, Mercado C, Galor A, Karp CL. Comparison of topical 5-fluorouracil and interferon alfa-2b as primary treatment modalities for ocular surface squamous neoplasia. Am J Ophthalmol. 2019;199:216–22.
13. Khong JJ, Muecke J. Complications of mitomycin C therapy in 100 eyes with ocular surface neoplasia. Br J Ophthalmol. 2006;90(7):819–22.
14. Kaliki S, Vempuluru VS, Ghose N, Gunda S, Vithalani NM, Sultana S, Ganguly A, Bejjanki KM, Jakati S, Mishra DK. Ocular surface squamous neoplasia in India: a study of 438 patients. Int Ophthalmol. 2022;42(6):1915–26.
15. Shields JA, Shields CL, De Potter P. Surgical management of conjunctival tumors. The 1994 Lynn B. McMahan lecture. Arch Ophthalmol. 1997;115(6):808–15.
16. Galor A, Karp CL, Oellers P, Kao AA, Abdelaziz A, Feuer W, Dubovy SR. Predictors of ocular surface squamous neoplasia recurrence after excisional surgery. Ophthalmology. 2012;119(10):1974–81.
17. Kusumesh R, Ambastha A, Kumar S, Sinha BP, Imam N. Retrospective comparative study of topical interferon α2b versus Mitomycin C for primary ocular surface squamous neoplasia. Cornea. 2017;36(3):327–31.
18. Meel R, Dhiman R, Sen S, Kashyap S, Tandon R, Vanathi M. Ocular surface squamous neoplasia with intraocular extension: clinical and ultrasound biomicroscopic findings. Ocul Oncol Pathol. 2019;5(2):122–7.
19. Kaliki S, Freitag SK, Chodosh J. Nodulo-ulcerative ocular surface squamous neoplasia in 6 patients: a rare presentation. Cornea. 2017;36(3):322–6.
20. Kaliki S, Jajapuram SD, Maniar A, Taneja S, Mishra DK. Ocular surface squamous neoplasia with intraocular tumour extension: a study of 23 patients. Eye (Lond). 2020;34(2):319–26.
21. Singh S, Mittal R, Ghosh A, Tripathy D, Rath S. High-resolution anterior segment optical coherence tomography in intraepithelial versus invasive ocular surface squamous neoplasia. Cornea. 2018;37(10):1292–8.
22. Meel R, Dhiman R, Kashyap S, Agrawal S, Pushker N, Bakhshi S. Systemic neoadjuvant chemotherapy in non-resectable invasive squamous cell carcinoma of ocular surface. Eur J Ophthalmol. 2022;32(2):1205–10.
23. Kapoor AG, Vempuluru VS, Laghimshetty S, Roy A, Sharma S, Mishra DK, Mohamed A, Kaliki S. Ocular surface squamous neoplasia with coexistent microbial keratitis: incidence, risk factors, clinical features, microbiological profile, and treatment outcome. Cornea. 2022;41(3):294–303.

Corneal Trauma

25

Anna Artymowicz, Armaan Shah, and Allison E. Rizzuti

25.1 Corneal Abrasion and Recurrent Corneal Erosion

25.1.1 Key Points

- Corneal abrasions are traumatic defects in the corneal epithelium.
- Topical anesthetic drops should not be prescribed for corneal abrasions, as their use can delay wound healing, resulting in corneal infection and ulceration.
- Recurrent corneal erosion syndrome is a complication of corneal trauma occurring in 5–25% of patients.
- Conservative management of recurrent corneal erosion syndrome includes lubricating agents, topical anti-inflammatories, and punctal occlusion.

25.1.2 Case Presentation

A 36-year-old female presented with pain and blurry vision in the left eye which occurred suddenly upon awakening that morning. Her past ocular history was notable for a scratch by her daughter's fingernail to the cornea of the same eye 2 years

A. Artymowicz · A. Shah
Department of Ophthalmology, SUNY Downstate Health Sciences University, Brooklyn, NY, USA
e-mail: Armaan.Shah@downstate.edu

A. E. Rizzuti (✉)
Department of Ophthalmology, SUNY Downstate Health Sciences University, Brooklyn, NY, USA

Department of Ophthalmology, New York City Health and Hospitals, Kings County Hospital Center, Brooklyn, NY, USA
e-mail: allison.rizzuti@downstate.edu

F. A. Woreta, R. B. Singh (eds.), *Cornea Casebook*, Current Practices in Ophthalmology, https://doi.org/10.1007/978-981-96-0495-1_25

prior, followed by two similar episodes of eye pain upon awakening. Visual acuity was 20/20 in the right eye and 20/50 in the left eye. The left conjunctiva was diffusely injected, and there was an epithelial defect in the central cornea (Fig. 25.1). The rest of the examination was within normal limits. The patient was diagnosed with recurrent corneal erosion syndrome secondary to her history of corneal trauma. She requested that we prescribe a topical anesthetic, as she had been given one during an emergency room visit the previous year. We explained the risks associated with this practice and instead prescribed fluoroquinolone eye drops to be used four times a day in the left eye for a total of 5 days in addition to long-term use of lubricating agents. We explained the chronic course of the condition and that a stepwise management approach may be necessary to prevent recurrences.

25.1.3 Discussion

Corneal abrasions, or traumatic defects in the corneal epithelium, are among the most common eye conditions seen in US emergency departments [1]. Common causes of corneal abrasions include injury by fingernails, animal claws, tree branches, makeup applicators, and other handheld tools. Corneal abrasions are managed conservatively with topical antibiotic prophylaxis, and most resolve spontaneously within 24–72 h without sequelae. Though there are studies that report that the short-term use of topical anesthetics for corneal abrasions is safe [2], the corneal analgesia prevents protective reflex tearing and blinking which can result in impaired wound healing, infection, and ulceration [3, 4].

Recurrent corneal erosion syndrome (RCES) is a complication of corneal trauma occurring in 5–25% of patients [5]. The syndrome is characterized by repeated disruption to the corneal epithelium resulting in recurrent epithelial defects. A history of corneal injury is the most common cause of RCES, but it can also occur spontaneously in patients with congenital dystrophies of the corneal epithelium. Patients present with acute eye pain, tearing, and blurry vision which typically occurs

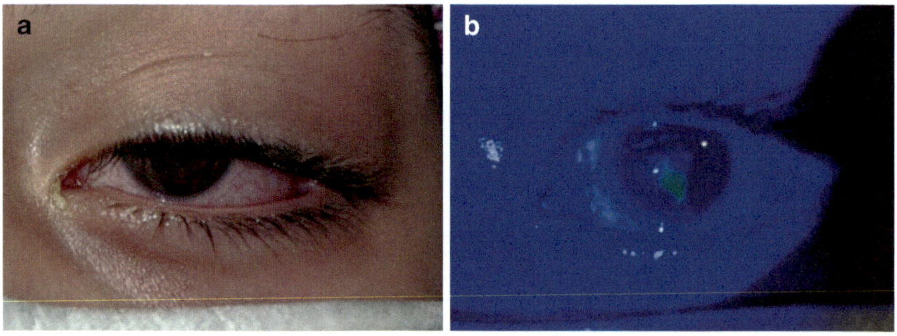

Fig. 25.1 (**a**) External photograph showing diffuse conjunctival injection and ptosis. (**b**) Slit lamp examination of the eye after application of topical anesthetic and fluorescein. Fluorescein staining reveals a central corneal epithelial defect

suddenly upon awakening [6]. Patients with an acute epithelial defect secondary to RCES should be treated with topical antibiotic drops or ointments for infection prophylaxis. Once the acute epithelial defect has healed, there are many available treatment options to prevent subsequent attacks. A stepwise approach may be necessary for adequate control. Medical management with hypertonic sodium chloride, artificial tears, and ointments is first-line therapy for RCES. Punctal occlusion, oral doxycycline, topical corticosteroids, and topical cyclosporine are used in moderate to severe cases. Surgical treatments should be reserved for patients who have failed aggressive medical therapies and include anterior stromal micropuncture, superficial keratectomy, or phototherapeutic keratectomy (PTK) [7].

25.2 Traumatic Injury to the Transplanted Cornea

25.2.1 Key Points

- Dehiscence of the corneal graft is common in patients with a history of corneal transplantation who sustain ocular trauma.
- Traumatic graft dehiscence of a deep anterior lamellar keratoplasty (DALK) graft is theoretically less common than that of a penetrating keratoplasty (PKP) graft due to the structural integrity provided by the host's Descemet's membrane, but studies report a similar incidence.
- Surgical options for graft dehiscence depend on the extent of the injury and include re-suturing the dislocated graft or transplanting new corneal tissue.

25.2.2 Case Presentation

A 28-year-old female with a history of keratoconus who underwent deep anterior lamellar keratoplasty (DALK) in the right eye 2 months prior presented with decreased vision in the right eye after being hit by a falling box. On examination, her visual acuity was counting fingers in the right eye and 20/20 in the left eye. Extraocular movements were full, and there was no relative afferent pupillary defect. Slit lamp examination was notable for 9 clock hours of corneal graft dehiscence, and there was a defect in the underlying Descemet's membrane with prolapsing uvea (Fig. 25.2). The patient underwent emergent penetrating keratoplasty (PK) with new donor tissue.

25.2.3 Discussion

A cornea that has undergone transplantation lacks the tensile strength of an intact cornea due to suboptimal wound healing and tissue remodeling at the graft–host junction [8]. This, compounded with factors such as corneal avascularity and prolonged topical corticosteroid use, leads to a reduction in corneal tensile strength that

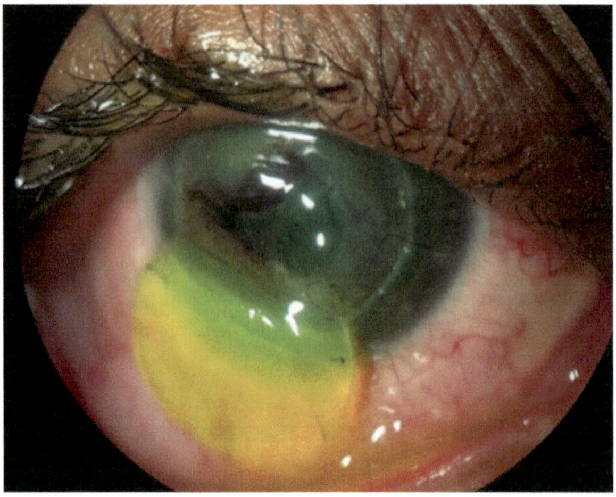

Fig. 25.2 Slit lamp examination of the right eye with ~210 degrees of DALK graft dehiscence. Seidel positivity in the central endothelium indicates the presence of a full-thickness corneal perforation

predisposes corneal transplant patients to an increased risk of wound dehiscence, particularly in the setting of trauma [9]. Graft dehiscence following full-thickness penetrating keratoplasty has been found to range from 0.6% to 5.8% [10]. Because the host's Descemet's membrane remains intact following DALK, the susceptibility to dehiscence is theoretically lower but in fact still occurs at a reported incidence of 0.5–3.2% [11].

The highest risk of traumatic dehiscence following PK or DALK is during the first 3 postoperative years [8, 11]. However, the risk remains elevated lifelong, and dehiscence occurring more than a decade after the surgery has been described [12]. Traumatic dehiscence is more common in young male transplant patients, likely due to increased incidents of human-induced trauma in this group. Falls are the leading cause of graft dehiscence in elderly patients [11]. Graft dehiscence involves the graft–host junction in virtually all cases, regardless of the presence or type of sutures [11].

Patients with traumatic wound dehiscence may present with pain or decreased vision after sustaining a blunt or penetrating injury to the eye. Because of the inherent weakness of the corneal wound, the extent of injury may seem out of proportion to the trauma described. Slit lamp examination may reveal a partially attached or completely absent corneal graft. Loose or broken sutures may be visible at the graft–host junction. A shallow anterior chamber, iris prolapse, lens extrusion, hyphema, and vitreous prolapse are other common findings. Retinal detachment or vitreous hemorrhage may be present in more severe injuries.

Management of a traumatic graft dehiscence should follow a similar protocol to a routine open globe injury. A fox shield should be placed over the eye and intravenous antibiotics administered with the plan for surgical repair within 24 h of the injury. Dehiscence of the graft–host interface can be re-sutured either by a running suture joined to the free ends of the remaining intact running suture or by placing new interrupted sutures [8]. Anterior vitrectomy should be performed in all cases of vitreous loss, and any prolapsed iris should be carefully repositioned. If the graft (or the Descemet's membrane in the case of a dehisced DALK graft) appears compromised, a penetrating keratoplasty with new donor tissue will achieve the best results [13].

Visual outcomes after traumatic wound dehiscence are generally poor but depend on the extent of dehiscence and the presence of complications such as lens injury, retinal detachment, and vitreous hemorrhage. Final best corrected visual acuity following dehiscence after penetrating keratoplasty ranges from no light perception to 20/50 [8]. There is less data available regarding visual outcomes after graft dehiscence following DALK, with some studies suggesting a trend for better visual outcomes compared to PK [14].

25.3 Corneal Laceration and Intraocular Foreign Body

25.3.1 Key Points

- A corneal laceration can be partial or full thickness. A partial-thickness corneal laceration does not violate the integrity of the globe. A full-thickness corneal laceration constitutes an open globe injury.
- Full-thickness corneal lacerations should be repaired within 24 h with the goals of watertight closure with minimal corneal distortion.
- Corneal lacerations are most commonly repaired with 10-0 nylon interrupted sutures placed at 90% corneal depth.
- An intraocular foreign body may result from a lacerating corneal injury, and its removal should take place at the time of globe closure if possible.

25.3.2 Case Presentation

A 19-year-old male presented with left eye pain and blurry vision after having been accidentally shot in the eye with a BB gun. Visual acuity was 20/20 in the right eye and hand motions in the left eye. The external exam revealed a corneal laceration with iris prolapsing through the wound (Fig. 25.3a and b). Applanation tonometry and dilated eye examination were within normal limits in the right eye and deferred in the left eye. Computed tomography (CT) scan of the orbits revealed the bullet located in the vitreous cavity (Fig. 25.3c). The patient was started on broad-spectrum intravenous antibiotics, given tetanus prophylaxis and pain control, and underwent emergent removal of the intraocular foreign body and corneal laceration repair.

25.3.3 Discussion

A corneal laceration is a traumatic injury through multiple layers of the cornea. A partial-thickness laceration involves the anterior layers of the cornea and does not violate the integrity of the globe. A full-thickness laceration constitutes an open

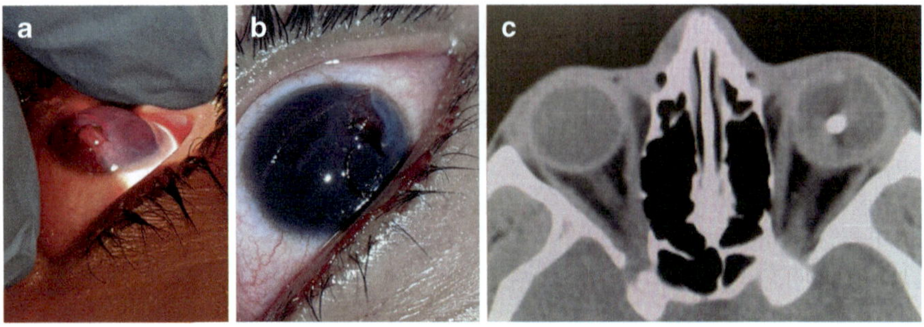

Fig. 25.3 (**a/b**) External photographs of the left eye demonstrating protrusion of uveal tissue through a corneal wound and a total hyphema. (**c**) CT orbit revealing a hyperintense foreign body (BB bullet) in the left orbit

globe injury unless the wound had self-sealed. Open globe injuries typically occur due to being struck by an object or person [15]. Bullets and other small foreign bodies projected from explosions or pressurized equipment most commonly enter the eye through the cornea, and the resulting intraocular foreign body can land in the anterior chamber, vitreous, or retina. Lacerations can also result after the dislodgement of a foreign body embedded in the cornea (such as a fishhook or piece of metal) [16]. Risk factors for sustaining corneal lacerations include male sex, age < 40 years, working in industrial settings, not wearing eye protection, and performing metal-on-metal tasks [17].

A careful history is important in all instances of corneal trauma, particularly to identify risk factors for an open globe and/or intraocular foreign body. Patients with corneal lacerations typically present with a history of trauma and are usually able to identify the characteristics of the object responsible for the injury. However, it is important to note that subtle injuries from small objects may not be recognized by the patient. Not all corneal lacerations are obvious, and all corneal trauma warrants a meticulous slit lamp examination. Eye pain, redness, decreased vision, and tearing are all common symptoms. The size, depth, and shape of the corneal laceration are best visualized on slit beam visualization of the cornea at the slit lamp. The laceration is often discrete and linear but can also be stellate or multiple. The injured layers will show a disruption of the normal corneal architecture. Corneal edema and anterior chamber inflammation is often, but not always, present.

It is important to differentiate a partial-thickness corneal laceration from a full-thickness, open globe injury. The Seidel test can be used to identify a full-thickness corneal injury by observing aqueous humor flow out from the anterior chamber [18]. This is best visualized under cobalt blue light after application of fluorescein dye. Leaking aqueous will dilute the surrounding fluorescein resulting in a dark stream flowing through green dye. Other signs of a full-thickness laceration include iris or vitreous prolapse, a flat anterior chamber, hyphema, and lens dislocation. Sometimes an embedded foreign body entering the anterior chamber can be visualized. In cases where the history and physical exam are suspicious for an open globe injury, a CT of the orbits should be obtained to assess for foreign bodies. If a patient in whom suspicion for open globe is high cannot cooperate with the exam, the patient should undergo an examination under anesthesia.

Partial-thickness corneal lacerations are typically observed and managed with topical antibiotics for infection prophylaxis. An extended wear bandage contact lens or tissue adhesives can be used for partial- or full-thickness self-sealing lacerations [19]. A full-thickness corneal laceration resulting in an open globe should be repaired in the operating room as soon as possible. The eye should be immediately covered by a protective eye shield to prevent inadvertent pressure on the globe and expulsion of intraocular contents. Intravenous antibiotics, antiemetics, pain control, and tetanus prophylaxis should be administered. Any foreign body believed to pose a risk for corneal perforation upon removal should not be removed until the patient is in the operating room.

The goal of surgery is to achieve a watertight closure with minimal corneal distortion and resulting astigmatism. Under sterile conditions, the laceration is first inspected and cleaned of any debris. Any prolapsing iris should be reposited if possible. A peritomy should be performed to evaluate for any scleral involvement. There are various suturing techniques, but most involve 10-0 interrupted sutures placed at 90% corneal depth [19, 20]. Each suture should be of equal length and depth on both sides of the laceration to prevent wound gape or overlay. Purse-string or mattress sutures may be needed for stellate corneal lacerations, and large lacerations with tissue loss may require transplantation of donor corneal tissue. The suture ends should be cut short, and the knots should be buried. Once the laceration is repaired and the globe closed, concurrent injuries such as hyphema and iris or lens injury can be addressed. Corneal sutures are typically removed 3–6 months postoperatively to allow for stable wound architecture [20].

IOFBs in the posterior segment and resulting retinal or vitreous pathology should be addressed at the same time as laceration repair if a vitreoretinal surgeon is available [21]. Organic material in the eye is associated with a high risk of endophthalmitis and should be removed without delay. Retained iron and copper should be removed to prevent metallosis. Inert substances such as glass, stone, and plastic are better tolerated, and their removal can be deferred.

The prognosis of a corneal laceration depends on its size, depth, location, and associated injuries. Wound leaks, suture abscesses, infectious keratitis, and endophthalmitis are potential complications. Small lacerations not involving the visual axis have the best outcomes. Large or central lacerations can result in decreased visual acuity secondary to central corneal scarring, and corneal transplantation may be indicated for these patients. Negative prognostic factors include a longer wound length (greater than 3.5 mm), poor initial visual acuity, and complications such as retinal detachment or endophthalmitis [22].

Acknowledgments Funding: none.

Financial Disclosures none.

References

1. Channa R, Zafar SN, Canner JK, Haring RS, Schneider EB, Friedman DS. Epidemiology of eye-related emergency department visits. JAMA Ophthalmol. 2016;134(3):312–9. https://doi.org/10.1001/JAMAOPHTHALMOL.2015.5778.
2. Puls HA, Cabrera D, Murad MH, Erwin PJ, Bellolio MF. Safety and effectiveness of topical anesthetics in corneal abrasions: systematic review and meta-analysis. J Emerg Med. 2015;49(5):816–24. https://doi.org/10.1016/J.JEMERMED.2015.02.051.
3. Patel M, Fraunfelder FW. Toxicity of topical ophthalmic anesthetics. Expert Opin Drug Metab Toxicol. 2013;9(8):983–8. https://doi.org/10.1517/17425255.2013.794219.
4. Pharmakakis NM, Katsimpris JM, Melachrinou MP, Koliopoulos JX. Corneal complications following abuse of topical anesthetics. Eur J Ophthalmol. 2002;12(5):373–8. https://doi.org/10.1177/112067210201200505.
5. Albert D, Miller J, Azar D. Recurrent corneal epithelial erosion. Albert & Jakobiec's principles and practice of ophthalmology. Philadelphia, PA: Saunders/Elsevier; 2008.
6. Miller DD, Hasan SA, Simmons NL, Stewart MW. Recurrent corneal erosion: a comprehensive review. Clin Ophthalmol. 2019;13:325–35. Published 2019 Feb 11. https://doi.org/10.2147/OPTH.S157430.
7. Watson SL, Leung V. Interventions for recurrent corneal erosions. Cochrane Database Syst Rev. 2018;7(7):CD001861. Published 2018 Jul 9. https://doi.org/10.1002/14651858.CD001861.pub4.
8. Rehany U, Rumelt S. Ocular trauma following penetrating keratoplasty: incidence, outcome, and postoperative recommendations. Arch Ophthalmol. 1998;116(10):1282–6. https://doi.org/10.1001/ARCHOPHT.116.10.1282.
9. Haddadin RI, Vora GK, Chodosh J. Corneal trauma following keratoplasty. Int Ophthalmol Clin. 2013;53(4):23–32. https://doi.org/10.1097/IIO.0B013E3182A12B3B.
10. Barut Selver Ö, Palamar M, Eğrilmez S, Yağcı A. Traumatic wound dehiscence after penetrating keratoplasty. Ulus Travma Acil Cerrahi Derg. 2016;22(5):437–40. https://doi.org/10.5505/tjtes.2016.26963.
11. Kawashima M, Kawakita T, Shimmura S, Tsubota K, Shimazaki J. Characteristics of traumatic globe rupture after keratoplasty. Ophthalmology. 2009;116(11):2072–6. https://doi.org/10.1016/J.OPHTHA.2009.04.047.
12. Pettinelli DJ, Starr CE, Stark WJ. Late traumatic corneal wound dehiscence after penetrating keratoplasty. Arch Ophthalmol. 2005;123(6):853–6. https://doi.org/10.1001/ARCHOPHT.123.6.853.
13. Feizi S, Javadi MA, Khajuee-Kermani P, Jafari R. Repeat keratoplasty for failed deep anterior lamellar keratoplasty in keratoconus: incidence, indications, and outcomes. Cornea. 2017;36(5):535–40. https://doi.org/10.1097/ICO.0000000000001169.
14. Sogutlu Sari E, Koytak A, Kubaloglu A, et al. Traumatic wound dehiscence after deep anterior lamellar keratoplasty. Am J Ophthalmol. 2013;156(4):767–772.e1. https://doi.org/10.1016/J.AJO.2013.05.014.
15. Mir TA, Canner JK, Zafar S, Srikumaran D, Friedman DS, Woreta FA. Characteristics of open globe injuries in the United States from 2006 to 2014. JAMA Ophthalmol. 2020;138(3):268–75. https://doi.org/10.1001/jamaophthalmol.2019.5823.
16. Ehlers JP, Kunimoto DY, Ittoop S, Maguire JI, Ho AC, Regillo CD. Metallic intraocular foreign bodies: characteristics, interventions, and prognostic factors for visual outcome and globe survival. Am J Ophthalmol. 2008;146(3):427–33. https://doi.org/10.1016/J.AJO.2008.05.021.
17. Hoskin AK, Low R, Sen P, Mishra C, Kamalden TA, Woreta F, Shah M, Pauly M, Rousselot A, Sundar G, Natarajan S, Keay L, Gunasekeran DV, Watson SL, Agrawal R. Epidemiology and outcomes of open globe injuries: the international globe and adnexal trauma epidemiology study (IGATES). Graefes Arch Clin Exp Ophthalmol. 2021;259(11):3485–99. https://doi.org/10.1007/s00417-021-05266-1.

18. Seidel E. Weitere experimentelle Untersuchungen über die Quelle und den Verlauf der intraokularen Saftströmung. Graefes Arhiv für Ophthalmologie. 1921;107:101–4. https://doi.org/10.1007/BF01864034.
19. Deshmukh R, Stevenson L, Vajpayee R. Management of corneal perforations: an update. Indian J Ophthalmol. 2020;68(1):7. https://doi.org/10.4103/IJO.IJO_1151_19.
20. Matalia HP, Nandini C, Matalia J. Surgical technique for the management of corneal perforation in brittle cornea. Indian J Ophthalmol. 2021;69(9):2521. https://doi.org/10.4103/IJO.IJO_2542_20.
21. Mukkamala LK, Soni N, Zarbin MA, Langer PD, Bhagat N. Posterior segment intraocular foreign bodies: a 10-year review. Ophthalmol Retina. 2017;1(4):272–7. https://doi.org/10.1016/j.oret.2017.01.007.
22. Bai HQ, Yao L, Meng XX, Wang YX, Wang DB. Visual outcome following intraocular foreign bodies: a retrospective review of 5-year clinical experience. Eur J Ophthalmol. 2011;21(1):98–103. https://doi.org/10.5301/EJO.2010.2210.

Chemical Corneal Injuries 26

Catherine Liu, Sana Qureshi, and Grayson W. Armstrong

Key Concepts

- Alkali and acidic chemical exposure can lead to serious ocular injury and result in permanent visual dysfunction.
- Prompt normalization of pH and initiation of protocolized management can maximize the chances of restoration of ocular health.
- Various medical and surgical treatment options exist to address alkali and acidic injuries of the cornea and periocular tissues.
- Topical and surgical therapies focus on control of inflammation, prevention of stromal breakdown, promotion of reepithelialization of the cornea and conjunctiva, and prevention of late complications.

26.1 Introduction

Chemical exposure to the ocular surface is an emergency requiring prompt attention, as resultant damage to superficial ocular tissues, intraocular structures, and periocular adnexa can lead to permanent visual dysfunction. Rapid normalization of pH and prompt treatment can lead to recovery of the eye, while delay or mismanagement can lead to complications including corneal clouding and neovascularization, glaucoma or hypotony, eyelid malposition, cataract formation, or disfigurement. Advances in therapeutics, surgical techniques, and an algorithmic approach to post-chemical exposure can improve patient outcomes.

C. Liu · S. Qureshi · G. W. Armstrong (✉)
Massachusetts Eye and Ear, Department of Ophthalmology, Harvard Medical School, Boston, MA, USA
e-mail: catherine_liu@meei.harvard.edu; sana_qureshi@meei.harvard.edu; grayson_armstrong@meei.harvard.edu

F. A. Woreta, R. B. Singh (eds.), *Cornea Casebook*, Current Practices in Ophthalmology, https://doi.org/10.1007/978-981-96-0495-1_26

Each year, an estimated 357,710 ophthalmic chemical burns occur worldwide, leading to an estimated 107,000 cases of resultant blindness annually [1]. These injuries often afflict males, younger populations, and patients with lower socioeconomic status and occur in the workplace, at home, or during assault [2–4]. Despite efforts to reduce the incidence of chemical-related eye injuries, such as protective glasses, these injuries still account for a substantial proportion of visual morbidity worldwide.

In this chapter, we will highlight treatment recommendations and algorithms, as well as representative patient cases that exemplify the wide range of patient outcomes that may be encountered.

26.2 Mechanism of Damage from Alkali and Acidic Injuries

Alkali and acidic chemicals each have the potential to cause severe damage to ocular and periocular structures. Alkali chemicals characteristically lead to the creation of hydroxide ions. These chemicals and ions tend to absorb through surface tissues of the eye and affect intraocular tissues more readily than acidic chemicals [5]. The hydroxide ions saponify fatty acids in cell walls and denature organic proteins, leading to loss of tissue structure and function. Corneal, conjunctival, and eyelid epithelia come into contact with alkali chemicals first, leading to frequent damage of these structures. However, the chemicals can penetrate the anterior chamber of the eye and cause damage to the iris, ciliary body, and lens [6]. The vitreous cavity has been shown to maintain its pH, though proinflammatory cytokines can lead to retinal damage [7].

Acidic chemicals, in contrast, lead to the creation of hydrogen ions that interact with and denature proteins. Direct damage to proteins upon exposure causes superficial tissue destruction and can lead to a layer of necrotic tissue [5]. This layer acts as a physical barrier, preventing further damage of underlying structures by preventing penetration of acidic chemicals into the eye.

Common alkali and acidic chemicals implicated in ocular disease are cited in Table 26.1 (adapted from Cornea, chapter "Chemical and Thermal Injuries of the Eye." Cornea, third edition, St Louis, Mo, Mosby/Elsevier, c2011).

26.3 Management of Chemical Injuries of the Eye

26.3.1 Initial Evaluation and Management

The extent and severity of injury following an acidic or alkali burn depends on several factors including concentration and pH of the solution, extent of exposure to ocular and adnexal structures, and the duration of time before treatment is initiated. Initial investigation should identify the responsible chemical agent and pH information, duration of exposure before irrigation was started, and presence or absence of

Table 26.1 Common alkali and acidic chemicals implicated in eye injuries

Alkali/ acid	Chemical	pH of 0.1 M solution	Sources/uses	Comments
Alkali	Ammonium hydroxide (NH_3)	11.1	Fertilizers, refrigerants, cleaning agents	Rapid penetration
Alkali	Sodium hydroxide (NaOH)—lye	13	Caustic soda, drain cleaner, manufacture of pulp, paper, textiles, and soaps	Rapid penetration
Alkali	Potassium hydroxide (KOH)	12	Caustic potash	Dissolution in water strongly exothermic; corrosive
Alkali	Magnesium hydroxide ($Mg[OH]_2$)	10.5	Fireworks	Combined chemical and thermal injury
Alkali	Calcium hydroxide ($Ca[OH]_2$)—lime	12.4	Cement, plaster, whitewash, industrial cleaners	Often found in composite mixtures. Poor penetration. Retained particulate matter provides sump for ongoing toxicity
Acid	Sulfuric acid (H_2SO4)	1.2	Battery acid, industrial cleaners	Diprotic acid
Acid	Sulfurous acid (H2SO3)	1.5	Fruit and vegetable preservatives, bleach, refrigerants	Good penetration
Acid	Hydrofluoric acid (HF)	2.1	Mineral refining and production, glass polishing and frosting, gasoline alkylation	Severe injury due to rapid penetration and chelation of calcium and magnesium ion
Acid	Acetic acid (CH3COOH)	2.9	Vinegar	Classified as a weak acid but corrosive in concentrated form
Acid	Hydrochloric acid (HCL)	1.1	Gastric acid, household cleaning, plastic production	Stable on storage
Acid	Chromic acid (H2CrO4)	1	Chrome plating	Diprotic acid

eye protection at the time of exposure. The presence of foreign material and debris or high velocity or explosive impact can further compound the injury.

Patients and first-line emergency medical responders should promptly irrigate the ocular surface as soon as a chemical injury is suspected. This often occurs well before an evaluation by an ophthalmologist. pH should be checked prior to initiation of irrigation if the proper tools are available; however, irrigation should never be delayed to try and evaluate pH. The goal of irrigation is to minimize the potential penetration of the chemical agent into the anterior chamber, quickly dilute the chemical, and flush away any particles or debris that can serve as a potential reservoir for ongoing injury. A chemical should never try to be neutralized with the opposite acid or base as this can cause significant worsening of the injury. In animal models, external irrigation of the ocular surface for 90 minutes can reduce the pH by 1.5 units [6]. Outside of a medical facility, any neutral irrigation fluid such as clean water can be used to flush the eye. In a hospital setting, either lactated Ringer's or normal saline with or without the assistance of a Morgan lens can be used. The Morgan lens is a sterile plastic device consisting of a contact lens connected to tubing that fits over the eye and allows for copious and continuous irrigation of the eye. Once inserted, the Morgan lens floats on the irrigating solution without directly touching the corneal or conjunctival surfaces. The pH can be rechecked after 2–3 L of fluid has been used to flush the eye. In some cases, more than 10–15 L may be needed to achieve a neutral pH.

When possible, the eyelids should be everted in order to evaluate for retained foreign bodies or particulate matter. All particles should be removed with either a cotton-tipped applicator or carefully with jeweler forceps as their presence may continue to cause ocular damage. Notably, the Morgan lens can sometimes hold foreign substances against the eye, which can lead to persistent pH abnormalities despite irrigation.

26.3.2 Ophthalmic Evaluation

After irrigation has taken place, a thorough ophthalmic examination of both eyes including dilated fundus exam should be performed to determine the extent of injury. Careful assessment for the degree of damage to the corneal epithelium, conjunctiva and sclera, and lid margins should be recorded. The Dua classification can be used to prognosticate outcomes based on the proportion of ocular tissue damaged [8].

26.3.3 Control of Inflammation

Topical corticosteroids have a central role in the management of ophthalmic chemical injuries. Animal studies have shown that treatment with topical or subconjunctival corticosteroids results in less corneal opacity, neovascularization, and inflammation in chemical injuries [9, 10]. Some controversy exists as to the timing and duration of corticosteroid use, as steroids have the advantageous effect of inflammation and collagenase activity suppression, though they have the disadvantage of suppression of keratocyte migration and collagen production which can lead to corneal thinning. In experimental models, the use of steroids in the first 10 days post-injury does not appear to have an adverse effect on outcomes or lead to sterile thinning of the cornea. Steroids should therefore be instituted rapidly and frequently and tapered after the first 7–10 days to prevent inhibition of wound healing. For additional anti-inflammatory treatment needed past 10–15 days, a topical progesterone steroid, such as medroxyprogesterone 1%, can be used to minimize adverse effects.

26.3.4 Prevention of Stromal Breakdown

Tetracycline antibiotics have been shown to be effective in reducing collagenase activity in experimental models of alkali injuries. Collagenases are enzymes involved in the breakdown of collagen, which accounts for 70% of the corneal total dry weight. Animal studies have shown slightly improved healing times and less corneal neovascularization in groups treated with doxycycline compared with controls. While data shows the effectiveness of tetracyclines in promoting healing of the cornea, additional studies are needed to confirm efficacy in humans. A dose of 100 mg of doxycycline BID is recommended as initial treatment in patients with ocular burns, though tetracyclines should be avoided in patients who are pregnant and under the age of 8.

Vitamin C (ascorbic acid) plays a critical role in the maintenance and production of a normal mature collagen. Vitamin C is a cofactor for prolyl hydroxylase and lysyl hydroxylase, enzymes that promote proper collagen protein folding [11, 12]. Vitamin C is also a powerful antioxidant that neutralizes reactive oxygen species [13]. The concentration of ascorbic acid is about 15–20 times greater in the aqueous humor of the eye than in plasma and is hypothesized to play an important role in wound healing after chemical injury to the ocular surface as its concentration in the aqueous humor has been found to fall to one-third of its normal level after alkali burn [14, 15]. Vitamin C can be administered orally or topically and may be more efficacious topically in severe chemical injuries where ciliary body dysfunction may lead to decreased penetration of systemic ascorbic acid into the eye [16, 17].

26.3.5 Promotion of Reepithelialization

Reepithelialization is key to prevent infection and corneal scarring. Bandage contact lenses can be used to promote reepithelialization of corneal defects and improve patient comfort in the acute period. These can include commercial contact lenses with low prescriptions, such as Acuvue Oasys or Air Optix Night and Day. Larger lenses, such as Kontur lenses, can be used as well but may be more uncomfortable due to the larger diameter. Patients should be educated on contact lens hygiene, placed on topical antibiotics, and evaluated at regular intervals to reduce the possibility of corneal ulceration or infection.

Amniotic membrane transplantation (AMT) can be used as an early and immediate surgical procedure to reduce pain and discomfort while promoting more rapid healing [18]. AMT provides a basement membrane which serves as a scaffold for epithelial cell regrowth and also contains growth factors including epidermal growth factor and keratocyte growth factor [19]. AMT also reduces inflammation and scarring by downregulating transforming growth factor-β signal transduction and the production of proinflammatory cytokines [19–21]. ProKera (Bio-Tissue, Inc.) is a biological corneal bandage that contains amniotic membrane fit between clear flexible plastic rings which has demonstrated success in the treatment of chemical injuries of the cornea [22]. The presence of the plastic ring in the forniceal spaces may also help to reduce symblepharon formation in patients with conjunctival injury. AmbioDisk is a processed dehydrated amniotic membrane graft containing extracellular matrix proteins and growth factors that will self-adhere to corneal epithelial defects, though it is often secured in place with a bandage contact lens. In cases of severe corneal thinning, multilayered AMT is an appropriate management technique [23].

Chemical burns can also damage the conjunctiva and mucus-producing goblet cells, which can lead to acute and chronic dry eye. The use of preservative-free artificial tears, gels, or ointments should be implemented early and used frequently to provide adequate ocular lubrication. Temporary or permanent punctal occlusion can also supplement the usage of topical lubrication and improve ocular surface wetting.

Topical antibiotics have been used for antimicrobial prophylaxis in the setting of epithelial defects. The choice of antibiotic should take into consideration the risk of microbial contamination with the mechanism of injury as well as the potential for preservative-induced epithelial toxicity. Commonly used antibiotics include trimethoprim/polymyxin and moxifloxacin, the latter being a non-preserved option. In the setting of microbial keratitis or a contaminated wound, fortified antibiotics may be required.

26.3.6 Pain Control

Topical cycloplegic agents promote ciliary body relaxation and can help reduce pain while also minimizing the formation of posterior synechiae. In milder injuries, cyclopentolate can be used, while longer-acting atropine sulfate may be preferred in more severe injuries. Phenylephrine and other adrenergic drugs should be avoided as much as possible, as these cause vasoconstriction and worsened limbal ischemia in severe injuries.

26.4 Acute Surgical Interventions

Surgical management following an acute chemical injury starts with the initial debridement of any necrotic material. In cases of impending perforation, descemetocele, or true corneal perforation, tissue glue may be used to preserve the integrity of the globe [24]. Tissue adhesives also help to decrease risk of further corneal melting and microbial keratitis as it decreases inflammation and has antimicrobial properties [25, 26]. Tissue glue with or without AMT, and with or without a bandage contact lens, can be used successfully for small to medium perforations (1–3 mm) [24, 27]. In larger perforations, a tectonic graft or a penetrating keratoplasty (PKP) may be required, though transplants have a high risk of failure and graft rejection in the acute phase of injury [28, 29].

26.5 Long-Term Management: Reconstruction of Fornices and Adnexa

Severe ocular burns can also damage adnexal structures, causing tear gland destruction and dysfunction, cicatricial lid changes, symblepharon, and scarring. In cases of symblepharon formation, early and mild stages may be amenable to lysis and/or treatment with AMT, whereas severe disease may necessitate oral mucous membrane transplantation [30–32]. Interdisciplinary surgical management may be required for eyelid and forniceal reconstruction, especially prior to limbal stem cell or corneal transplantation to maximize chances of graft survival. Ocular exposure can be treated with temporary or permanent tarsorrhaphy, while more complex lid procedures may be needed to correct entropion or ectropion.

26.6 Long-Term Management: Limbal Stem Cell Deficiency

Limbal stem cell deficiency (LSCD) resulting from chemical injury can result in persistent or recurrent epithelial defects, chronic stromal inflammation, corneal conjunctivalization and neovascularization, and scarring. Fortunately, there are multiple limbal stem call transplant (LSCT) techniques available.

In cases of unilateral injury where the contralateral eye is healthy, successful reconstruction can be achieved with a conjunctival limbal autograft (CLAU) [33]. The procedure typically involves the removal of two large free grafts spanning 60 degrees from the healthy eye, though smaller grafts have also shown success [34, 35]. An autologous source leads to a decreased risk of rejection, with CLAU survival rates of 76% and 62% at 3 and 6 years, respectively [36]. Ex vivo cultured limbal epithelial transplantation (CLET), using smaller amounts of donor limbal epithelium co-cultured with 3T3 fibroblasts, has demonstrated success rates up to 76% [37]. However, CLET is limited by high cost, the need for manufacturing clean-room facilities, and complex surgical and laboratory techniques and is presently not FDA approved.

Yet another procedure, simple limbal epithelial transplant (SLET), uses small amounts of autologous donor limbal epithelium to treat LCSD [38]. This technique dissects a 2 × 2 mm limbal biopsy into many small pieces which are evenly distributed over an amniotic membrane affixed to the ocular surface with fibrin glue [38]. In a large case series, 76% of patients undergoing SLET maintained a positive outcome, with 67% of patients attaining vision of 20/60 or better [39].

In cases of bilateral injury, allograft procedures can be utilized [40–42]. Allografts carry a lifetime risk of rejection and require systemic immunosuppression [43]. To circumvent the risk of allograft rejection and need for systemic immunosuppression, the cultivated oral mucosal epithelial transplantation (COMET) can be used to stabilize the ocular surface with demonstrated improvement in visual acuity in 53% of eyes at 36 months in one study [44, 45].

26.7 Long-Term Management: Keratoplasty and Keratoprosthesis

In patients with significant stromal scarring or large perforation corneal transplantation, either PKP or deep anterior lamellar keratoplasty (DALK) should be considered. The status of the cornea as well as the adjacent limbus should be taken into consideration when deciding on treatment modality. Larger-diameter grafts carry the advantage of transplanting donor corneal limbal stem cells as well as the disadvantage of higher risk of rejection. Smaller grafts performed after or concomitantly with LSCT have a higher likelihood of survival [46, 47]. Keratoplasty should be delayed at least 3 months after limbal stem cell surgery.

Traditionally, keratoprosthesis surgery was reserved for patients with multiple failed PKPs as a last resort for visual rehabilitation. Innovations in the design and surgical technique of this device have increased its clinical relevance. The Boston keratoprosthesis (KPro) type 1 is the more commonly used keratoprosthesis but is limited by the need for a well-lubricated surface with normal fornices. The Boston KPro type 2 can be used in patients with severe dryness and keratinization and is used for visual rehabilitation in end-stage disease. Complications of keratoprosthesis include infection, corneal melt, glaucoma, retinal detachment, and retroprosthetic membrane.

26.8 Alkali Cases

26.8.1 Case 1: Mild Alkali Injury—Corneal Involvement (Single Epithelial Defect)

A 54-year-old female was cleaning a table at work when bleach solution splashed in her face and eyes. She was brought to a local emergency room and evaluated within the hour following the incident. The pH was measured to be 7.0 in the right eye and 8.0 in the left eye. Morgan lenses were used and the eyes irrigated with lactated Ringer's solution. After 4 L of irrigation, the pH improved to 7.0 in both eyes. The patient was subsequently transferred to Massachusetts Eye and Ear (MEE).

At MEE, the patient noted her pain level at 10/10 with photophobia. Visual acuity was 20/80 in the right eye (OD) and 20/125 in the left (OS). The pH was 7.2 in the upper and lower fornices of the right eye and 7.6 in the upper and lower fornices of the left eye. Additional irrigation was performed using 1 L of normal saline solution on the right and 2 L on the left. After irrigation, the pH was normalized to 7.0 in both eyes. On slit lamp examination, there were diffuse peripheral punctate erosions on the right eye and a left-sided 5 mm × 2 mm corneal epithelial defect. There was no conjunctival staining and no limbal whitening.

For initial management, a drop of atropine was instilled in both eyes in the emergency department. The patient was instructed to start trimethoprim/polymyxin drops QID, prednisolone acetate 1% q1h while awake, and preservative-free artificial tears as needed in both eyes. Doxycycline 100 mg PO daily and vitamin C 1 g by mouth BID were also started. On follow-up with the cornea service 2 days later, the left-sided corneal epithelial defect had near-complete resolution. The patient was instructed to continue trimethoprim/polymyxin drops QID and to decrease prednisolone to QID for 5 more days and then stop. Two months later, the patient was feeling much better. The patient's best corrected visual acuity returned to 20/20 in both eyes, and the corneal epithelial defect had completely healed with no significant sequelae.

26.8.2 Case 2: Moderate-Severe Alkali Injury—Corneal and Conjunctival Involvement (Multiple Epithelial Defects)

A 75-year-old male presented following exposure to a household drainage cleaner containing sodium hypochlorite (bleach) and sodium hydroxide (lye). The eyes had been immediately rinsed at home and then irrigated at a community hospital with 3 L of normal saline solution. The reported pH by the outside institution was 7.0 OU after irrigation. Upon transfer to the MEE, the pH of bilateral upper and lower fornices were measured to be elevated at 8.0. An additional 2 L of irrigation was performed, and the pH normalized to 7.0 in both eyes.

On examination, visual acuity was 20/60 OD and 20/25 OS. Total corneal epithelial defects were noted bilaterally, with extensive bulbar and palpebral conjunctival staining on the right side and inferior bulbar conjunctival staining on the left side. There was 360 degrees of limbal whitening on the right and inferior limbal whitening on the left. ProKera corneal bandages were placed in both eyes. In addition, a drop of atropine was instilled in both eyes, and trimethoprim/polymyxin drops QID, prednisolone acetate 1% q1h while awake, and preservative-free artificial tears as needed were initiated in both eyes. Doxycycline 100 mg PO daily and vitamin C 1 gram by mouth BID were also started.

The patient was followed up the next day and subsequently every 2 days by the cornea service. The measurements of intraocular pressure (IOP) were noted to be within normal limits. Of note, 4 days after the initial injury, the cornea attending felt the limbal whitening to be minimal in both eyes (Fig. 26.1). Prednisolone was tapered to 6×/day at day 4 and then to QID at day 12 from injury. The ProKera was replaced every 4–5 days upon dissolution of the amniotic membrane until complete healing of the corneal epithelial defect was achieved. Tobramycin and dexamethasone ointment BID was added to address right eyelid margin and tarsal conjunctiva staining. No symblepharon or membranes were noted on follow-up. The patient was eventually followed up by a local cornea specialist in his home state.

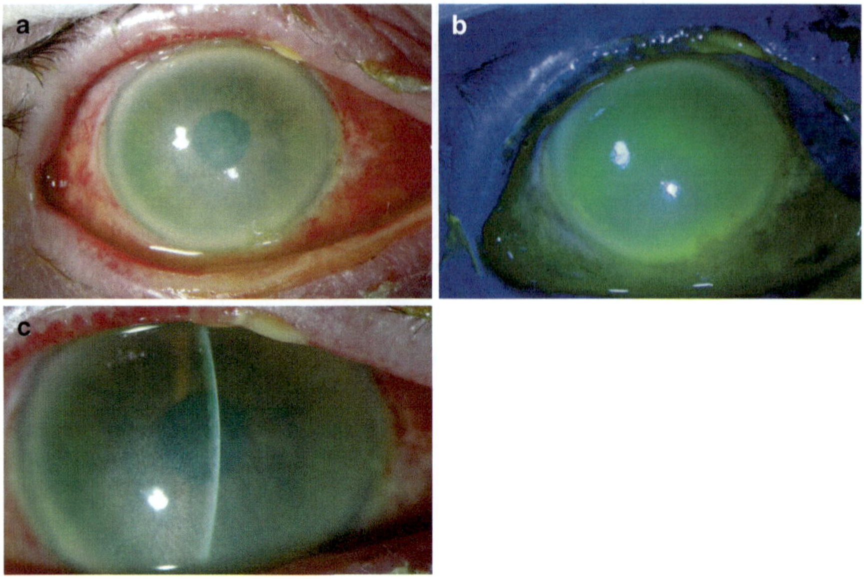

Fig. 26.1 (**a**) Complete epithelial defect, diffuse conjunctival epithelial defect, and lid margin involvement in the right eye. (**b**) Complete epithelial defect, diffuse bulbar conjunctival epithelial defect, and lid margin involvement in the right eye. (**c**) Corneal subepithelial haze in the right eye

26.8.3 Case 3: Severe Alkali Injury—Corneal and Conjunctival Involvement (Stromal Opacification, Epithelial Defect) and Elevated IOP

A 60-year-old man had sodium hydroxide (lye) sprayed into his left eye while working in the kitchen. After rinsing his eye for 10 min, he presented to the MEE emergency department. He described 10/10 pain in his left eye. On presentation, the pH of his left upper and lower fornices were noted to be 8.0, normalizing to 7.0 after greater than 5 L of normal saline solution irrigation.

The patient's visual acuity was decreased to counting fingers at 6 feet OS, with an IOP of 43.2. On examination, he had a total corneal epithelial defect, with diffuse stromal haze obscuring iris details (Fig. 26.2). Limbal whitening was noted temporally from 3 to 5 o'clock and nasally from 9 to 10 o'clock. His conjunctiva was diffusely chemotic and injected, with diffuse staining of his inferior palpebral conjunctiva. His elevated IOP was addressed initially with several rounds of IOP-lowering medications including brimonidine, dorzolamide/timolol, and latanoprost. After several rounds of topical medication, oral acetazolamide was added, and the IOP was eventually lowered to 35. A ProKera corneal bandage was placed. A drop of atropine was instilled in both eyes, and trimethoprim/polymyxin drops QID, prednisolone acetate 1% q1h while awake, and preservative-free artificial tears as needed were initiated in both eyes. Doxycycline 100 mg PO daily and vitamin C 1 g by mouth BID were also started.

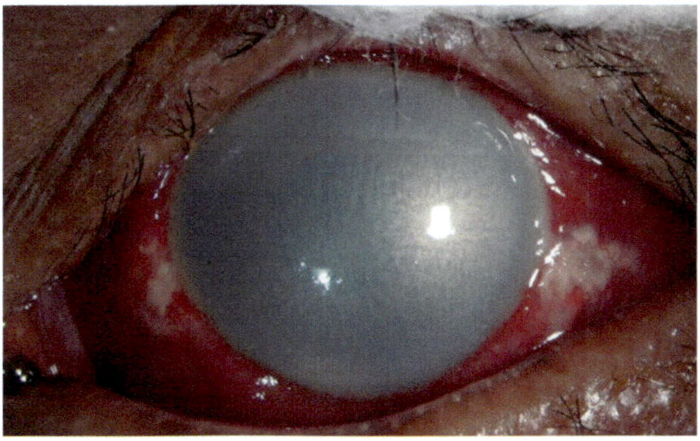

Fig. 26.2 Total corneal epithelial defect, with diffuse stromal haze obscuring iris details (2 weeks after injury)

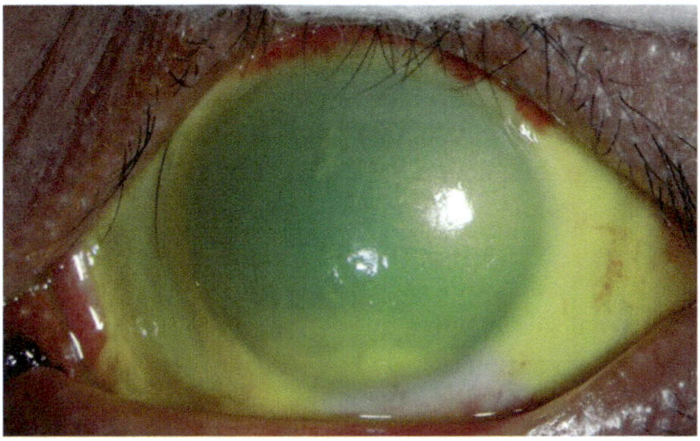

Fig. 26.3 Extensive perilimbal ischemia (1 month after injury)

The patient was closely followed by the cornea service. At 1 month after initial injury, the patient's visual acuity only marginally improved to 20/300. His examination was remarkable for a persistent total corneal epithelial defect, severe diffuse stromal haze, and limbal ischemia (Fig. 26.3). His corneal surface did not reepithelialize despite the use of multiple ProKera bandages, though his IOP improved to 22 on maximal topical therapy. After discussion, the patient agreed to proceed with an ocular surface reconstruction.

In the operating room, ischemic conjunctiva was dissected away. A 10 cm × 5 cm sheet of cryopreserved amniotic membrane was used to cover the entire area of ischemia and secured into place using fibrin glue. A Kontur bandage contact lens (DIA 16.0/BC 8.0) was placed over the membrane, followed by a 22 mm symblepharon ring. One week later, the patient was noted to have a small amount of corneal epithelialization and neovascularization inferiorly, which continued to progress on subsequent visits (Fig. 26.4). Serum tears were added to his treatment regimen. Unfortunately, his visual acuity remained poor due to the opacified stroma.

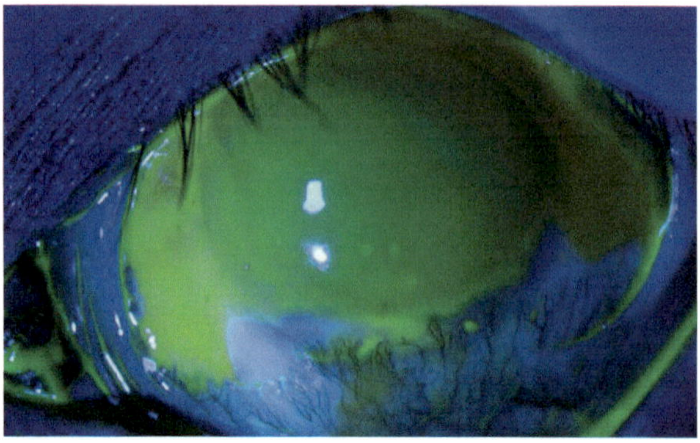

Fig. 26.4 Corneal epithelialization and neovascularization (2 months after ocular surface reconstruction/AMT placement)

26.9 Acidic Cases

A 42-year-old female mistakenly instilled toenail antifungal medication containing of 1% terbinafine and 0.1% glycyrrhetinic acid in her eye thinking it was an artificial tear. Immediately after installation, the patient began experiencing significant pain and proceeded to flush the eye for several minutes. Upon presentation to the emergency department, pH was noted to be 6.8 and the eye was irrigated with 2 L of normal saline with a return to pH of 7. On exam, visual acuity was 20/25, and slit lamp examination revealed a conjunctival defect from 3 o'clock to 7 o'clock extending from the limbus to the inferior fornix, as well as a 6 mm × 3 mm corneal epithelial defect with areas of overlying necrotic epithelium. The fornices were swept, and whitish material along the upper tarsal conjunctiva was noted and easily removed with a cotton swab without creating a conjunctival defect. No limbal or corneal whitening was noted. A ProKera was placed on the right eye, and the patient was started on moxifloxacin QID, prednisolone acetate q1h, atropine daily, doxycycline 50 mg daily, and vitamin C 1000 mg BID. The following day, the patient was seen in the cornea clinic where the ProKera was removed and necrotic corneal epithelium was debrided. No membranes or symblepharon was noted, and the ProKera was replaced. Doxycycline was discontinued due to nausea and vomiting. On day 6, the ProKera was removed and the conjunctiva and corneal epithelium was healed, with trace stromal haze noted in the temporal cornea. Atropine was stopped, moxifloxacin was planned to be discontinued 3 days later, vitamin C was continued, and prednisolone acetate was tapered weekly at a rate of 6–4–3–2–1–0 drops daily. The patient completed her subsequent follow-ups at an outside institution.

26.10 Conclusion

Exposure of the ocular surface to alkali and acidic chemicals has the potential for poor clinical outcomes. These cases highlight the varying severity of clinical pathology and the different treatment approaches that can be instituted.

Prompt normalization of pH, identification and removal of foreign bodies, and institution of proper medical and surgical therapies can improve the changes of visual recovery.

References

1. White ML, Chodosh J, Jang J, Dohlman C. Incidence of Stevens-Johnson syndrome and chemical burns to the eye. Cornea. 2015;34(12):1527–33. https://doi.org/10.1097/ICO.0000000000000646.
2. Hong J, Qiu T, Wei A, Sun X, Xu J. Clinical characteristics and visual outcome of severe ocular chemical injuries in Shanghai. Ophthalmology. 2010;117(12):2268–72. https://doi.org/10.1016/j.ophtha.2010.03.050.
3. Haring RS, Sheffield ID, Channa R, Canner JK, Schneider EB. Epidemiologic trends of chemical ocular burns in the United States [published correction appears in JAMA Ophthalmol. 2017;135(4):404]. JAMA Ophthalmol. 2016;134(10):1119–24. https://doi.org/10.1001/jamaophthalmol.2016.2645.
4. Morgan SJ. Chemical burns of the eye: causes and management. Br J Ophthalmol. 1987;71(11):854–7. https://doi.org/10.1136/bjo.71.11.854.
5. Wagoner MD. Chemical injuries of the eye: current concepts in pathophysiology and therapy. Surv Ophthalmol. 1997;41(4):275–313. https://doi.org/10.1016/s0039-6257(96)00007-0.
6. Paterson CA, Pfister RR, Levinson RA. Aqueous humor pH changes after experimental alkali burns. Am J Ophthalmol. 1975;79(3):414–9. https://doi.org/10.1016/0002-9394(75)90614-5.
7. Paschalis EI, Zhou C, Lei F, et al. Mechanisms of retinal damage after ocular alkali burns. Am J Pathol. 2017;187(6):1327–42. https://doi.org/10.1016/j.ajpath.2017.02.005.
8. Dua HS, King AJ, Joseph A. A new classification of ocular surface burns. Br J Ophthalmol. 2001;85(11):1379–83. https://doi.org/10.1136/bjo.85.11.1379.
9. Donshik PC, Berman MB, Dohlman CH, Gage J, Rose J. Effect of topical corticosteroids on ulceration in alkali-burned corneas. Arch Ophthalmol. 1978;96(11):2117–20. https://doi.org/10.1001/archopht.1978.03910060497024.
10. Saud EE, Moraes HV Jr, Marculino LG, Gomes JA, Allodi S, Miguel NC. Clinical and histopathological outcomes of subconjunctival triamcinolone injection for the treatment of acute ocular alkali burn in rabbits. Cornea. 2012;31(2):181–7. https://doi.org/10.1097/ICO.0b013e318221ce99.
11. Manela-Azulay M, Bagatin E. Cosmeceuticals vitamins. Clin Dermatol. 2009;27(5):469–74. https://doi.org/10.1016/j.clindermatol.2009.05.010.
12. Phillips CL, Combs SB, Pinnell SR. Effects of ascorbic acid on proliferation and collagen synthesis in relation to the donor age of human dermal fibroblasts. J Invest Dermatol. 1994;103(2):228–32. https://doi.org/10.1111/1523-1747.ep12393187.
13. Kaźmierczak-Barańska J, Boguszewska K, Adamus-Grabicka A, Karwowski BT. Two faces of vitamin C-antioxidative and pro-oxidative agent. Nutrients. 2020;12(5):1501. Published 2020 May 21. https://doi.org/10.3390/nu12051501.
14. Hah YS, Chung HJ, Sontakke SB, et al. Ascorbic acid concentrations in aqueous humor after systemic vitamin C supplementation in patients with cataract: pilot study. BMC Ophthalmol. 2017;17(1):121. Published 2017 Jul 11. https://doi.org/10.1186/s12886-017-0515-2.
15. Li M, Chen Z, Liu L, Ma X, Zou J. Topical vitamin C promotes the recovery of corneal alkali burns in mice. J Ophthalmol. 2021;2021:2406646. Published 2021 Dec 23. https://doi.org/10.1155/2021/2406646.
16. Pfister RR, Paterson CA, Spiers JW, Hayes SA. The efficacy of ascorbate treatment after severe experimental alkali burns depends upon the route of administration. Invest Ophthalmol Vis Sci. 1980;19(12):1526–9.

17. Al-Namaeh M, Andersson R. Effects of ascorbic acid on chemical and thermal corneal burns: a comprehensive literature review. Med Hypothesis Discov Innov Optom. 2020;1(2):44–51.
18. Tandon R, Gupta N, Kalaivani M, Sharma N, Titiyal JS, Vajpayee RB. Amniotic membrane transplantation as an adjunct to medical therapy in acute ocular burns. Br J Ophthalmol. 2011;95(2):199–204. https://doi.org/10.1136/bjo.2009.173716. Epub 2010 Jul 31
19. Kim JS, Kim JC, Na BK, Jeong JM, Song CY. Amniotic membrane patching promotes healing and inhibits proteinase activity on wound healing following acute corneal alkali burn. Exp Eye Res. 2000;70(3):329–37. https://doi.org/10.1006/exer.1999.0794.
20. Fish R, Davidson RS. Management of ocular thermal and chemical injuries, including amniotic membrane therapy. Curr Opin Ophthalmol. 2010;21(4):317–21. https://doi.org/10.1097/ICU.0b013e32833a8da2.
21. Shimmura S, Shimazaki J, Ohashi Y, Tsubota K. Anti-inflammatory effects of amniotic membrane transplantation in ocular surface disorders. Cornea. 2001;20(4):408–13. https://doi.org/10.1097/00003226-200105000-00015.
22. Suri K, Kosker M, Raber IM, Hammersmith KM, Nagra PK, Ayres BD, Halfpenny CP, Rapuano CJ. Sutureless amniotic membrane ProKera for ocular surface disorders: short-term results. Eye Contact Lens. 2013;39(5):341–7. https://doi.org/10.1097/ICL.0b013e3182a2f8fa.
23. Hanada K, Shimazaki J, Shimmura S, Tsubota K. Multilayered amniotic membrane transplantation for severe ulceration of the cornea and sclera. Am J Ophthalmol. 2001;131(3):324–31. https://doi.org/10.1016/s0002-9394(00)00825-4.
24. Yin J, Singh RB, Al Karmi R, Yung A, Yu M, Dana R. Outcomes of cyanoacrylate tissue adhesive application in corneal thinning and perforation. Cornea. 2019;38(6):668–73. https://doi.org/10.1097/ICO.0000000000001919.
25. Eiferman RA, Snyder JW. Antibacterial effect of cyanoacrylate glue. Arch Ophthalmol. 1983;101(6):958–60. https://doi.org/10.1001/archopht.1983.01040010958022.
26. Sharma A, Sharma N, Basu S, Sharma R, Aggarwal S, Gupta PC, Ram J, Nirankari VS. Tissue adhesives for the Management of Corneal Perforations and Challenging Corneal Conditions. Clin Ophthalmol. 2023;17:209–23. https://doi.org/10.2147/OPTH.S394454. PMID: 36685088; PMCID: PMC9851054
27. Kara S, Arikan S, Ersan I, Taskiran CA. Simplified technique for sealing corneal perforations using a fibrin glue-assisted amniotic membrane transplant-plug. Case Rep Ophthalmol Med. 2014;2014:351534. https://doi.org/10.1155/2014/351534. Epub 2014 Jun 18. PMID: 25045563; PMCID: PMC4087251
28. Vanathi M, Sharma N, Titiyal JS, Tandon R, Vajpayee RB. Tectonic grafts for corneal thinning and perforations. Cornea. 2002;21(8):792–7. https://doi.org/10.1097/00003226-200211000-00013.
29. Sharma N, Kaur M, Agarwal T, Sangwan VS, Vajpayee RB. Treatment of acute ocular chemical burns. Surv Ophthalmol. 2018;63(2):214–35. https://doi.org/10.1016/j.survophthal.2017.09.005. Epub 2017 Sep 19
30. Kheirkhah A, Ghaffari R, Kaghazkanani R, Hashemi H, Behrouz MJ, Raju VK. A combined approach of amniotic membrane and oral mucosa transplantation for fornix reconstruction in severe symblepharon. Cornea. 2013;32(2):155–60. https://doi.org/10.1097/ICO.0b013e318247983d.
31. Martinez-Osorio H, Schellini SA, Marin-Muñoz LS. Long-term follow up of oral mucosa autograft sutured to the sclera in severe symblepharon. Am J Ophthalmol Case Rep. 2021;23:101099. Published 2021 May 25. https://doi.org/10.1016/j.ajoc.2021.101099.
32. Kate A, Doctor MB, Shanbhag SS. Management of Symblepharon Prior to Keratoprosthesis in chronic ocular burns: a sequential approach. Cureus. 2022;14(4):e24611. Published 2022 Apr 29. https://doi.org/10.7759/cureus.24611.
33. Kenyon KR, Tseng SC. Limbal autograft transplantation for ocular surface disorders. Ophthalmology. 1989;96(5):709–23. https://doi.org/10.1016/s0161-6420(89)32833-8.
34. Holland EJ, Schwartz GS. The evolution of epithelial transplantation for severe ocular surface disease and a proposed classification system. Cornea. 1996;15(6):549–56.

35. Kheirkhah A, Raju VK, Tseng SC. Minimal conjunctival limbal autograft for total limbal stem cell deficiency. Cornea. 2008;27(6):730–3. https://doi.org/10.1097/QAI.0b013e31815cea8b.
36. Wylegala E, Dobrowolski D, Tarnawska D, et al. Limbal stem cells transplantation in the reconstruction of the ocular surface: 6 years experience. Eur J Ophthalmol. 2008;18(6):886–90. https://doi.org/10.1177/112067210801800605.
37. Baylis O, Figueiredo F, Henein C, Lako M, Ahmad S. 13 years of cultured limbal epithelial cell therapy: a review of the outcomes. J Cell Biochem. 2011;112(4):993–1002. https://doi.org/10.1002/jcb.23028.
38. Sangwan VS, Basu S, MacNeil S, Balasubramanian D. Simple limbal epithelial transplantation (SLET): a novel surgical technique for the treatment of unilateral limbal stem cell deficiency. Br J Ophthalmol. 2012;96(7):931–4. https://doi.org/10.1136/bjophthalmol-2011-301164.
39. Basu S, Sureka SP, Shanbhag SS, Kethiri AR, Singh V, Sangwan VS. Simple Limbal epithelial transplantation: long-term clinical outcomes in 125 cases of unilateral chronic ocular surface burns. Ophthalmology. 2016;123(5):1000–10. https://doi.org/10.1016/j.ophtha.2015.12.042.
40. Bhalekar S, Basu S, Sangwan VS. Successful management of immunological rejection following allogeneic simple limbal epithelial transplantation (SLET) for bilateral ocular burns. BMJ Case Rep. 2013;2013:bcr2013009051. Published 2013 Mar 14. https://doi.org/10.1136/bcr-2013-009051.
41. Daya SM, Ilari FA. Living related conjunctival limbal allograft for the treatment of stem cell deficiency. Ophthalmology. 2001;108(1):126–34. https://doi.org/10.1016/s0161-6420(00)00475-9.
42. Tsai RJ, Tseng SC. Human allograft limbal transplantation for corneal surface reconstruction. Cornea. 1994;13(5):389–400. https://doi.org/10.1097/00003226-199409000-00003.
43. Yin J, Jurkunas U. Limbal stem cell transplantation and complications. Semin Ophthalmol. 2018;33(1):134–41. https://doi.org/10.1080/08820538.2017.1353834.
44. Nakamura T, Endo K, Cooper LJ, et al. The successful culture and autologous transplantation of rabbit oral mucosal epithelial cells on amniotic membrane. Invest Ophthalmol Vis Sci. 2003;44(1):106–16. https://doi.org/10.1167/iovs.02-0195.
45. Nakamura T, Takeda K, Inatomi T, Sotozono C, Kinoshita S. Long-term results of autologous cultivated oral mucosal epithelial transplantation in the scar phase of severe ocular surface disorders. Br J Ophthalmol. 2011;95(7):942–6. https://doi.org/10.1136/bjo.2010.188714.
46. Shi W, Gao H, Wang T, Xie L. Combined penetrating keratoplasty and keratolimbal allograft transplantation in comparison with corneoscleral transplantation in the treatment of severe eye burns. Clin Experiment Ophthalmol. 2008;36(6):501–7. https://doi.org/10.1111/j.1442-9071.2008.01802.x.
47. Basu S, Mohamed A, Chaurasia S, Sejpal K, Vemuganti GK, Sangwan VS. Clinical outcomes of penetrating keratoplasty after autologous cultivated limbal epithelial transplantation for ocular surface burns. Am J Ophthalmol. 2011;152(6):917–924.e1. https://doi.org/10.1016/j.ajo.2011.05.019.

Pediatric Cornea Cases

27

Abdelrahman M. Elhusseiny, Hajirah N. Saeed, and Aisha S. Traish

27.1 Case 1

27.1.1 Key Points

- Dupilumab is an effective biologic agent in the management of atopic conditions such as eczema.
- Several ocular manifestations such as conjunctivitis and keratitis have been associated with its use.
- Ocular adverse events range in severity from mild conjunctivitis to severe cicatrization, limbal stem cell deficiency, and uveitis.
- Regular ophthalmic examination is necessary before and after the start of dupilumab for early detection and proper management of the ophthalmic manifestations, which may be challenging.

A. M. Elhusseiny
Department of Ophthalmology, Harvey and Bernice Jones Eye Institute, University of Arkansas for Medical Sciences, Little Rock, AR, USA

Department of Ophthalmology, Boston Children's Hospital, Harvard Medical School, Boston, MA, USA

H. N. Saeed
Department of Ophthalmology, Illinois Eye and Ear Infirmary, University of Illinois at Chicago, Chicago, IL, USA

A. S. Traish (✉)
Department of Ophthalmology, Boston Children's Hospital, Harvard Medical School, Boston, MA, USA

Department of Ophthalmology, Massachusetts Eye and Ear Infirmary, Harvard Medical School, Boston, MA, USA
e-mail: Aisha_Traish@meei.harvard.edu

F. A. Woreta, R. B. Singh (eds.), *Cornea Casebook*, Current Practices in Ophthalmology, https://doi.org/10.1007/978-981-96-0495-1_27

27.1.2 Case Presentation

A 17-year-old boy with a past medical history of Tourette's syndrome, depression, and atopic dermatitis presented with redness, crusting, mild itching, and irritation of both eyes (OU) 10 months after the initiation of dupilumab (Dupixent®, Regeneron Pharmaceuticals, Inc., NY, and Sanofi-Aventis US, NJ, USA) for treatment of atopic dermatitis. He had a past ocular history of keratoconus OU for which he had undergone corneal collagen cross-linking OU 2 years earlier. His best corrected visual acuity (BCVA) with spectacles was 20/30 in the right eye (OD) and left eye (OS). Slit lamp examination demonstrated 2+ conjunctival injection and large papillae of the palpebral conjunctiva in both eyes. The corneal evaluation showed 1+ superficial punctate keratopathy (SPK) OD and a clear cornea OS. He was diagnosed with dupilumab-associated conjunctivitis and was started on topical fluorometholone (FML) three times daily (TID) with gradual tapering over 3 weeks, topical olopatadine hydrochloride 0.1% twice daily (BID) (which he did not end up using), and artificial tears (ATs). Six weeks later, conjunctival and corneal signs improved but were not completely resolved, and a small reactive inferior fornix conjunctival lesion was noted in the left eye (Fig. 27.1). The patient was switched to a stronger topical steroid (prednisolone acetate 1% BID) and encouraged to start olopatadine 0.7% once daily and continue ATs. One month later, conjunctival inflammation had resolved, and the patient had rare corneal SPKs; however, he developed bilateral temporal palpebral conjunctival lesions (Fig. 27.2). The tapering of topical steroids resulted in recurrent inflammation. Topical cyclosporine 0.05% (Restasis®, Allergan Inc., Irvine, CA, USA) BID was added to the treatment for steroid-sparing effect, and he was switched back to topical loteprednol etabonate once daily for reduced steroid potency. At the last follow-up 5 months later, BCVA was 20/20 OD and OS, and ocular examination demonstrated trace conjunctival injection with few SPKs and slowly resolving conjunctival lesions.

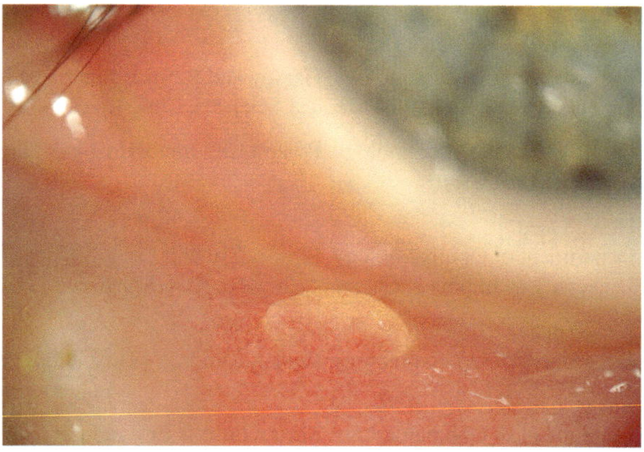

Fig. 27.1 External photograph with palpebral conjunctival injection and reactive lesion

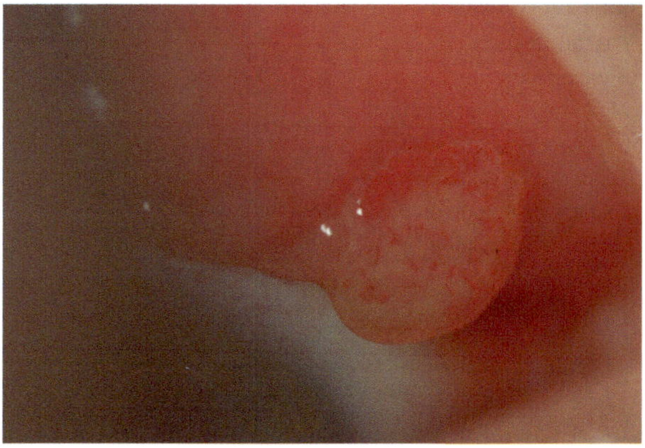

Fig. 27.2 External photograph demonstrating temporal left upper eyelid palpebral conjunctival lesion

27.1.3 Discussion

Dupilumab is the first biologic agent approved for the management of several atopic conditions including atopic dermatitis/eczema, asthma, and chronic rhinosinusitis [1]. Several ocular adverse events have been associated with the use of dupilumab (Table 27.1), the most common of which is conjunctivitis and has been reported in 3.7–22.1% of atopic dermatitis patients using dupilumab [2, 3]. Although the exact mechanism of conjunctivitis is unknown, several hypotheses have been proposed. Dupilumab binds to the IL-4 receptor alpha subunit, which is expressed in conjunctival and corneal cells, inhibiting IL-4 and IL-13. This prevents the release of pro-inflammatory cytokines, increasing the risk of *Malassezia* and *Demodex* colonization resulting in conjunctival and corneal inflammation. Other possible theories include reduction of goblet cell density and subsequent mucin production, increased OX40 ligand activity, and eosinophilia [2, 4]. It has been proposed that dupilumab is secreted in tears, inducing an inflammatory reaction and punctal stenosis. Proliferative conjunctival lesions, as in our case, have been rarely reported in the literature with dupilumab use; however, the mechanism responsible for this is unknown [5].

The risk of dupilumab-associated ocular adverse events is increased in patients with a previous history of conjunctivitis, dry eye, more severe atopic dermatitis at baseline, food allergy, and inadequate or low dose of dupilumab [2, 6].

Table 27.1 Summary of dupilumab-associated ocular adverse events

Punctal stenosis
Blepharitis
Meibomian gland dysfunction
Conjunctivitis
Subconjunctival hemorrhage
Cicatrizing conjunctivitis
Cicatricial ectropion
Keratitis
Limbal stem cell deficiency
Reactivation of latent infections, e.g., herpes infection
Uveitis

Mild cases of conjunctivitis can be managed by topical lubricant drops and antihistamines. However, in moderate to severe cases, as in our patient, a short course of topical steroids is usually necessary. Discontinuation of topical steroids may result in the recurrence of symptoms. We recommend starting a topical steroid-sparing agent such as cyclosporine or tacrolimus while tapering the steroids to maintain regression. In severe cases of conjunctivitis that is refractory to all other treatments, discontinuation of dupilumab may need to be discussed with the prescribing provider.

Presently, there is no consensus on the management of dupilumab-associated ocular adverse events. However, Wu and colleagues have proposed a management algorithm (Fig. 27.3) [2].

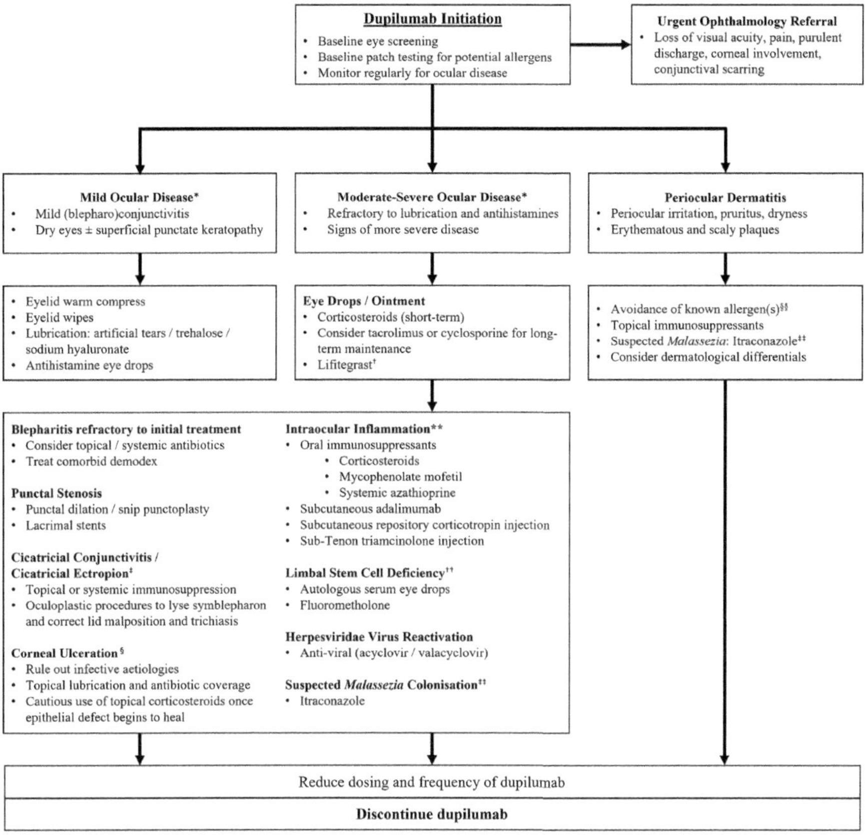

Fig. 27.3 Summary of reported dupilumab-induced ocular manifestations, treatments, and our proposed management algorithm. *No official guidelines exist on grading the severity of the dupilumab-induced ocular disease. (Reprinted with permission from Wu D, Daniel BS, Lai AJX, et al. Dupilumab-associated ocular manifestations: A review of clinical presentations and management. Surv Ophthalmol. 2022)

27.2 Case 2

27.2.1 Key Points

- Keratitis, ichthyosis, and deafness (KID) syndrome is a rare ectodermal dysplasia with reported ocular involvement in up to 95% of cases.
- Ophthalmic manifestations are of variable severity, the most common of which are corneal epithelial defects, neovascularization, and keratoconjunctivitis sicca.
- Mild cases are managed with ATs, topical antibiotics, steroids, and contact lenses. However, more severe cases may need limbal stem cell transplantation (LSCT) or keratoprosthesis (KPro).

27.2.2 Case Presentation

A 4-year-old boy with a past medical history of KID syndrome presented with recurrent epithelial erosions for which bilateral punctal plugs were inserted. The patient was lost to follow-up and presented 5 years later to our clinic. The ocular examination revealed bilateral thickened lids, loss of lashes, conjunctival hyperemia, dry eye, and left eye band keratopathy with extensive corneal scarring and neovascularization (Fig. 27.4). The patient underwent EDTA chelation, amniotic membrane transplantation (AMT) OS, and punctal cautery OS. The patient was fitted with scleral contact lenses (SCL), which improved his BCVA from 20/60 OD and counting fingers OS to 20/30 OD and 20/600 OS; however, he could not tolerate them. He was scheduled to have bilateral upper and lower lid punctal cautery; however, he was lost to follow-up for 11 months. The patient later presented with a right corneal ulcer OD and decreased BCVA to 20/125 OD. The left eye was stable in examination and vision. The corneal ulcer was managed medically (topical moxifloxacin and ATs) with improved BCVA to 20/70. The patient then underwent bilateral upper and lower punctal cauterization and was managed with aggressive lubrication, topical steroids, and erythromycin ointment postoperatively. At the last

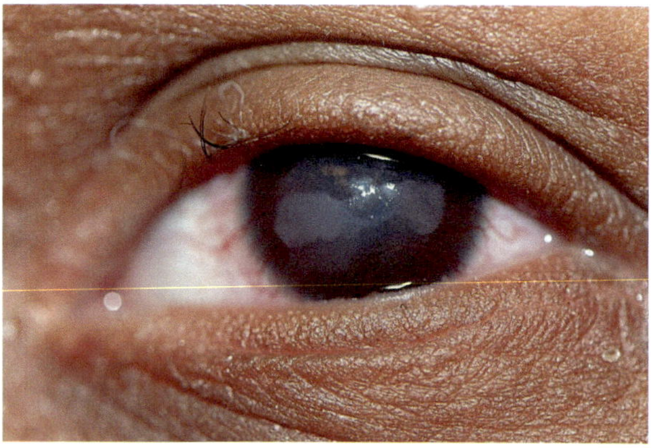

Fig. 27.4 Ocular image of the left eye showing loss of lashes, thickened lids, and extensive corneal opacification and neovascularization

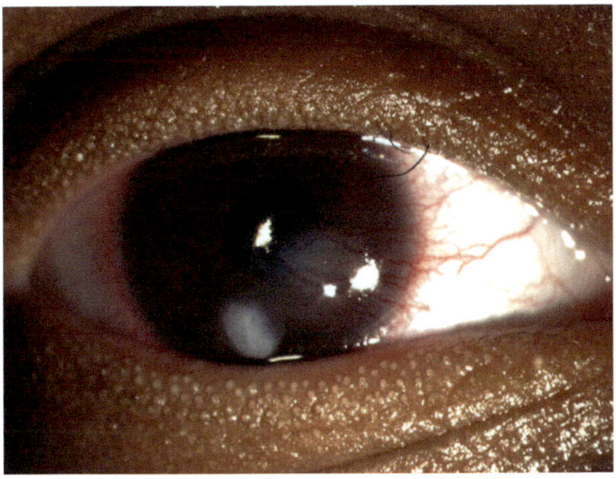

Fig. 27.5 Ocular image of the right eye demonstrating corneal conjunctivalization nasally at 3 o'clock, early keratinization, and an inferior scar

follow-up 8 months later, the BCVA had improved to 20/25 OD and 20/500 OS. However, the ocular evaluation (OD) at that time demonstrated corneal conjunctivalization nasally at 3 o'clock, early keratinization, and a faded inferior subepithelial scar (Fig. 27.5) without epithelial defect; thus, disease was progressing in his better eye despite improved visual acuity. Therapeutic focus thus shifted to promotion of ocular surface lubrication and ocular surface protection. Topical cyclosporine 0.05% (Restasis®) was prescribed but denied by insurance due to age; he did not tolerate compounded 0.1% cyclosporine. He is now undergoing an updated SCL fitting, initiating serum tears, and subconjunctival bevacizumab (Avastin®, Genentech, Inc., CA, USA) for active neovascularization is being considered.

27.2.3 Discussion

KID syndrome is a rare congenital ectodermal dysplasia characterized by corneal involvement, hyperkeratotic skin, and neurosensory hearing loss [7]. It has been hypothesized to occur as a result of genetic mutations in the genes encoding for connexin 26 [8]. The prevalence of KID syndrome has been estimated to be <1/1,000,000 people [7]. Connexins are important components of the tight junctions between epithelial cells facilitating the transfer of different molecules between cells. They also act as a tumor suppressor, which explains the high risk of squamous neoplasia of skin and mucous membranes in up to 15% of patients with KID syndrome [9]. Serrano-Ahumada and colleagues reported on a 30-year-old patient with severe KID syndrome presenting with ocular surface squamous neoplasia [10].

Ocular involvement has been reported in up to 95% of patients with KID syndrome. Most common manifestations include keratoconjunctivitis sicca, recurrent corneal epithelial defects, limbal stem cell deficiency, corneal neovascularization, and increased risk of infectious keratitis [11, 12]. The term "keratitis" is a misnomer because corneal pathology is mainly due to ectodermal and corneal basal epithelium maturation dysfunction rather than inflammation [12].

Management of ophthalmic manifestations of KID is challenging and depends on the severity of the condition. Mild cases are usually managed with ATs, topical antibiotics, and bandage contact lenses in cases of epithelial defects. Strul and Straughn demonstrated successful management of a KID syndrome patient with gas-permeable contact lenses with improved BCVA from 20/200 to 20/40 [13]. Punctal plugs and cauterization are good options to increase lubrication. In severe corneal involvement, several surgical options including superficial keratectomy, AMT (as in our patient), LSCT, and KPro have been attempted; however, results are generally disappointing [12, 14–16]. Cheung and colleagues have reported better outcomes with living-related conjunctival limbal allograft compared to keratolimbal allograft [14]. Brown and colleagues described a case of Boston KPro surgery in a patient with KID syndrome who initially presented with severe corneal opacification and had undergone three prior failed penetrating keratoplasties. They reported improved visual acuity from hand motion to 20/70 33 months after the surgery [15].

27.3 Case 3

27.3.1 Key Points

- Increasing tear quantity with aggressive lubrication and punctal occlusion is the mainstay of management of exposure keratopathy (EK).
- Scleral contact lens is an excellent option to improve the ocular surface, reduce discomfort, and improve visual acuity.
- Inducing ptosis to protect the ocular surface by gold weight placement, botulinum toxin injection, or tarsorrhaphy may be needed.

27.3.2 Case Presentation

An 8-year-old girl with a history of surgical resection of embryonic rhabdomyosarcoma involving right Meckel's diverticulum and cavernous sinus presented with lagophthalmos, right total ophthalmoplegia, decreased corneal sensation, and EK for which she underwent permanent lateral tarsorrhaphy 5 years prior to presenting to our service. Left eye examination was unremarkable. Right eye examination revealed conjunctival injection, non-confluent epithelial staining involving the central visual axis primarily inferonasally with mild underlying corneal haze, and inferior corneal neovascularization. After consulting the oculoplastic and contact lenses services, she underwent gold weight placement, punctal plug insertion of both puncta, SCL placement, and aggressive lubrication of the right eye (Fig. 27.6). The patient tolerated SCL well with proper fitting as demonstrated by anterior segment optical coherence tomography (AS-OCT) showing proper landing zone and an adequate saline-filled space between the lens and the cornea (Fig. 27.7). At the final

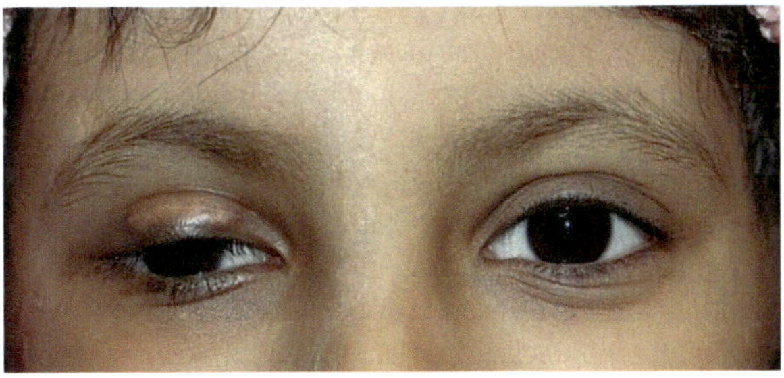

Fig. 27.6 External postoperative photograph after gold weight placement in the right upper eyelid

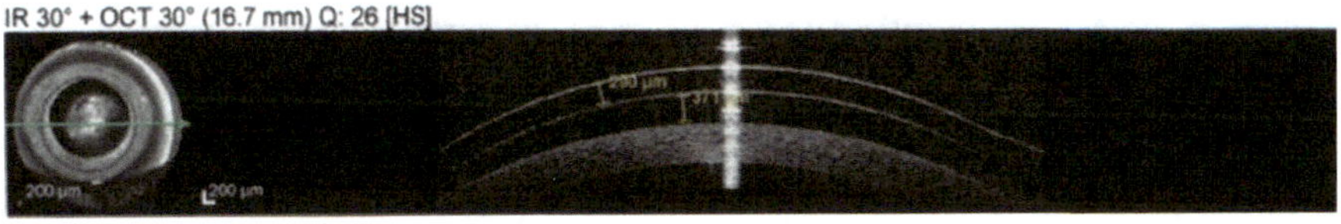

Fig. 27.7 Anterior segment optical coherence tomography illustrating adequate spacing between the cornea and the contact lens

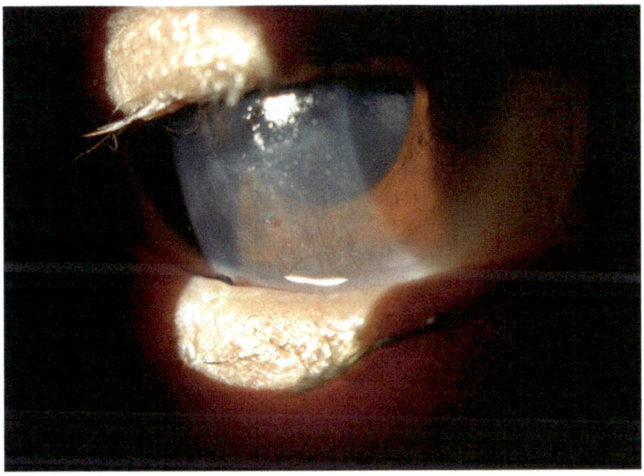

Fig. 27.8 Slit lamp photograph of the right eye demonstrating corneal haze involving the inferior one-third with fine corneal neovascularization between 4 and 6 o'clock and faint inferoparacentral anterior stromal scar with no epithelial defect or infiltrates

follow-up 7 months later, there was marked improvement in the visual acuity to 20/40 OD, and corneal examination showed corneal haze involving the inferior one-third of the cornea with fine corneal neovascularization between 4 and 6 o'clock that had improved through the course of treatment and faint inferoparacentral anterior stromal scar with no epithelial defect or infiltrates (Fig. 27.8).

27.3.3 Discussion

Our patient had multiple cranial nerve palsies, including facial nerve palsy with subsequent lagophthalmos and EK. Another contributing factor to the corneal pathology was trigeminal nerve palsy with subsequent decreased corneal sensation and neurotrophic keratopathy (NK). Management of EK consists of two main approaches. The first is to increase the quantity of tears to improve ocular surface lubrication. This can be achieved by punctal plug insertion or, for more definitive treatment, cautery of puncta. In the pediatric population, the ability to perform plug placement and cautery depends on the appropriate location, given the child's age and comfort. The former can often be done at the slit lamp, but the latter largely requires general anesthesia or sedation in the operating room. In addition, aggressive lubrication using preservative-free ATs is highly recommended [17]. The second main approach is ocular surface protection. In our experience, we have found SCL to be an excellent option. A properly fitted SCL vaults over the cornea to create space for continued surface lubrication, thus promoting reepithelialization and reducing corneal irregularities, which can improve visual acuity. In a retrospective study conducted by Schornack and colleagues evaluating SCL in patients with different corneal pathologies, including EK and NK, they reported a significant improvement in the logMAR visual acuity from 0.32 ± 0.37 prior to SCL use to 0.12 ± 0.19 after SCL use [18]. The challenge with SCL use in children is training patients and parents in insertion and removal techniques. Schornack and colleagues reported that only 115 out of 212 patients were able to complete the SCL fitting process.

A special type of SCL is the Prosthetic Replacement of the Ocular Surface Ecosystem (PROSE) (Fig. 27.9) which is an FDA-approved rigid gas-permeable SCL with high O_2 permeability. A study by Gervasio and colleagues included 27 eyes with EK managed with PROSE. They reported significant improvement in the visual acuity of three lines compared to baseline vision [19].

In severe cases of EK, inducing ptosis by botulinum toxin injection, gold weight placement, or partial or total tarsorrhaphy may be needed to cover the ocular surface and protect the eye. After the surface has healed, the surface may be maintained with aggressive lubrication and copious use of ointment at night when no SCL is in place.

It is common for EK to have a concurrent NK component in a case of trigeminal nerve involvement. There have been recent advances in the medical and surgical management of pediatric NK. Elhusseiny and colleagues recently reported

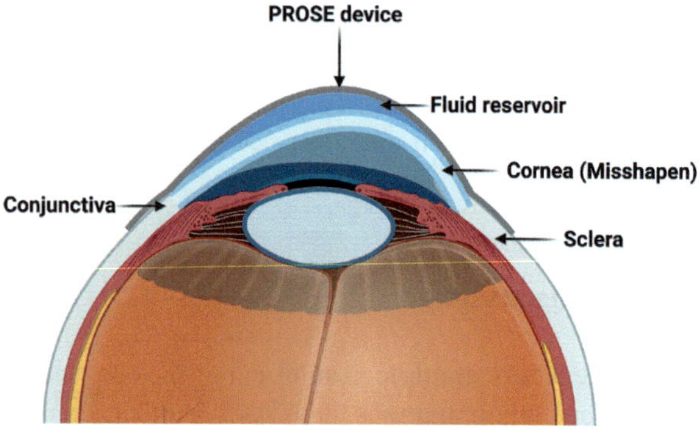

Fig. 27.9 Schematic illustration of the PROSE device position on the sclera with the fluid reservoir in between the lens and the cornea. (Courtesy of BostonSight®, Needham, MA)

successful management of pediatric NK with topical cenegermin 0.002% in five eyes with improved visual acuity and corneal healing [20]. In more severe cases, corneal neurotization has been reported as an effective surgical intervention [21]. However, these interventions do not address the incomplete lid closure seen in cases such as ours, and this must be addressed after intervention to maintain the ocular surface.

27.4 Case 4

27.4.1 Key Points

- Thygeson's superficial punctate keratitis (TSPK) is a rare bilateral corneal disorder characterized by recurrent attacks of exacerbations and remissions that may last over several years.
- Topical steroids can be very successful in managing disease, but steroid cessation often results in recurrences.
- Scleral contact lens is effective for resolution of ocular symptoms for several years after stopping steroid drops.

27.4.2 Case Presentation

A 7-year-old girl was referred to our clinic with a history of bilateral recurrent steroid-dependent TSPK over the past year. She had three previous attacks of TSPK, which were controlled by FML eye drops; however, she had recurrences soon after, even with slow tapers. On initial presentation to our clinic, she was complaining of bilateral tearing and intermittent photosensitivity without ocular redness or pain. She had not used any eye drops for a few days. Uncorrected visual acuity was 20/20 in each eye. Anterior segment evaluation revealed bilateral multiple elevated snowflake-shaped corneal lesions (OD > OS) (Fig. 27.10). The right cornea had a

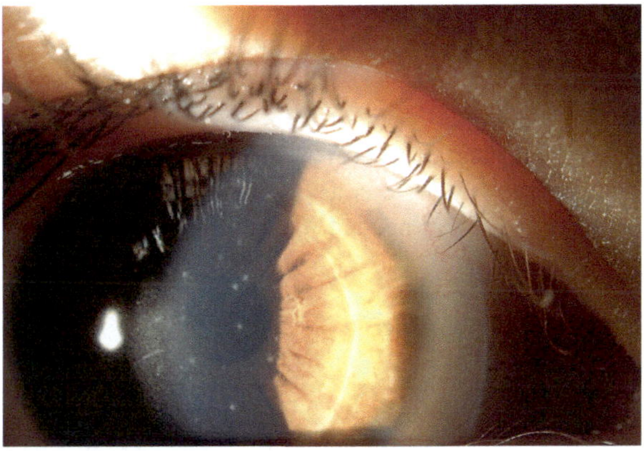

Fig. 27.10 Slit lamp photography of the right eye illustrating multiple snowflake-shaped, elevated corneal lesions

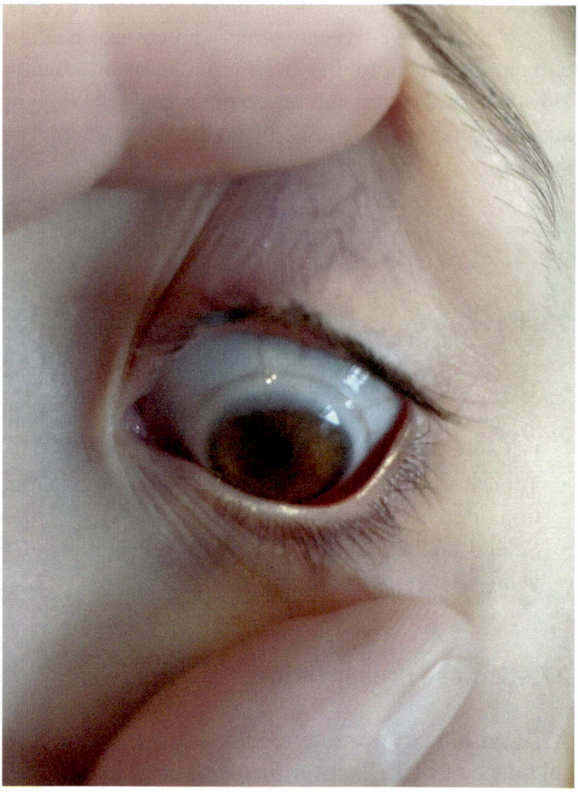

Fig. 27.11 External photograph demonstrating a properly fit scleral contact lens

patch of five lesions nasally, with multiple other lesions forming a paracentral ring of about 10–12 corneal lesions. The left cornea had a paracentral patch of four lesions. The rest of the ocular examination was unremarkable. Topical FML BID OU and topical prednisolone/sulfacetamide drops once daily were prescribed with gradual tapering over a month. Bandage soft contact lenses were tried for symptomatic relief; however, the fitting was poor. The patient was referred to the contact lens service for SCL fitting (Fig. 27.11). At the 3-month follow-up visit, the patient reported resolution of tearing and photosensitivity with SCL despite stopping all eye drops for 2 months. AS-OCT showed adequate area between the lens and the cornea with fluid present (Fig. 27.12). Although corneal examination revealed the same bilateral corneal opacities, we decided not to restart the steroid drops because the patient was asymptomatic. She remained symptom-free without eye drops except for as needed ATs for over 3 years of follow-up.

27.4.3 Discussion

TSPK is characterized by recurrent attacks of exacerbations and remissions that may last over several years [22]. Diagnosis is mainly clinical, based on the classic

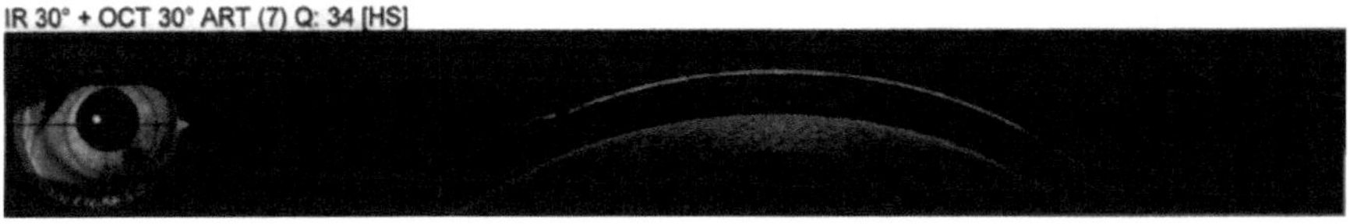

Fig. 27.12 Anterior segment optical coherence tomography demonstrating adequate spacing between the cornea and the contact lens

features of multiple grayish white raised corneal epithelial lesions without stromal involvement [23]. Lesions are usually paracentral with minimal or no conjunctival inflammation or injection. Patients usually complain of photosensitivity, ocular irritation, and tearing [23]. Although the exact etiology of TSPK is not known, several theories have been proposed. Thygeson suggested a viral etiology [24]; however, Connell and colleagues have demonstrated an absence of viral particles in the corneal epithelium of TSPK patients using polymerase chain reaction [25]. Darrell and Foca have reported a genetic association with HLA-DR3 with an associated immune response as a possible cause of TSPK [26]. There is no consensus on the optimal treatment for these patients. Topical steroids are recognized to be successful; however, recurrences are common once steroids are withdrawn [27]. Gagrani and colleagues reported the largest series to date of pediatric TSPK including 15 patients (30 eyes) with a mean age of 8 ± 4 years at presentation. All patients were managed initially with topical FML, and topical prednisolone acetate was used only in cases of poor response to topical FML. They recommended very slow tapering of topical steroids every 4–6 weeks to reduce the risk of recurrence. In cases of recurrence, they recommended increasing the frequency of topical steroids and adding cyclosporine (9 out of 15 patients in their cohort). At the final follow-up, 13 out of 15 patients were still on topical FML of varying frequencies ranging from once weekly to TID [28]. In our case, we present the successful use of SCL for TSPK patients to relieve discomfort and symptoms without the need for the chronic topical steroid use, thus reducing future risks of steroid-induced cataract and glaucoma.

27.5 Case 5

27.5.1 Key Points

- Keratoconus can be found in up to 71% of patients with Down syndrome.
- Diagnosis can be challenging in some cases due to difficulty in obtaining corneal topography. An autokeratometer can aid in the assessment of keratometric (K) readings and detection of progression.
- Corneal cross-linking (CXL) under general anesthesia is a safe and effective method which can halt the progression of keratoconus in children and developmentally delayed patients.
- Accelerated CXL has similar results to the standard CXL with less procedure time.

27.5.2 Case Presentation

A 9-year-old girl with a past history of Down syndrome, high myopia, astigmatism, and large angle esotropia for which she had undergone strabismus surgery was referred to our service for corneal evaluation. Her cycloplegic refraction was −9.00 + 1.50 × 090 OD and −11.00 + 4.00 × 095 OS. Corneal topography was obtained but was unreliable. Keratometry values of 42.5/45.25 diopters (D) × 009 OD and 43.5/45.75 D × 159 OS were obtained from the autokeratometer. Anterior segment examination demonstrated no signs of keratoconus. One year later, there was a progressive increase in the keratometry to 43.16/46.55 D × 168 OD and 42.03/46.55 D × 001 OS with evidence of keratoconus on slit lamp evaluation with Vogt's striae. Uncorrected visual acuity was 20/200 OD and 20/400 OS. The patient underwent CXL OU under general anesthesia. At the last follow-up 15 months later, the keratometry was stable (42.75/47.0 D × 178 OD and 42.0/46.75 D × 160 OS) with uncorrected visual acuity of 20/150 OD and 20/300 OS.

27.5.3 Discussion

Several studies have reported an increased prevalence of keratoconus in patients with Down syndrome that is 6–30 times higher than the rest of the population [29–31]. Haugen and Hovding demonstrated thinner corneas, higher K-readings, and thinner crystalline lenses in patients with Down syndrome compared to the general population [32]. Alio and colleagues studied 112 patients with Down syndrome and found corneal features similar to keratoconus in >70% of their cohort, suggesting a strong association between the two conditions [33]. Topographical screening has been recommended for early detection of keratoconus [34]; however, this is often infeasible, as with our patient, because of limited cooperation. The autokeratometer can be useful in such cases, but even then it often needs to be done under general anesthesia in the operating room. Other challenges in the pediatric population include compulsive eye-rubbing behavior, communication limitations, and low tolerance for contact lenses.

Cross-linking is the only treatment modality with the potential to slow or halt the progression of keratoconus. The procedure is usually performed under topical anesthesia; however, young children and developmentally delayed patients require general anesthesia. Soeters and colleagues have suggested using a clinical decision tool based on several factors such as eye-rubbing behavior, abrupt movements, and spectacle tolerance to determine whether CXL can be performed under local anesthesia versus general anesthesia [35]. Even with this clinical decision tool, general anesthesia may eventually be necessary for safe and effective treatment. Several studies have evaluated the efficacy of CXL under general anesthesia. Ahmad and colleagues retrospectively evaluated 14 eyes of pediatric and developmentally delayed patients who underwent CXL and demonstrated stable BCVA and K-values at 6 months postoperatively with no reported anesthesia or surgical complications [36]. Fung and colleagues developed a technique for pediatric keratoconus patients undergoing bilateral CXL aimed at reducing the total anesthesia time by 25% compared to the standard technique. They proposed performing CXL on both eyes simultaneously in a staggered fashion [37]. Shareef and colleagues have compared the outcomes of CXL in developmentally delayed patients (9 patients) who underwent CXL under general anesthesia to non-developmentally delayed patients who underwent CXL under topical anesthesia (13 patients). They reported no statistically significant differences in the postoperative K-readings, refractive errors, or corneal thicknesses between both groups [38].

In a recent systematic review by Achiron and colleagues, 9.9% of pediatric keratoconus had progression, defined as increased Kmax, Kmean, or Ksteep by at least 1D, after CXL [39]. Sarac and colleagues reported that pediatric keratoconus patients with paracentral cone and corneal thickness at thinnest point <450 μ are more likely to progress after CXL [40].

Acknowledgments Funding: None.

Financial Disclosures No financial disclosures.

References

1. Johnson H, Adler BL, Yu J. Dupilumab for allergic contact dermatitis: an overview of its use and impact on patch testing. Cutis. 2022;109(5):265–7.
2. Wu D, Daniel BS, Lai AJX, et al. Dupilumab-associated ocular manifestations: a review of clinical presentations and management. Surv Ophthalmol. 2022;67(5):1419–42.
3. Neagu N, Dianzani C, Avallone G, et al. Dupilumab ocular side effects in patients with atopic dermatitis: a systematic review. J Eur Acad Dermatol Venereol. 2022;36(6):820–35.
4. Jia QN, Qiao J, Fang K, Zeng YP. Ocular adverse effects in atopic dermatitis patients treated with dupilumab: a bibliometric analysis. Front Med (Lausanne). 2022;9:802036.
5. Fukuda K, Ishida W, Kishimoto T, Fukushima A. Development of conjunctivitis with a conjunctival proliferative lesion in a patient treated with dupilumab for atopic dermatitis. Allergol Int. 2019;68(3):383–4.
6. Halling AS, Loft N, Silverberg JI, Guttman-Yassky E, Thyssen JP. Real-world evidence of dupilumab efficacy and risk of adverse events: a systematic review and meta-analysis. J Am Acad Dermatol. 2021;84(1):139–47.
7. Panteliadis CP. KID/HID Syndrome. In: Panteliadis CP, Benjamin R, Hagel C, editors. Neurocutaneous disorders: a clinical, diagnostic and therapeutic approach. Cham: Springer International Publishing; 2022. p. 413–5.
8. Alvarez A, del Castillo I, Pera A, et al. De novo mutation in the gene encoding connexin-26 (GJB2) in a sporadic case of keratitis-ichthyosis-deafness (KID) syndrome. Am J Med Genet A. 2003;117a(1):89–91.
9. Madariaga J, Fromowitz F, Phillips M, Hoover HC Jr. Squamous cell carcinoma in congenital ichthyosis with deafness and keratitis. A case report and review of the literature. Cancer. 1986;57(10):2026–9.
10. Serrano-Ahumada AS, Cortes-González V, González-Huerta LM, Cuevas S, Aguilar-Lozano L, Villanueva-Mendoza C. Severe phenotype of keratitis-ichthyosis-deafness syndrome with presumed ocular surface squamous neoplasia. Cornea. 2018;37(2):252–4.
11. Perez-Rueda A, Melero-Giménez R, Valero-Marcos A, Fernández-Castro J, Martín-Molina J, Castro-Luna G. Keratitis–ichthyosis–deafness (KID) syndrome: ocular manifestations and management. Indian J Ophthalmol Case Rep. 2021;1(4):619.

12. Messmer EM, Kenyon KR, Rittinger O, Janecke AR, Kampik A. Ocular manifestations of keratitis-ichthyosis-deafness (KID) syndrome. Ophthalmology. 2005;112(2):e1–6.
13. Strul S, Straughn P. Successfully improving visual acuity in keratitis-ichthyosis-deafness syndrome utilizing gas-permeable lenses: a case report. Eye Contact Lens. 2018;44(Suppl 1):S330–s332.
14. Cheung AY, Patel S, Kurji KH, et al. Ocular surface stem cell transplantation for treatment of keratitis-ichthyosis-deafness syndrome. Cornea. 2019;38(1):123–6.
15. Brown C, Rowlands M, Lee D, Geffin JA, Huang J. Keratoprosthesis in pediatric keratitis-icthyosiform-deafness syndrome. J AAPOS. 2016;20(1):73–5.
16. Djalilian AR, Kim JY, Saeed HN, Holland EJ, Chan CC. Histopathology and treatment of corneal disease in keratitis, ichthyosis, and deafness (KID) syndrome. Eye (Lond). 2010;24(4):738–40.
17. Moshirfar M, Pierson K, Hanamaikai K, Santiago-Caban L, Muthappan V, Passi SF. Artificial tears potpourri: a literature review. Clin Ophthalmol. 2014;8:1419–33.
18. Schornack MM, Pyle J, Patel SV. Scleral lenses in the management of ocular surface disease. Ophthalmology. 2014;121(7):1398–405.
19. Gervasio KA, Godfrey KJ, Marlow ED, Lee MN, Lelli GJ Jr. Prosthetic replacement of the ocular surface ecosystem (PROSE) versus standard of care for postsurgical lagophthalmos and exposure keratopathy: trends in visual outcomes. Ophthalmic Plast Reconstr Surg. 2019;35(3):281–5.
20. Elhusseiny AM, Traish AS, Saeed HN, Mantagos IS. Topical cenegermin 0.002% for pediatric neurotrophic keratopathy. Eur J Ophthalmol. 2022;32(6):3420–4.
21. Solyman O, Elhusseiny AM, Ali SF, Allen R. A review of pediatric corneal neurotization. Int Ophthalmol Clin. 2022;62(1):83–94.
22. Chan TCY, Chau HHT, Bhat AK, Nischal KK, Jhanji V. Thygeson's superficial punctate keratitis. J EuCornea. 2019;3(3):5–8.
23. Nagra PK, Rapuano CJ, Cohen EJ, Laibson PR. Thygeson's superficial punctate keratitis: ten years' experience. Ophthalmology. 2004;111(1):34–7.
24. Thygeson P. Clinical and laboratory observations on superficial punctate keratitis. Am J Ophthalmol. 1966;61(5, Part 2):1344–9.
25. Connell PP, O'Reilly J, Coughlan S, Collum LMT, Power WJ. The role of common viral ocular pathogens in Thygeson's superficial punctate keratitis. Br J Ophthalmol. 2007;91(8):1038.
26. Darrell RW, Suciu-Foca N. HLA DR3 in Thygeson's superficial punctate keratitis. Tissue Antigens. 1981;18(3):203–4.
27. Priyadarshini SR, Roy A, Das S. Thygeson's superficial punctate keratopathy: a review and case series. Indian J Ophthalmol. 2021;69(4):806–11.
28. Gagrani M, Conner EA, Scanga H, Hiasat JG, Tripi KS, Pihlblad MS, Jhanji V, Nischal KK. Thygeson's superficial punctate keratitis in children. Eye (Lond). 2023;37(16):3455–60.
29. Woodward MA, Blachley TS, Stein JD. The association between sociodemographic factors, common systemic diseases, and keratoconus: an analysis of a nationwide heath care claims database. Ophthalmology. 2016;123(3):457–465.e452.
30. Kristianslund O, Drolsum L. Prevalence of keratoconus in persons with down syndrome in a national registry in Norway. JAMA Netw Open. 2021;4(3):e210814.
31. Haseeb A, Huynh E, ElSheikh RH, et al. Down syndrome: a review of ocular manifestations. Therap Adv Ophthalmol. 2022;14:25158414221101718.
32. Haugen OH, Høvding G. Strabismus and binocular function in children with down syndrome. A population-based, longitudinal study. Acta Ophthalmol Scand. 2001;79(2):133–9.
33. Alio JL, Vega-Estrada A, Sanz P, et al. Corneal morphologic characteristics in patients with down syndrome. JAMA Ophthalmol. 2018;136(9):971–8.
34. Asgari S, Mehravaran S, Aghamirsalim M, Hashemi H. Tomography-based definition of keratoconus for down syndrome patients. Eye Vis (Lond). 2020;7:49.
35. Soeters N, Bennen E, Wisse RPL. Performing corneal crosslinking under local anaesthesia in patients with down syndrome. Int Ophthalmol. 2018;38(3):917–22.

36. Ahmad TR, Pasricha ND, Rose-Nussbaumer J, Oatts JT, Schallhorn JM, Indaram M. Corneal collagen cross-linking under general anesthesia for pediatric patients with keratoconus and developmental delay. Cornea. 2020;39(5):546–51.
37. Fung SSM, Mason M, Gore DM, Mireskandari K, Ali A. Technique for pediatric corneal crosslinking under general anesthesia. J AAPOS. 2020;24(3):162–4.
38. Shareef O, Elhusseiny A, Kwan JT, Saeed HN. Corneal collagen cross-linking in children and developmentally delayed populations. Invest Ophthalmol Vis Sci. 2021;62(8):785.
39. Achiron A, El-Hadad O, Leadbetter D, et al. Progression of pediatric keratoconus after corneal cross-linking: a systematic review and pooled analysis. Cornea. 2022;41(7):874–8.
40. Sarac O, Caglayan M, Cakmak HB, Cagil N. Factors influencing progression of keratoconus 2 years after corneal collagen cross-linking in pediatric patients. Cornea. 2016;35(12):1503–7.

GPSR Compliance

The European Union's (EU) General Product Safety Regulation (GPSR) is a set of rules that requires consumer products to be safe and our obligations to ensure this.

If you have any concerns about our products, you can contact us on ProductSafety@springernature.com

In case Publisher is established outside the EU, the EU authorized representative is:

Springer Nature Customer Service Center GmbH
Europaplatz 3
69115 Heidelberg, Germany

Batch number: 10726133

Printed by Printforce, the Netherlands